METHODS IN MOLECULAR BIOLOGY™

Series Editor
John M. Walker
School of Life Sciences
University of Hertfordshire
Hatfield, Hertfordshire, AL10 9AB, UK

For other titles published in this series, go to
www.springer.com/series/7651

METHODS IN MOLECULAR BIOLOGY™

Tumor Biomarker Discovery

Methods and Protocols

Edited by

Michael A. Tainsky

Department of Molecular Biology and Genetics, Barbara Ann Karmanos Cancer Institute, Wayne State University, Detroit, MI, USA

Humana Press

Editors
Michael A. Tainsky
Department of Molecular Biology and Genetics
Barbara Ann Karmanos Cancer Institute
Wayne State University
Detroit, MI
USA

ISSN: 1064-3745   e-ISSN: 1940-6029
ISBN: 978-1-60327-810-2   e-ISBN: 978-1-60327-811-9
DOI: 10.1007/978-1-60327-811-9

Library of Congress Control Number: 2008943240

Preface

Biomarkers are molecular indicators of a biological status and, as biochemical species, can be interrogated to evaluate disease status and therapeutic interventions. Biomarkers may be detectable in the blood, other body fluids, or tissues. The expectation is that the level of an informative biomarker is related to the specific type of disease present in the body. Hence, disease-relevant biomarkers can be used to measure the presence, progress, or intensity of disease.

Through a variety of mechanisms, cancer cells provide the biomarker material for their own detection. Tumor biomarkers include cancer-specific mutations or changes in gene expression, both of which can result in aberrant protein expression. These variant or abundant proteins can be detectable in the circulation as the free proteins or as novel autoantibodies to those proteins, the latter indicating that the immune system can provide an exquisitely sensitive sensor of disease. Because cancer cells shed DNA in the circulation, an event rarely seen in healthy individuals, tumor-specific genetic changes, such as promoter methylation or gene mutations, are detectable in DNA prepared from plasma or other body fluids. Cancer-related biochemical changes often effect measurable metabolic variations within a cell or organism. In addition, these biochemical changes result in posttranslational modification of proteins via glycosylation or phosphorylation providing a plethora of opportunity for biomarker discovery.

An emerging theme in biomarker research and the perspective of this volume is the expectation that panels of biomarker analytes rather than single markers will be needed to have sufficient sensitivity and specificity for the presymptomatic detection of cancer. This realization became apparent from the failure of single biomarker discoveries to be suitable for clinical practice. A requirement for panels of biomarkers for each cancer is consistent with the observations from two decades of molecular oncology research that demonstrated mechanistic heterogeneity in the critical events in human carcinogenesis even within single cancer sites. With this quest for accurate panels of biomarkers comes the need for robust computational methods that are capable of reducing large-scale biomarker discovery projects to smaller panels of analytes suitable for clinical diagnostics. Those employing novel technologies for biomarker discovery must focus on the real goal, the development of diagnostic tests that can be implemented in a true clinical setting whether a large reference lab, a hospital lab, or a point-of-care health care provider.

This volume begins with chapters on methods to harness the human immune system as a biosensor of the presence of cancer using technologies to clone the cDNAs of tumor-associated antigens from cDNA libraries followed by immune detection using a variety of platforms including western blotting, ELISAs, or protein microarrays (chapters by Zhang et al., Gnjatic et al., and Chatterjee et al.). Posttranslational modifications are frequently different between normal and cancer cells and technologies exploiting these changes are described for analyzing glycosylation using antibody microarrays, 2D gels or mass spectroscopy (chapters by Chen and Haab, Comunale and Mehta, and Patwa et al.), and phosphorylation on reverse phase protein microarrays (chapter by Espina et al.). Serum proteomes are highly amenable to tumor biomarker discovery using mass spectroscopy techniques (chapter by Hood et al.). Another technology for the analysis of panels of tumor proteins in serum or extracts of tissues is the ELISA method as recently adapted to multianalyte platforms. Panels of protein biomarkers can be evaluated in parallel ELISA tests on bead array-based XMAP technology (chapter by Linkov et al.) or on spotted microarrays (chapter by Servoss et al.). The quantitative validation of expression of tumor biomarkers on an independent platform is now possible in high throughput on tissue microarrays (chapters by Hewitt and Moeder et al.). Nucleic acids, such as RNA expression profiling (chapter by Cronin et al.) and somatic genetic changes (chapters by Shi and Landers, Farwell and Joshi, and Nakamura et al.), provide fundamental technologies for biomarker discovery and validation especially in this fast-moving era of high-throughput genomic-wide genetic techniques. The identification of biomarkers of response to therapeutic agents, "Pharmacogenomics" (chapter by Zhong and Romkes), utilizes many of these genomics approaches. Of fundamental importance in biomarker discovery is appropriate study design and this is addressed for genetic epidemiology, genomics and proteomics studies (chapters by Cote and Tarca et al.). Metabolomics, the global analysis of metabolic changes resulting from oncogenic transformation, in living tissues holds great promise for noninvasive disease detection employing MRI and MRS (chapters by Serkova and Glunde, Hou and Hu, and Serkova et al.).

Given these advances in bioanalytical methods and their lifesaving possibilities for the early and accurate detection of cancer, the field of tumor biomarkers has tremendous opportunities to impact cancer survival rates. The analysis of body fluids and noninvasively evaluating tissues offers promise as sources of surrogate analytes indicative of the presence of tumors or the level of tumor burden. These methods are at the cutting edge of analytic technologies and therefore we have produced a volume for the Methods in Molecular Biology series that can provide a rapid introduction to the most appropriate technology. This volume on *Tumor Biomarker Discovery* is targeted to both researchers interested in the identification and development of new tumor biomarkers and clinicians who need to be familiar with these new technologies as they enter the clinical setting. The chapters presented cover nucleic acids and protein-based technologies, metabolic profiling by analytic means or spectroscopy, as well as study designs for biomarker discovery and validation. If there is bias in the choice of subject matter in this volume, it is slanted toward technologies that can be used to discover and validate tumor biomarker panels suitable for presymptomatic detection of cancer at stages that the patients can easily be cured, thereby focusing on early detection.

The authors of each chapter within this volume have provided extraordinary levels of detailed information, and their insight into each technology and their outstanding contributions are greatly appreciated. In addition, the exceptional organizational and editorial skills of Megan Stojcevski made this volume possible.

Detroit, MI   *Michael A. Tainsky*

Contents

Contributors

WILLIAM L. BIGBEE • *Department of Pathology, University of Pittsburgh School of Medicine, University of Pittsburgh Cancer Institute, Pittsburgh, PA, USA*

MADHUMITA CHATTERJEE • *Department of Molecular Biology and Genetics, Barbara Ann Karmanos Cancer Institute, Wayne State University, Detroit, MI, USA*

SONGMING CHEN • *Van Andel Research Institute, Grand Rapids, MI, USA*

YAO-TSENG CHEN • *Department of Pathology, Weill Cornell Medical College, New York, NY, USA*

MARY ANN COMUNALE • *Department of Microbiology and Immunology, Drexel University College of Medicine, Doylestown, PA, USA*

THOMAS P. CONRADS • *Department of Pharmacology & Chemical Biology, University of Pittsburgh School of Medicine, University of Pittsburgh Cancer Institute, Pittsburgh, PA, USA*

MICHELE L. COTE • *Department of Epidemiology, Karmanos Cancer Institute, Wayne State University, Detroit, MI, USA*

MAUREEN T. CRONIN • *Research Department, Genomic Health, Inc., Redwood City, CA, USA*

SORIN DRAGHICI • *Department of Computer Science, Wayne State University, Detroit, MI, USA*

DEBJANI DUTTA • *Operations Department, Genomic Health, Inc., Redwood City, CA, USA*

VIRGINIA ESPINA • *Center for Applied Proteomics and Molecular Medicine, George Mason University, Manassas, VA, USA*

LISA M. FARWELL • *Partners HealthCare Center for Genetics and Genomics, Harvard Medical School, Boston, MA, USA*

JENNIFER M. GILTNANE • *Department of Pathology, Vanderbilt Medical School, Nashville, TN, USA*

KRISTINE GLUNDE • *Department of Radiology and Radiological Sciences, The Johns Hopkins University, Baltimore, MD, USA*

SACHA GNJATIC • *Ludwig Institute for Cancer Research, New York Branch at Memorial Sloan-Kettering Cancer Center, New York, NY, USA*

RACHEL GONZALEZ • *Biological Sciences Division, Pacific Northwest National Laboratory, Richland, WA, USA*

BRIAN B. HAAB • *Van Andel Research Institute, Grand Rapids, MI, USA*

KENDRA M. HASEBROOCK • *Department of Anesthesiology, University of Colorado at Denver and Health Sciences Center, Aurora, CO, USA*

STEPHEN M. HEWITT • *Tissue Array Research Program, Laboratory of Pathology, Center for Cancer Research, National Cancer Institute, National Institutes of Health, Bethesda, MD, USA*

BRIAN L. HOOD • *Clinical Proteomics Facility, University of Pittsburgh Cancer Institute, Pittsburgh, PA, USA*

DAVE S.B. HOON • *Department of Molecular Oncology, John Wayne Cancer Institute, Saint John's Health Center, Santa Monica, CA, USA*

BOB L. HOU • *Departments of Medical Physics and Radiology, Memorial Sloan-Kettering Cancer Center, New York, NY, USA*

JIANI HU • *Department of Radiology, Wayne State University, Detroit, MI, USA*

JENNIE JEONG • *Research Department, Genomic Health, Inc., Redwood City, CA, USA*

VICTORIA A. JOSHI • *Partners HealthCare Center for Genetics and Genomics, Harvard Medical School, Boston, MA, USA; Department of Pathology, Massachusetts General Hospital, Boston, MA, USA*

SUSAN L. KRAFT • *Department of Radiological Sciences, Colorado State University, Fort Collins, CO, USA*

JOHN E. LANDERS • *Cecil B. Day Laboratory for Neuromuscular Research, Massachusetts General Hospital East, Charlestown, MA, USA*

FAINA LINKOV • *Department of Medicine, University of Pittsburgh, Pittsburgh, PA, USA*

LANCE A. LIOTTA • *Center for Applied Proteomics and Molecular Medicine, George Mason University, Manassas, VA, USA*

MEI-LAN LIU • *Research Department, Genomic Health, Inc., Redwood City, CA, USA*

ANNA E. LOKSHIN • *Department of Medicine, Pathology, Ob/Gyn RS, University of Pittsburgh, Pittsburgh, PA, USA*

KOK SUN LOOI • *Department of Biological Sciences, The University of Texas at El Paso, El Paso, TX, USA*

DAVID M. LUBMAN • *Department of Chemistry, University of Michigan, Ann Arbor, MI, USA*
Department of Surgery and Comprehensive Cancer Center, University of Michigan Medical Center, Ann Arbor, MI, USA

DAVID E. MALEHORN • *Department of Pathology, University of Pittsburgh School of Medicine, University of Pittsburgh Cancer Institute, Pittsburgh, PA, USA*

ANAND MEHTA • *Department of Microbiology and Immunology, Drexel University College of Medicine, Doylestown, PA, USA*

CHRISTOPHER B. MOEDER • *Department of Pathology, Yale University School of Medicine, New Haven, CT, USA*

SHARON POZNER MOULIS • *Merrimack Pharmceuticals, Cambridge, MA, USA*

TAKESHI NAKAMURA • *Department of Molecular Oncology, John Wayne Cancer Institute, Saint John's Health Center, Santa Monica, CA, USA*

ANHTHU NUGYEN • *Operations Department, Genomic Health, Inc., Redwood City, CA, USA*

LLOYD J. OLD • *Ludwig Institute for Cancer Research, New York Branch at Memorial Sloan-Kettering Cancer Center, New York, NY, USA*

TASNEEM H. PATWA • *Department of Chemistry, University of Michigan, Ann Arbor, MI, USA*

EMANUEL F. PETRICOIN III • *Center for Applied Proteomics and Molecular Medicine, George Mason University, Manassas, VA, USA*

MYLAN PHO • *Research Department, Genomic Health, Inc., Redwood City, CA, USA*

YINGHUA QIU • *Department of Chemistry, University of Michigan, Ann Arbor, MI, USA*

DAVID L. RIMM • *Department of Pathology, Yale University School of Medicine, New Haven, CT, USA*

ROBERTO ROMERO • *Perinatology Research Branch, NIH/NICHD/DHHS, Detroit, MI, USA*

MARJORIE ROMKES • *Department of Medicine, Center for Clinical Pharmacology, University of Pittsburgh, Pittsburgh, PA, USA*

NATALIE J. SERKOVA • *Department of Anesthesiology and Radiology, University of Colorado at Denver and Health Sciences Center, Aurora, CO, USA*

SHANNON L. SERVOSS • *Biological Sciences Division, Pacific Northwest National Laboratory, Richland, WA, USA*

LIJIA SHI • *Cecil B. Day Laboratory for Neuromuscular Research, Massachusetts General Hospital East, Charlestown, MA, USA*

DIANE M. SIMEONE • *Department of Surgery, The University of Michigan Medical Center, Ann Arbor, MI, USA*

EIJI SUNAMI • *Department of Molecular Oncology, John Wayne Cancer Institute, Saint John's Health Center, Santa Monica, CA, USA*

MICHAEL A. TAINSKY • *Department of Molecular Biology and Genetics, Barbara Ann Karmanos Cancer Institute, Wayne State University, Detroit, MI, USA*

ENG M. TAN • *Department of Molecular and Experimental Medicine, The Scripps Research Institute, La Jolla, CA, USA*

ADI LAURENTIU TARCA • *Department of Computer Science, Wayne State University, Detroit, MI, USA*

SUSAN VARNUM • *Biological Sciences Division, Pacific Northwest National Laboratory, Richland, WA, USA*

JERZY WOJCIECHOWSKI • *Department of Molecular Biology and Genetics, Barbara Ann Karmanos Cancer Institute, Wayne State University, Detroit, MI, USA*

ZOYA YURKOVETSKY • *Department of Medicine, University of Pittsburgh, Pittsburgh, PA, USA*

RICHARD C. ZANGAR • *Biological Sciences Division, Pacific Northwest National Laboratory, Richland, WA, USA*

JIAN-YING ZHANG • *Department of Biological Sciences, The University of Texas at El Paso, El Paso, TX, USA*

JIA ZHAO • *Department of Chemistry, University of Michigan, Ann Arbor, MI, USA*

SHILONG ZHONG • *Department of Medicine, Center for Clinical Pharmacology, University of Pittsburgh, Pittsburgh, PA, USA*

Chapter 1

Identification of Tumor-Associated Antigens as Diagnostic and Predictive Biomarkers in Cancer

Jian-Ying Zhang, Kok Sun Looi, and Eng M. Tan

Summary

Many studies demonstrated that cancer sera contain antibodies which react with autologous cellular antigens generally known as tumor-associated antigens (TAAs). In our laboratories, the approach used in the identification of TAAs has involved initially examining the sera of cancer patients using extracts of tissue culture cells as source of antigens in Western blotting and by indirect immunofluorescence on whole cells. With these two techniques, we identify sera which have high-titer fluorescent staining or strong signals to cell extracts on Western blotting and subsequently use these sera as probes in immuno-screening cDNA expression libraries, and also in proteomic approaches to isolate and identify targeted antigens which might potentially be involved in malignant transformation. In this manner, several novel TAAs including HCC1, p62, p90, and others have been identified. In extension of these studies, we evaluate the sensitivity and specificity of different antigen-antibody systems as markers in cancer in order to develop "tumor-associated antigen array" systems for cancer diagnosis, cancer prediction, and for following the response of patients to treatment.

Key words: Autoantibodies, Tumor-associated antigens, cDNA expression library screening, Two-dimensional SDS-polyacrylamide gel electrophoresis, Proteomic approach, Cancer marker.

1. Introduction

It is well established that cancer sera contain antibodies that react with a unique group of autologous cellular antigens called TAAs (1–3). The types of cellular proteins that induce these autoantibody responses are quite varied and include the tumor suppressor p53 (4, 5), oncogene products such as HER-2/neu and ras (6), proteins that protect mRNAs from degradation such as p62 (7) and CRD-BP (8), onconeural antigens (9), differentiation-antigens such as tyrosinase and the cancer/testis antigens (10), and

Michael A. Tainsky, *Methods in Molecular Biology, Tumor Biomarker Discovery, Vol. 520*
© Humana Press, a part of Springer Science + Business Media, LLC 2009
DOI: 10.1007/978-1-60327-811-9_1

antiapoptotic proteins such as survivin *(11)* and LEDGF *(12)*. Factors leading to the production of such autoantibodies are not completely understood, but the available data show that many of the target antigens are cellular proteins whose aberrant regulation or overexpression could lead to tumorigenesis, such as p53 *(4, 5)*. A highly informative study showed that lung tumors contained several types of p53 gene mutations including missense, stop codon and frameshift mutations, but it was the missense mutations with overexpression of protein which altered function and increased protein stability that correlated with antibody production *(13)*. In the case of the mRNA-binding protein p62, a fetal protein absent in adult tissues, immunogenicity appears to be related to abnormal expression of p62 in tumor cells *(14)*. The immune system in certain cancer patients appears to have the capability of sensing these abnormalities in cellular proteins and responding by producing autoantibodies. Importantly, it has been shown that the patients' immune system is capable of sensing abnormalities in cellular proteins involved in malignant transformation earlier than clinical diagnostic procedures *(5, 15)*. An emerging concept is that autoantibodies associated with a specific type of cancer are directed against aberrantly regulated or activated protein components of molecular pathways involved in the malignant transformation process in that particular type of cancer *(1, 16)*. Thus, cancer-associated autoantibodies might be regarded as reporters identifying aberrant cellular mechanisms in tumorigenesis. In recent years, research on humoral immunity to TAAs has received significant attention, and investigators are now beginning to address specific clinical questions such as the potential utility of TAA-autoantibody systems as early cancer biomarkers, tools to monitor therapeutic outcomes, or indicators of disease prognosis *(17)*.

2. Materials

2.1. Cell Culture and Cell Extracts

1. HepG2 (human hepatocellular carcinoma) cell lines were obtained from the American Type Culture Collection (ATCC) and cultured following the specific protocol.

2. Cells grown in monolayers were solubilized directly in Laemmli's sample buffer containing protease inhibitors (Boehringer, Mannheim). Solubilized lysates were briefly sonicated and then electrophoresed on SDS-PAGE and transferred to nitrocellulose paper.

2.2. cDNA Expression Library Cloning

1. Amplified premade hepatocellular carcinoma (HepG2) cDNA library constructed in the Uni-ZAP® XR vector (Stratagene, La Jolla, CA).

2. *Host strains.* Bacterial glycerol stock of XL1-Blue MRF' strain and SOLR™ strain (Stratagene, La Jolla, CA).

3. ExAssist® interference-resistant helper phage (Stratagene, La Jolla, CA).

4. Isopropyl-1-thio-β-D-galactopyranoside (IPTG) (Fisher Scientific, Houston, TX).

5. Nitrocellulose membrane (Osmonics Inc. MA).

6. Chemiluminescent reagent (Pierce Biotechnology, Rockford, IL).

7. Additional reagents include:
   1 M MgSO$_4$ 20% maltose, tryptone, yeast extract, antibiotics (tetracycline, ampicillin), SM buffer (5.8 g NaCl; 2.0 g MgSO$_4$; 50 mL Tris, pH 7.4, 1 M; 5 mL 2% gelatin, add H$_2$O to 1 L and autoclave), PBS-Tween (PBST) solution, 3% nonfat dry milk in PBST, horseradish peroxidase (HRP)-conjugated goat antihuman IgG (Caltag Laboratories, San Francisco, CA).

2.3. Proteomic Approach

1. Protein assay Bradford dye reagent. (Bio-rad, Hercules, CA)

2. Immobilized pH gradient IPG gel strip. (Bio-rad, Hercules, CA)

3. Dithiothreitol (DTT) equilibration buffer 1 for sulfhydryl group reduction: 2% DTT, 6 M Urea, 20% SDS, 1.5 M Tris–HCl, pH 8.8, 50% glycerol, nanopure water

4. Iodoacetamide equilibration buffer 2 for sulfhydryl group alkylation: 2.5% Iodoacetamide, 6 M Urea, 20% SDS, 1.5 M Tris-HCl, pH 8.8, 50% glycerol, nanopure water

5. Nitrocellulose membrane: Osmonics Inc. MA

6. Chemiluminescent reagent: Pierce Biotechnology, Rockford, IL

7. Sequencing-grade modified trypsin: Promega, Madison, WI

8. C18 bead zip-tips: POROS R2 from Applied Biosystems, CA.

9. Additional reagents include proteomics-grade water, mineral oil, PBS-Tween (PBST) solution, 3% nonfat dry milk in PBST, horseradish peroxidase (HRP)-conjugated goat antihuman IgG (Caltag Laboratories, San Francisco, CA), HPLC-grade Acetonitrile, ammonium bicarbonate, formic acid (FA), Methanol, Trifluoroacetic acid (TFA).

3. Methods

The methods which we have used in the identification of putative TAAs has involved initially examining the sera from cancer patients using extracts of tissue culture cells as source of antigens in Western blotting and by indirect immunofluorescence on whole cells. With these two techniques, we identify sera which have high-titer fluorescent staining or strong signals to cell extracts on Western blotting and subsequently use the antibodies in these sera to isolate cDNA clones from cDNA expression libraries. In this manner, several novel TAAs including HCC1 *(18)*, SG2NA *(19)*, CENP-F *(20)*, p62 *(7)*, and p90 *(21)* have been identified. Several novel as well as previously defined tumor antigens have been recently identified with autoantibodies from patients with different types of cancer *(2)* using a methodology called SEREX (serological analysis of recombination cDNA expression libraries) *(22)*, which is essentially a modification of our previous approach *(18, 19)*. Immunoscreening of cDNA libraries with serum antibodies for identifications of autoantigens is a well-established method and has been used not only to identify TAAs but also antigens in autoimmune diseases *(23)*. This methodology was the basis of the methods described in SEREX (serological analysis of recombination cDNA expression libraries) with the difference that cDNA expression libraries constructed from autologous patient tumor were used as substrate in immunoscreening. Subsequent reports using the SEREX technique have shown that the TAAs identified are no different from standard methods using cDNA expression libraries from cell lines derived from different sources, so that there did not appear to be any advantage to using cDNA libraries from autologous patients. A proteome-based approach has been recently implemented for identifying tumor-associated antigens in cancer patients *(24, 25)*. The proteome-based technology allows individual screening of a large number of sera, as well as potential identification of a large number of autoantigens. Proteome-based approach can also distinguish isoforms and the detection of autoantibodies directed against post-translational modifications of specific targets. The practical utility of this approach remains to be established with the proviso that efforts should be made to identify tumor-associated from tumor-irrelevant antigens. In this chapter, we will use the hepatocellular carcinoma (HCC)-associated antigens as examples to describe how to isolate and identify TAAs as markers in cancer. The schematic representation of TAA identification is shown in **Fig. 1**.

Fig. 1. Schematic representation of TAA identification. (**a**) TAA identification using cDNA library immunoscreening. In brief, the sera from cancer patients were initially examined using extracts of tissue culture cells as source of antigens in Western blot and by indirect immunofluorescence (IIF) on whole cells. With these two techniques, we identify sera which have high-titer fluorescent staining or strong signals to cell extracts on Western blot and subsequently use the antibodies in these sera to isolate cDNA clones from cDNA expression libraries. (**b**) TAA identification using proteomic approach. In brief, cell extract of cultured cancer cells was applied onto the first-dimension gel (isoelectro-focusing gel), and subsequently loaded onto the second-dimension gel (2D-SDS-PAGE). The protein was transferred to the nitrocellulose membrane or visualized by silver staining. High-titer sera from cancer patients and sera from normal individuals (used as controls) were selected for the study. Reactivity with cancer cells for all selected serum samples was confirmed by Western blotting analysis and immunofluorescence assay. After immunoblotting with cancer sera and normal human sera, a number of protein spots of interest were excised from the 2-D gels, digested by trypsin, and subsequently analyzed

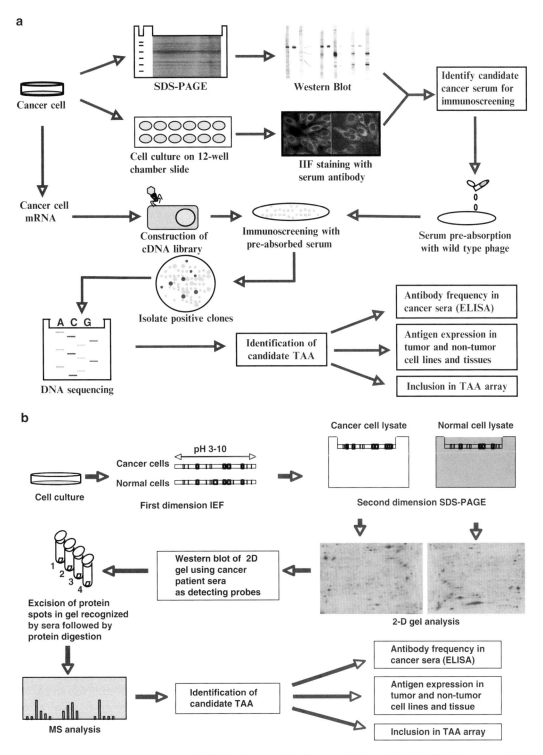

Fig. 1. (continued) by mass spectrometry (MS). In subsequent studies, we will characterize identified tumor-associated antibody-antigen systems that are potentially useful for the early detection of cancer, and then evaluate the sensitivity and specificity of different antigen-antibody systems as markers in cancer for further developing "TAA array" systems for cancer diagnosis, prediction, and for following the response of patients to treatment (*See Color Plates*).

3.1. Methods for cDNA Expression Library Immunoscreening

1. Immunoscreening HepG2 cDNA expression library: The HepG2 cDNA expression library constructed in the Uni-ZAP XR vector system was purchased from the company (Stratagene, La Jolla, CA). One selected HCC serum was diluted 1:200 and used as a probe for initial immunoscreening of the cDNA library. Before screening the cDNA library, the HCC serum was extensively adsorbed against wild-type Uni-ZAP XR phage-infected *E. coli* mixture to reduce nonspecific antibody binding (*see* **Notes 1–5**). All screenings were performed on duplicate isopropyl β-D-thiogalactoside (IPTG) preimpregnated nitrocellulose filters. Horseradish peroxidase (HRP)-conjugated goat antihuman IgG (CALTAG, Burlingame, CA) at 1:3,000 dilution was used as secondary antibody; immunoreactive clones were detected by chemiluminescence. Double positive phages in first screening were subsequently screened to 100% purity. At least, 400,000 phage recombinants need to be screened in each screening. Positive cDNA clones were isolated and converted to pBluescript phagemid by in vivo excision using the EXAssist helper phage (Stratagene Inc.) with SOLR strain. The phagemids were purified by Qiaprep spin columns (Qiagen, Valencia, CA), and the size of insert was determined by restriction enzyme digestion with *Eco*R1 and *Xho*1.

2. Sequencing of the positive cDNA clones derived from library screening: The cDNA inserts of the pBluescript phagemid were sequenced with T3 and T7 primers by the dideoxy chain termination method using SequiTherm EXCEL™ II DNA Sequencing Kit (Epicentre Technologies, Madison, WI, USA). All sequence data were analyzed by BLAST search with known sequence databases.

3.2. Methods for Proteomic Approach

1. Two-dimensional SDS-polyacrylamide gel electrophoresis (2D-SDS-PAGE) analysis: Cells were briefly sonicated with lysis buffer (10 mM Tris 5 mM EDTA, 50 mM Nacl, 30 mM Na pyrophosphate, 50 mM Na fluoride, 1 mM Na orthovanadate, 1% Triton, pH 7.6). Protein concentration was measured with Bradford assay (Bio-Rad). For the first-dimensional gel analysis, total protein of 200 µg was mixed with denatured buffer and applied on pH 3–10 11 cm isoelectric-focusing strip (IEF) from Bio-Rad. IEF was performed at a current of 50 mA per gel for 300 V 30min, followed by 8,000 V for 2.5 h and additional 5 h (*see* **Note 6**). The total volt-hour-product was 45 kvh. Strips were immediately stored at –80°C for SDS-PAGE analysis. The second dimension was carried out using 15% polyacrylamide gels and 200 V under an appropriate cooling system (*see* **Note 7**).

2. Immunoblotting analysis: Proteins separated by first and second dimensions were transferred to pure nitrocellulose membranes (Osmonics Inc.). After preblocking with phosphate-buffered saline containing 0.05% Tween-20 (PBST) and 5% nonfat milk for 30 min at room temperature, the nitrocellulose membranes were incubated for 2 h at room temperature with 1:300 dilution of serum. Horseradish peroxidase-conjugated goat antihuman IgG (Caltag Laboratories, San Francisco, CA) was applied as secondary antibody using 1:3,000 dilution. Immunoreactive spots were visualized by the ECL kit (Amersham, Arlington Heights, IL) according to the manufacturer's instructions.

3. In-gel protein Digestion: The proteins of interest were excised from a Coomassie stained preparative gel (*see* **Note 8**) and then washed with HPLC-grade water, followed by destaining with acetonitrile (ACN) for 15 min to remove Coomassie blue staining, and dried in a SpeedVac concentrator as described previously *(26)*. After the reduction (with 5 mM DTT) and alkylation (with 10 mM iodoacetoamide) of cysteine residues, digestion was performed by addition of 12.5 ng/μL of trypsin (Promega, Madison,WI) in 50 mM ammonium bicarbonate containing 5 mM $CaCl_2$ (*see* **Note 9**). Following the enzymatic digestion overnight at 37°C, the peptides were extracted with 25 mM ammonium bicarbonate/50% ACN and with 5% formic acid (FA) in 50% ACN solution. After removal of acetonitrile by SpeedVac concentrator, the sample was desalted by C18 bead ziptips (POROS R2, Applied Biosystems). The samples were dried out by SpeedVac concentrator before mass spectrometry analysis.

4. LC-MS/MS Analysis: Samples were resuspended in 0.1% FA before running the LC-MS/MS analysis. The liquid chromatography mass spectrum (LC-MS/MS) analysis was carried using a nano-HPLC (LC packings system, Ultimate) coupled to the ESI-QUAD-TOF-MS (Micromass). Peptides were separated with the following gradient: 100% solvent A for 5 min, 0–50% solvent B in 25 min, 50–90% solvent B in 1 min, and 90% solvent B for 5 min (solvent A = 5% ACN/0.1% FA; solvent B = 80% ACN/0.1% FA). The mass spectrometry (MS) spectra were collected for 2 s in a range between 400 and 1,800 amu. Each peptide with intensity higher than 10 counts was submitted only once to fragmentation, using ramp collision energy (22–60 eV). The MS/MS spectra were collected for 3 s in a range between 50 and 2,050 amu.

5. Protein Identification: Protein identification was performed using MASCOT software (http://www.matrixscience.com(, and all tandem mass spectra were searched against the IPI

Human database. The following search parameters were used: trypsin is used as the cutting enzyme, carbamidomethyl (C) and Oxidation (M) are chosen as fixed and variable modifications, mass tolerance for monoisotopic peptide is set to 500 ppm, fragment mass tolerance is set to 0.8 Da, protein mass is unrestricted, one missed cleavage is allowed. Briefly, the algorithm searches candidate sequences from the database by intact peptide masses. After this step, all candidates were submitted to an in silico fragmentation, and the resulting theoretical fragments were compared with the fragments from experimental spectrum. Finally a statistical analysis was used to validate the sequences. Mascot validates its results based on the probability of the identification being a random event.

4. Notes

1. All sera, even "normals," may have antibacterial and antiphage antibodies. Sera used for screening must therefore be absorbed against bacteria and phages.

2. Use wild-type λ phage, specific clone(s), or a mixture of clones from the same library being screened.

3. Plating as described earlier, using ~20,000 pfu per small plate or 200,000 pfu per large square plate. After 4–6 h when the plagues are visible, overlay plate with corresponding filter presoaked in IPTG. After several hours or overnight, flip nitrocellulose filter upside down for several more hours of incubation at 37°C so that both sides of the filter will be coated with phage/*E. coli*. The number and size of nitrocellulose filter required for absorption depends on the background signal for each screening serum.

4. Proceed as for immunoblotting earlier, block filters with 3% milk/PBST, use 15 mL of 1:50 diluted serum in 3% milk in PBST against eight filters. Incubate primary antibody with filters for 1–2 h with occasional mixing.

5. Remove absorbed sera and add equal volume of 3% milk PBST to generate 30 mL of 1:100 preabsorbed antibody. Use immediately or store at –20°C. Save filters for stripping and reuse.

6. The current of IEF strips should be maintained below 100 mA. All proteins should be run through the desalt procedures if the voltage of the gel cannot go up to the desired setting.

7. Before starting the second dimension the strips are equilibrated in DTT equilibration buffer 1 for 15 min. Afterward, they were briefly rinsed in double distilled water and equilibrated in Iodoacetamide equilibration buffer 2 for an additional 15 min.

The IEF strips were overlayered with a solution containing agarose (0.5% w/v) on the top of second-dimension gels. The second dimension was carried out using 10% or 15% polyacrylamide gels and current is nonlimited per gel in a cooling system.

8. Spot patterns on each membrane are matched to an equivalent spot on original 2D-PAGE gel. This gel analysis can be done by using PDQuest 2-D Analysis Software (Bio-Rad, Hercules, CA).

9. If the gel pieces still have Coomassie blue staining, the gel pieces need to be rehydrated again in an equal volume of ammonium bicarbonate and acetonitrile.

Acknowledgments

This work was supported by grants from National Institutes of Health (2S06GM008012-37, 5G12RR08124, CA56956).

References

1. Tan, E.M. (2001) Autoantibodies as reporters identifying aberrant cellular mechanisms in tumorigenesis. *J Clin Invest* 108, 1411–1415

2. Old, L.J. and Chen, Y.T. (1998) New paths in human cancer serology. *J Exp Med* 187, 1163–1167

3. Zhang, J.Y., Casiano, C.A., Peng, X. X., Koziol, J. A., Chan, E. K. L., and Tan, E. M. (2003) Enhancement of antibody detection in cancer using panel of recombinant tumor-associated antigens. *Cancer Epidemiol Biomarkers Prev* 12:136–143

4. Crawford, L. V., Pim, D. C. and Bulbrook, R. D. (1982) Detection of antibodies against the cellular protein p53 in sera from patients with breast cancer. *Int J Cancer* 30, 403–408

5. Soussi, T. (2000) p53 antibodies in the sera of patients with various types of cancer. A review. *Cancer Res* 60, 1777–1788

6. Disis, M.L., Pupa, S.M., Gralow, J.R., Dittadi, R., Menard, S., Cheever, M.A. (1997) High-titer HER-2/neu protein-specific antibody can be detected in patients with early-stage breast cancer. *J Clin Oncol* 15, 3363–7

7. Zhang, J. Y., Chan, E. K. L., Peng, X. X., and Tan, E. M. (1999) A novel cytoplasmic protein with RNA-binding motifs is an autoantigen in human hepatocellular carcinoma. *J Exp Med* 189, 1101–1110

8. Doyle, G.A., Bourdeaux-Heller, J.M., Coulthard, S., Meisner, L.F. and Ross, J. (2000) Amplification in human breast cancer of a gene encoding a c-myc mRNA binding protein. *Cancer Res* 60, 2756–2759

9. Keene, J. D. (1999) Why is Hu where? Shuttling of early response gene messenger RNA subsets. *Proc Natl Acad Sci USA* 96, 5–7

10. Stockert, E., Jager, E., Chen, Y.T., Scanlan, M.J., Gout, I., Karbach, J., Arand, M., Knuth, A., and Old, L.J. (1998) A survey of humoral immune response of cancer patients to a panel of human tumor antigens. *J Exp Med* 187, 1349–1354

11. Ambrosini, G., Adida, C. and Altieri, D.C. (1997) A novel anti-apoptosis gene, survivin, expressed in cancer and lymphoma. *Nat Med* 3, 917–992

12. Daniels, T., Zhang, J., Gutierrez, I., Elliot, M.L., Yamada B, Heeb MJ, Sheets SM, Wu X, and Casiano CA.(2005) Antinuclear autoantibodies in PCa: Immunity to LEDGF/p75, a survival protein highly expressed in prostate tumors and cleaved during apoptosis. *Prostate* 62, 14–26

13. Winter, S.F., Minna, J.D., Johnson, B.E., Takahashi, T., Gazdar, A.F., and Carbone, D.P. (1992) Development of antibodies against p53 in lung cancer patients appears to

be dependent on the type of p53 mutation. *Cancer Res* 52, 4168–4174

14. Lu, M., Nakamura, R.M., Dent, E.D., Zhang, J.Y., Nielsen, F.C., Christiansen, J., Chan, E.K., and Tan, E.M. (2001) Aberrant expression of fetal RNA-binding protein p62 in liver cancer and liver cirrhosis. *Am J Pathol* 159, 945–953

15. Imai, H., Nakano, Y., Kiyosawa, K., and Tan, E.M. (1993) Increasing titers and changing specificities of antinuclear antibodies in patients with chronic liver disease who develop hepatocellular carcinoma. *Cancer* 71, 26–35

16. Anderson, K. S., and LaBaer, J. (2005) The sentinel within: exploiting the immune system for cancer biomarkers. *J Proteome Res* 4, 1123–1133

17. Disis, M.L., Montgomery, R.B., Goodell, V., dela Rosa, C., and Salazar, L.G. (2005) Antibody immunity to cancer-associated proteins. *The Education Book of the 96th Annual AACR Meeting, Anaheim, CA*, p166–169

18. Imai H, Chan EKL, Kiyosawa K, Fu XD, Tan EM. (1993) Novel nuclear antoantigen with splicing factor motifs identified with antibody from hepatocellular carcinoma. *J Clin Invest* 92, 2419–2426

19. Landberg G, Tan EM. (1994) Characterization of a DNA-binding nuclear autoantigen mainly associated with S phase and G2 cells. *Exp Cell Res* 212, 255–261

20. Casiano CA, Landberg G, Ochs R, Tan EM. (1993) Autoantibodies to a novel cell cycle-regulated protein that accumulates in the nuclear matrix during S phase and is localized in the kinetochores and spindle midzone during mitosis. *J Cell Sci* 106, 1045–1056

21. Soo Hoo L, Zhang JY, Chan EKL. (2002) Cloning and characterization of a novel 90kDa 'companion' auto-antigen of p62 overexpressed in cancer. *Oncogene* 21, 5006–5015

22. Sahin U, Tureci O, Schmitt H, Cochlovius B, Johannes T, Schmits R, Stenner F, Luo G, Schobert I, Pfreundschuh M. (1995) Human neoplasms elicit multiple specific immune responses in the autologous host. *Proc Natl Acad Sci USA* 92, 11810–11813

23. Chambers JC, Keene JD. (1985) Isolation and analysis of cDNA clones expressing human lupus La antigen. *Proc Natl Acad Sci USA* 82, 2115–2119

24. Le Naour, F., Brichory, F., Beretta, L., Hanash, S.M. (2002) Identification of tumor-associated antigens using proteomics. *Technol Cancer Res Treat* 1, 257–262

25. Le Naour, F., Brichory, F., Misek, D.E., Brechot, C., Hanash, S.M., Beretta, L. (2002) A distinct repertoire of autoantibodies in hepatocellular carcinoma identified by proteomic analysis. *Mol Cell Proteomics* 1, 197–203

26. Shevchenko, A., Wilm, M., Vorm, O., Mann, M. (1996) Mass spectrometric sequencing of proteins silver-stained polyacrylamide gels. *Anal Chem* 68, 850–858

Chapter 2

Autoantibodies Against Cancer Antigens

Sacha Gnjatic, Lloyd J. Old, and Yao-Tseng Chen

Summary

With the identification of tumor antigens, the host immune response to various types of cancers can now be studied with a high degree of specificity in large cohorts of patients, in the hope of correlating immunity with clinical events and defining immunotherapeutic strategies. Several antigens, such as NY-ESO-1, p53, or SOX2, have attracted attention because of their frequent spontaneous immunogenicity in cancer patients, notably in their ability to induce humoral responses. We describe in this chapter a simple implementation of a serological monitoring platform for autoantibody measurement in cancer patients, from production of recombinant antigens to ELISA testing and interpretation.

Key words: Humoral immunity, Enzyme-linked immunosorbent assay, Immunoglobulin (IgG, IgM, IgG1, IgG2, IgG3, IgG4), Tumor antigen, Protein purification, Serum, Plasma, Antibody titration and titer calculation, Serological screening, Immunoediting, Immunosurveillance.

1. Introduction

It has been established that cancer develops in a dynamic process that is significantly influenced by the immune system (1). The adaptive immune response edits the antigenic content of the tumor and may affect its course. Understanding the nature of this immune response would help to establish benchmarks that are required for each step of this interactive process (a) Immune recognition during early carcinogenesis (2), potentially yielding antigenic signatures of diagnostic value in early detection; (b) equilibrium phase between tumor and immune system (3), during which the immune responses to immunogenic antigens may confer some degree of protection and be of prognostic significance; and (c) eventual tumor escape from the immune system

Michael A. Tainsky, *Methods in Molecular Biology, Tumor Biomarker Discovery, Vol. 520*
© Humana Press, a part of Springer Science+Business Media, LLC 2009
DOI: 10.1007/978-1-60327-811-9_2

(4), where immune responses may indicate progressive burden of disease and the analysis of such responses may help identify subset of patients for targeted therapies.

The host immune response to various types of cancer has led to the identification of many tumor antigens. Among those, several have attracted attention because of their frequent and spontaneous immunogenicity in cancer patients, notably NY-ESO-1 *(5)* and p53 *(6)*. Spontaneously occurring antibody and/or T cell responses to tumor antigens NY-ESO-1 or p53 have been observed in various tumor types *(6–9)*. Presence of serum antibodies to these self-antigens has been extensively studied by ELISA and Western blot and in some cases has been found to be a surrogate for the presence of T cell responses. For example, we and others *(5, 8, 9)* have found that the presence of specific anti-NY-ESO-1 antibodies in patients correlated strongly with the presence of both CD8$^+$ and CD4$^+$ T cell responses to NY-ESO-1, indicating that antibody and T cell responses act together in an integrated manner *(5)*. Changes in antibody titers to NY-ESO-1 have also been associated with clinical events in cancer patients during the course of their disease *(10)*.

Therefore, a robust detection method of autoantibodies against cancer antigens is an important research tool that could potentially be useful in the clinical arena in the future. Although the presence of such antibodies, such as anti-p53 antibodies, has been documented earlier, a systematic analysis of antibody response to tumor antigens was not attempted until the development of SEREX technology by which serum samples from cancer patients were used to immunoscreen expression cDNA phage libraries constructed from autologous tumor samples *(11–13)*. Using this technique, we and others *(14, 15)* have identified a large panel of immunogenic tumor antigens, including cancer/testis (CT) antigens (e.g., NY-ESO-1, SSX2, CT7), mutational antigens (p53), differentiation antigens (tyrosinase, SOX2, ZIC2, etc.), and retroviral antigens (HERV-K), etc. This discovery that human humoral immune system is capable of reacting to a plethora of protein antigens elicited a major interest in serological survey studies of cancer patients *(7)*, to seek whether any of the autoantibody responses are indeed tumor specific, and whether these responses might be correlated to other clinical parameters, such as tumor stage and grade, response to treatment, and prognosis. However, although the SEREX technique was useful in identifying tumor antigens, it is not ideal for screening a large number of serum samples against a specific antigen. For that purpose, ELISA assay against the recombinant protein antigen is the method of choice, and it also has the additional advantage in that it could easily be set up across different laboratories, and standardization of the technique can potentially be achieved. The methodology that we present in the following protocol, modified from Stockert et al. *(7)*, has been implemented and validated in three laboratories independently, with highly reproducible results *(8, 9, 16)*.

2. Materials

2.1. Protein Preparation

1. *QIAexpress* type IV Kit (Qiagen, Valencia, CA).

2.2. Preparation of Serum/Plasma Samples

1. Red-top tubes: BD Vacutainer, Silica coated, #367815, (BD, Franklin Lakes, NJ).
2. Green-top tubes: BD Vacutainer, Sodium Heparin coated, #367878 (BD).
3. 15-mL centrifuge tubes: Fisher Scientific 05-538-59A, Corning #430790 (BD).
4. Cryotubes conical 1.0 mL, Nunc #375353 (Nalge Nunc, Rochester, NY).

2.3. Elisa

1. ELISA reader (Perseptive Biosystems, Cytofluor Series 4000, Foster City, CA), set for Excitation 450/50, Emission 580/50, gain 25 (*see* **Note 1**).
2. Microplate Washer ELx405 (BioTek, Winooski, VT) set for delivery volume of 150 µl/well at flow rate of 5.
3. 2 × 12-channel pipetter 5–50 µl and 50–300 µl; Fisher #21-377-828 and #21-377-830 (Thermo Fisher Scientific, Hampton, NH).
4. Finnpipette 0.5–10 µl Fisher #21-377-816.
5. Finnpipette 5–50 µl Fisher #21–377–818.
6. *Pipette tips.* Fisher Scientific 07-200-302 Corning #4865 (Corning, Lowell, MA).
7. *15-mL centrifuge tubes.* Fisher Scientific 05-538-59A, Corning #430790.
8. *50-mL centrifuge tubes.* Fisher Scientific 05526B, Corning #430828.
9. *96-well plates.* Costar half area, Corning #07-200-37.
10. *96-well lids.* Costar, Corning #07-200-597.
11. 96-well dilution trays, Assay Block, 0.5 mL, V-bottom: Costar, Corning #3957.
12. *Disposable pipetter basins.* Fisher #13-681-100.
13. *Secondary antibody.* Southern Biotech (Birmingham, AL) #2040-04, goat antihuman IgG-AP (1:2000–1:4000,

pretest each new lot). Store at –20°C, keep working aliquot at 4°C (*see* **Note 2**).

14. *Substrate*. Promega (Madison, WI) #S1013 or JBL Scientific Inc (San Luis Obispo, CA) #JBL 1670A, Attophos 1g. Stored at –20°C (can be refrozen).

15. *Attophos buffer*. Fisher #NC9780498, 60 mL per bottle. Store at 4°C.

16. *Ready-to-use substrate*. Weigh 36 mg substrate, add to 60 mL buffer, store 1 month at 4°C.

17. *Protein antigen*. Supplied in urea or PBS, always dilute in PBS. Store at –20°C, keep working aliquot at 4°C.

18. *Blocking buffer (5% NF milk in PBS)*. 500 mL PBS + 150 µg sodium azide + 25 g nonfat-dry-milk (any brand). Make fresh weekly. Store at 4°C.

19. *Wash buffers*. PBS and PBS + 0.1% Tween-20. Store at RT.

20. *Stop solution*. 3N NaOH (in distilled water). Store at RT.

3. Methods

3.1. Protein Preparation

Several prokaryotic expression systems are commercially available. We have used the Qiagen 6X-His tag expression system that allows purification of the recombinant protein by nickel affinity chromatography. Of the various vectors, we have used pQE30 vector with 6X His tag at the N-terminus.

For protein of interest, primers are designed to amplify the entire amino acid-encoding portion of the cDNA sequence. These primers are designed so that they contain the appropriate restriction cloning sites immediately flanking the translational initiation codon (ATG) and the termination codon. This design allows the production of a full-length protein with the 6X-His tag in the N-terminus, separated only by the 6-bp restriction enzyme site of choice, e.g., BamHI (GAATTC), which would encode two amino acid residues. The final protein product thus consists almost entirely of the protein sequence of interest, with a short 5′ tag of ~10 residues.

The cloning and induction of recombinant protein synthesis is performed following manufacturer's protocols, using *E. coli* strain M15 (pREP4) as the host cells. Large-scale protein production was performed using 1 l culture, with cells harvested after overnight IPTG induction (~20 h). The bacteria are lysed using 8 M Guanidinium HCl-based buffer, and the protein is purified over a nickel ion affinity column, under denaturing condition in 8 M urea buffer system. Column binding, washing, and protein elution are performed using a pH gradient (of 8.0, 6.3, 5.9, and 4.5), essentially as described in the manufacturer's manual. We have found the recombinant proteins to be eluted in the pH 4.5 fractions in most cases. The eluted protein fractions are pooled and dialyzed against a step gradient of PBS solutions that contain 6 M, 4 M, 2 M, 1 M, and 0 M urea, respectively. This allows at least partial renaturalization of the proteins. The final protein preparation is quantified and ready for ELISA. If desired, the purity of the protein can be evaluated by silver staining and/or Western blotting, using commercially available anti-His tag antibodies.

3.2. Preparation of Serum/Plasma Samples

This method measures the antibody (IgG, IgM, or IgG1–4) response to tumor antigens from either PLASMA or SERUM samples, as one chooses, without significant differences in results.

1. The collection of plasma samples is preferred if the amount of blood collection is limiting, as in the case of patients from clinical studies subjected to multiple bleedings. For plasma, separate a couple of heparin-coated green-top tubes (7–10 mL) intended for PBMC separation. Spin them at $350 \times g$ for 5 min and collect the yellow phase (1–4 mL: plasma). The rest of the tube can be used for PBMC separation if needed. The collected plasma is then spun again 10 min at ($900 \times g$) to remove platelets. The supernatant is aliquoted and stored at –70°C in polypropylene cryovials until use.

   For serum, collect 5–10 mL blood in a red-top tube (without heparin) and let it sit at room temperature for a few hours until it clots. Pipette the yellow phase (1–4 mL: serum) and spin it 10 min at 2,000 rpm ($900 \times g$) to remove possible debris. Collect the supernatant and store aliquots at –70°C in polypropylene cryovials until use.

3.3. ELISA

The following method is designed to allow high-throughput assays while minimizing amounts needed for serum or plasma.

A minimum of three antigens should be tested in each assay for determining specificity, and positive and negative control sera should be used for validation on each plate.

A negative control pool should be prepared from pretested sera from 5 to 6 healthy donors, without reactivity to the antigens tested, and pooled together. The same negative control pool should be used for standardization and reproducibility throughout an entire study, since titers will be calculated based on this control.

1. Coating plates with antigens: Add 1 μg/mL of desired antigen diluted in PBS, 30 μl/well.
   Incubate overnight at 4°C or at RT for 2 h.

2. Shake off contents and perform two cycles of four washes with PBS.

3. Block with 5% NF milk in PBS, 30 μl/well, incubate overnight at 4°C or 2 h at RT.

4. Shake off contents and wash as in **step 2**.

5. Prepare serum dilution in blocking buffer in 96-well dilution trays. Usual serum dilutions are in 4 × increments, starting from 1:100: 1:100, 1:400, 1:1,600, 1:6,400, etc (*see* **Note 3**).

6. Shake off last wash, blot dry, and add serum dilutions 30 μl/well, incubate at 4°C overnight.

7. Shake off contents and perform one cycle of four washes with PBS + 0.1% Tween 20 followed by one cycle of four washes with PBS.

8. Shake off last wash, blot dry, and add secondary antibody (goat antihuman IgG-AP, (*see* **Note 2**) at appropriate dilution in blocking buffer, 30 μl/well and incubate for 1 h at RT.

9. Shake off contents and wash as in **step 7**.

10. Shake off last wash, blot dry, and add 30 μl substrate, incubate in dark for 30 min at RT.

11. Stop color development by adding 15 μl stop solution (3N NaOH).

12. Read on ELISA reader at Excitation 450/50 and Emission 580/50 with gain of 25. Representative values from control and sample sera are shown in **Fig. 1**.

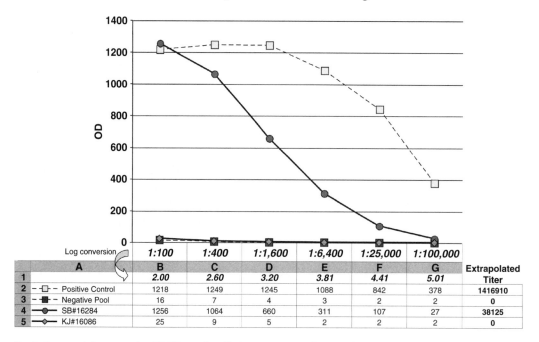

	A	B	C	D	E	F	G	Extrapolated Titer
Log conversion		*1:100*	*1:400*	*1:1,600*	*1:6,400*	*1:25,000*	*1:100,000*	
1		*2.00*	*2.60*	*3.20*	*3.81*	*4.41*	*5.01*	
2	– ☐ – Positive Control	1218	1249	1245	1088	842	378	1416910
3	– ■ – Negative Pool	16	7	4	3	2	2	0
4	● SB#16284	1256	1064	660	311	107	27	38125
5	◆ KJ#16086	25	9	5	2	2	2	0

Fig. 1. Representative example of ELISA results with four serum samples tested in serial dilutions, shown in OD values, against full-length protein antigen NY-ESO-1. All samples were obtained with informed consent under IRB approved protocols: positive control serum is from melanoma patient NW-29 (from Dr. E. Jäger, Frankfurt, Germany), negative control is from a pool of 6 healthy donor sera from the blood bank, and serum samples SB#16284 and KJ#16086 are from ovarian cancer patients (from Dr. K. Odunsi, Buffalo, NY) (*See Color Plates*).

3.4. Interpretation

ELISA results are expressed in titers, which is a standardized and comparable value, regardless of OD readings obtained.

As shown in **Fig. 2**, in order to calculate a titer, it is first necessary to determine a cutoff value above which a serum is considered reactive. This cutoff value is based on the reactivity of the negative control serum pool and is defined as: 10 × average OD of the first 4 dilutions of the negative control serum pool.

In the example from **Fig. 2**, the cutoff is calculated as: $10*AVERAGE(22,11,6,3) = 105$.

Then, the reciprocal titer of a specific serum/plasma sample is defined as the minimal dilution factor for which an OD greater than the cutoff can be measured **(Fig. 2)**. An approximation of this titer value can be performed using a simple function from Microsoft Excel® named FORECAST. This function will extrapolate the linear part of a dilution curve and determine the dilution factor at which the curve meets the cutoff.

The Excel® function is written as follows: $10^\wedge FORECAST$ (Cutoff, DilutionRange, DilutionCurve), where Cutoff is the value defined earlier, DilutionRange is the range of dilutions in a logarithmic scale, and DilutionCurve is the series of OD values for a particular sample.

In the example from **Fig. 1**:
- Cutoff is $10*AVERAGE(B3:E3) = 10*(16 + 7 + 4 + 3)/4 = 75$

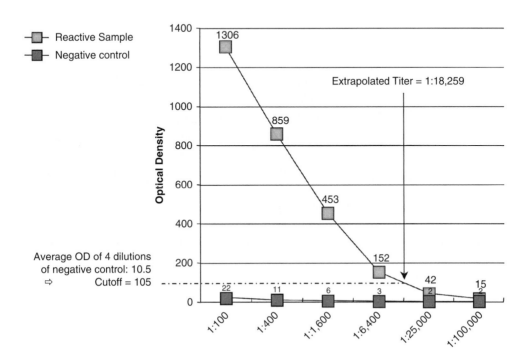

Fig. 2. Example of ELISA results to illustrate method for calculating titers (*See Color Plates*).

- DilutionRange is [B1:G1]
- DilutionCurve for sample SB#16284 is [B4:G4]
  The titer for sample SB#16284 is calculated as:
  =10^FORECAST(10*AVERAGE($B$3:$E$3),$B$1:$G$1, B4:G4), which yields an estimated reciprocal titer of 38,125.

If the actual titer has not been reached within the experimental titration, as in the case of the positive control in **Fig. 1**, a value is still extrapolated but may not be very accurate. The formula works best when the titer is actually within the linear part of the dilution range used.

One still needs to be careful, since there are quite a lot of false positive and artifacts that can come up. Notably, a single aberrant value can dramatically affect the aspect of the curve. Each titer should therefore be visually quality controlled!

Reactivity of a serum sample is considered negative if the reciprocal titer is < 100, weakly positive (±) from 100 to 1,000, positive (+) from 1,000 to 10,000, strongly positive (++) from 10,000 to 100,000, and very strongly positive (+++) above 100,000

4. Notes

1. Other fluorescence-detection microplate readers can be used. Results presented here are with the instrument cited, giving a dynamic range of OD readings from 0 to 3,000.
2. Instead of antihuman IgG, other secondary antibodies can be used for measuring for example IgM content, or subclasses of immunoglobulin (IgG1, IgG2, etc.)
3. Alternatively, especially for large series of sera, it is possible to proceed in two steps: screening samples at 2 dilutions only (for example 1:100 and 1:1,000) and then titrate these samples in the number of dilutions necessary to best estimate their actual titers.

Acknowledgments

The authors would like to thank Dr. Lin-Chi Chen and Erika Ritter for helping establish the method and Dr. Gerd Ritter for helpful discussions. The authors also acknowledge the Cancer Research Institute for its support.

References

1. Dunn, G. P., Old, L. J., and Schreiber, R. D. (2004) The three Rs of cancer immunoediting. *Annu. Rev. Immunol.* 22, 329–60

2. Smyth, M. J., Dunn, G. P., and Schreiber, R. D. (2006) Cancer immunosurveillance and immunoediting: the roles of immunity in suppressing tumor development and shaping tumor immunogenicity. *Adv. Immunol.* 90, 1–50

3. Koebel, C. M., Vermi, W., Swann, J. B., Zerafa, N., Rodig, S. J., Old, L. J. Smyth, M. J., and Schreiber, R. D. (2007) Adaptive wimmunity maintains occult cancer in an equilibrium state. *Nature* 450, 903–07

4. Zitvogel, L., Tesniere, A., and Kroemer, G. (2006) Cancer despite immunosurveillance: immunoselection and immunosubversion. *Nat. Rev. Immunol.* 6, 715–27

5. Gnjatic, S., Nishikawa, H., Jungbluth, A. A., Güre, A. O., Ritter, G., Jäger, E.,Knuth, A., Chen, Y. T., and Old, L. J. (2006) NY-ESO-1: review of an immunogenic tumor antigen. *Adv. Cancer Res.* 95, 1–30

6. Soussi, T. (2000) p53 Antibodies in the sera of patients with various types of cancer: a review. *Cancer Res.* 60, 1777–88

7. Stockert, E., Jäger, E., Chen, Y. T., Scanlan, M. J., Gout, I., Karbach, J., Arand, M., Knuth, A., and Old, L. J. (1998) A survey of the humoral immune response of cancer patients to a panel of human tumor antigens. *J. Exp. Med.* 187, 1349–54

8. Gnjatic, S., Atanackovic, D., Jäger, E., Matsuo, M., Selvakumar, A., Altorki, N. K., Maki, R. G., Dupont, B., Ritter, G., Chen, Y. T., Knuth, A., and Old, L. J. (2003) Survey of naturally occurring CD4+ T cell responses against NY-ESO-1 in cancer patients: correlation with antibody responses. *Proc. Natl Acad. Sci. U S A* 100, 8862–67

9. Jäger, E., Nagata, Y., Gnjatic, S., Wada, H., Stockert, E., Karbach, J., Dunbar, P. R., Lee, S. Y., Jungbluth, A., Jager, D., Arand, M., Ritter, G., Cerundolo, V., Dupont, B., Chen, Y. T., Old, L. J., and Knuth, A. (2000) Monitoring CD8 T cell responses to NY-ESO-1: correlation of humoral and cellular immune responses. *Proc. Natl Acad. Sci. U S A* 97, 4760–65

10. Jäger, E., Stockert, E., Zidianakis, Z., Chen, Y. T., Karbach, J., Jäger, D., Arand, M., Ritter, G., Old, L. J., and Knuth, A. (1999) Humoral immune responses of cancer patients against "Cancer-Testis" antigen NY-ESO-1: correlation with clinical events. *Int. J. Cancer* 84, 506–10

11. Chen, Y. T., Scanlan, M. J., Obata, Y., and Old, L. J. (2000) Humoral immune responses of cancer patients against "Cancer-Testis" antigen NY-ESO-1: correlation with clinical events in "Biologic therapy of cancer" (de Vita, V. T., Hellman, S., and Rosenberg, S. A., Eds.), pp. 557–70, J. B. Lippincott Company, Philadelphia, PA

12. Sahin, U., Tureci, O., Schmitt, H., Cochlovius, B., Johannes, T., Schmits, R., Stenner, F., Luo, G., Schobert, I., and Pfreundschuh, M. (1995) Human neoplasms elicit multiple specific immune responses in the autologous host. *Proc. Natl Acad. Sci. U S A* 92, 11810–3

13. Chen, Y. T., Gure, A. O., and Scanlan, M. J. (2005) Serological analysis of expression cDNA libraries (SEREX): an immunoscreening technique for identifying immunogenic tumor antigens. *Methods Mol. Med.* 103, 207–16

14. Chen, Y. T., Scanlan, M. J., Sahin, U., Türeci, Ö., Güre, A. O., Tsang, S., Williamson, B., Stockert, E., Pfreundschuh, M., and Old, L. J. (1997) A testicular antigen aberrantly expressed in human cancers detected by autologous antibody screening. *Proc. Natl. Acad. Sci. U S A* 94, 1914–18

15. Güre, A. O., Stockert, E., Scanlan, M. J., Keresztes, R. S., Jäger, D., Altorki, N. K., Old, L. J., and Chen, Y. T. (2000) Serological identification of embryonic neural proteins as highly immunogenic tumor antigens in small cell lung cancer. *Proc. Natl Acad. Sci. U S A* 97, 4198–203

16. Atanackovic, D., Arfsten, J., Cao, Y., Gnjatic, S., Schnieders, F., Bartels, K., Schilling, G., Faltz, C., Wolschke, C., Dierlamm, J., Ritter, G., Eiermann, T., Hossfeld, D. K., Zander, A. R., Jungbluth, A. A., Old, L. J., Bokemeyer, C., and Kroger, N. (2007) Cancer-testis antigens are commonly expressed in multiple myeloma and induce systemic immunity following allogeneic stem cell transplantation. *Blood* 109, 1103–12

Chapter 3

Discovery of Antibody Biomarkers Using Protein Microarrays of Tumor Antigens Cloned in High Throughput

Madhumita Chatterjee, Jerzy Wojciechowski, and Michael A. Tainsky

Summary

Development of humoral and cellular immunity against self-cellular proteins in cancer patients is a phe-
nomenal observation. The ability of immune system to sense the presence of the disease and to fight
of the disease by generating autoantibodies against tumor antigens makes it a natural biosensor. Several
screening technologies have been employed for the identification of tumor-specific antibodies in cancer
patients. We have developed a multidimensional approach for the identification of diagnostic antigens
that utilizes a combination of high-throughput antigen cloning and protein microarray-based serological
detection of complex panels of antigens by exploiting the serum autoantibody repertoire directed toward
tumor-associated antigens in cancer patients. Furthermore, validation of these antigens by different bioinformatics and biological approaches will reveal the diagnostic/prognostic utility of these antigens for
personalized immunotherapy.

Key words: Immune response, Tumor biomarkers, Autoantibodies, Epitopes, Protein microarrays,
Immunotherapy.

1. Introduction

The early diagnosis of cancer has been a challenging field of
research for many years. Early-stage diagnosis increases the probability of cure, and therefore diagnostic screening tests that can
detect these early stages are crucial. Some cellular proteins elevated in sera from cancer subjects are also found in individuals
suffering from other diseases such as inflammatory diseases and
autoimmune disorders. Tumor-specific proteins are identified as
elevated in primary tumor tissue, metastatic lesions, or ascites
fluid are only true tumor biomarkers suitable for early detection

Michael A. Tainsky, *Methods in Molecular Biology, Tumor Biomarker Discovery, Vol. 520*
© Humana Press, a part of Springer Science + Business Media, LLC 2009
DOI: 10.1007/978-1-60327-811-9_3

if they are elevated in blood (plasma, serum), saliva, or urine from cancer patients. These biomarkers are found to be specific and sensitive reporters of disease that are able to indicate a change in expression or state of a protein that correlates with the risk or progression of a disease, or with the susceptibility of the disease to various therapeutic interventions. In comparison to secreted tumor proteins that may be present in circulation for a short time because of transient shedding from tumors in the tumor microenvironment or degradation in serum, serum antibodies are stable, present in the serum for a long time, and are readily detectable with an enzyme-conjugated secondary antibody (1). The idea of using serum antibody for diagnosis of cancer is supported by the vast evidence of generation of humoral immune responses against tumor-associated antigens (TAA) in different cancers (2). It has been observed that 30% of patients with DCIS in which the protooncogene HER2/neu was overexpressed had serum autoantibodies specific to this protein (3, 4). In addition, autoantibodies to p53 have been reported in patients with early-stage ovarian and colorectal cancers (5, 6). Autoantibodies against heat shock protein HSP90 were also found to correlate with patient's survival and metastasis (7, 8). Autoantibodies against ribosomal proteins may constitute a novel serological marker. In this regard, autoantibodies to ribosomal protein S3 were detected in 10% of patients with breast cancer, whereas no reactivity was found in normal sera (9). Occurrence of autoantibodies to ubiquitin C-terminal hydrolase L3 in colon cancer had also been reported (10). Changes in the level of gene expression in cancer (3, 11–13) and aberrant expression of tissue-restricted gene products in cancer (14, 15) are factors in the development of a humoral immune response in cancer patients. Various technologies have been reported for the detection of antigens/TAAs on the basis of large repertoire of serum antibodies that are generated because of humoral immune responses in different cancers.

Serological analysis of tumor antigens by recombinant cDNA expression cloning (SEREX) was developed by the group of Michael Pfreundschuh at the University of Saarland, Germany, in 1995 (2). A SEREX/Cancer Immunome database (http://www2.licr.org/CancerImmunomeDB) has been organized and lists more than 2,000 antigens (16). The SEREX approach includes the construction of cDNA libraries from fresh tumor specimens and cloning into lambda phage expression vectors. The recombinant phages are used to infect E. coli cells. Recombinant proteins expressed during lytic infection of the bacteria are replica-plated onto nitrocellulose membranes and immunoscreened with autologous serum. Clones reactive with high-titer IgG antibodies are identified using enzyme-conjugated secondary antibody specific for human IgG. The identity of the reactive antigens is revealed by sequence results of the cDNA inserts.

The underlying mechanism for immunogenicity of cancer antigens is often overexpression of normal gene products or mutation in cancer. The immune response to cancer testis (CT) antigens is clearly related to the anomalous expression of gene products in cancer tissues that are normally only expressed in primitive germ cells (17). CT antigen expression in cancer has been ascribed to abnormal demethylation (18). Humoral immune response to SEREX-defined CT antigens, MAGE, tyrosinase, and NY-ESO-1 has been detected in melanoma patients (19). Amplified expression appears to be one of the most frequent reasons for the immunogenicity of antigens isolated by SEREX, and many examples of antibodies to overexpressed gene products in cancer have been detected in SEREX analysis, e.g.,, eIF-4 gamma in lung cancer (20); HER-2/neu in breast cancer (13). With regard to mutations as a basis for immunogenicity, the tumor suppressor gene p53 is a classic example of mutational antigen that was detected by SEREX analysis of ovarian cancer (21). The CT antigens are immunogenic and highly restricted to tumors. Therefore, they are considered as excellent targets for immunotherapy. Jager et al. have reported that immunization with peptides obtained from MAGE-1 and MAGE-3 when used alone or in combination with adjuvants have resulted in regression of tumor in more than 30% of patients diagnosed with melanoma (22). Although the SEREX approach has been successful in identifying tumor antigens from many different cancers, this technology has some limitations. First, this technology is based on screening tumor-derived cDNA libraries made from a particular patient with serum obtained from autologous patient. As a result, the identified TAAs in most cases do not show high reactivity with allogeneic patients' sera. Second, this approach tends to identify antigens that were overexpressed in the tumor and thus highly abundant in tumor-derived cDNA libraries. Thus low abundant messages that may be encoding for tumor relevant antigens are generally missed. Third, as prokaryotic system is used in this biopanning, post-translational modifications such as glycosylation cannot be found as novel cancer antigens. As a result, humoral immune responses directed toward glycosylated residues in TAA can remain unidentified. Thus, several modifications have been introduced to improve this technology. The first variation involves established tumor cell lines instead of fresh tumor specimen as a source of cDNA. Thus, contaminating normal cell types present in tumor specimens will not be included in cDNA preparation, and cDNA cloning of IgG sequences expressed by tumor infiltrating B cells giving rise to false-positives will be prevented (23). Second, the screening of sera from cancer patients on allogeneic cDNA libraries including testicular cDNA libraries may result in identification of TAA and CT antigens that will show higher reactivity with serum IgGs obtained from many different cancers.

1.1. Global Profiling of Cancer Antigen Epitopes (Epitomics)

1.1.1. Protein Microarrays

A new high-throughput technology has been recently developed by our group based on serological identification of tumor antigens by profiling humoral immune responses in cancer patients. We refer to this approach as "Epitomics." Our technology detects antibodies that are produced by cancer patients in reaction to proteins overexpressed or mutated in their tumors and uses them as diagnostic biomarkers. Our multidimensional strategy comprised high-throughput antigen cloning using phage display technology coupled with serological identification of tumor antigens and profiling humoral immune responses in cancer patients on protein microarrays. For high-throughput antigen cloning, our group has developed an undirected approach using T7 phage display techniques ("differential biopanning") to identify the cancer antigen space within the human proteome *(24, 25)*. T7 phages have several advantages over lambda phage in that one can screen 2–3 log more phage clones in a single experiment, several libraries can be pooled and screened in parallel, and the life cycle of the T7 phage is far faster so that the process of cloning is more rapid. Our lab has established a bar coding strategy for the identification of T7 phage cDNA clones from a pool of T7 phage cDNA libraries that are constructed with mRNAs obtained from multiple sources (cancer cell lines or tumor specimens) to maximize representation and heterogeneity of cDNA (**Fig. 1a–d**) also described in **Subheading 3.4**). Differential bioppaning involves immunoscreening of T7 phage tumor-derived cDNA libraries using a two-step process, starting with protein-G beads bound with serum IgGs pooled from different age-matched normal healthy individuals (as described **Subheading 3**). This step helps in the removal of nontumor/common antigens that bind to IgGs in normal sera. Next, serum IgGs from cancer patients also bound to protein-G beads are used as the bait in biopanning in order to enrich for clones of tumor antigens. The bound antigens are eluted and the resulting phage clones are amplified for the next round of biopanning. A graphical representation of output eluant phage enrichments/phage titers after each cycle of biopanning resembles the general shape of an exponential function with a trend to approach saturation curve in the last two stages of biopanning. That may be explained by the nature of T7 phage selection and its enrichment process retaining the diversity of the reactive phage clones (**Fig. 2a**). However, for certain biopannings, we have observed a variety of possible shapes for the curves. First, this may indicate a kinetic complexity of gradual enrichment of the eluant in specifically bound and selected T7 phage as well as complex equilibrium of reversible adsorption of phage to the beads and antibodies. We postulate that interactions between beads, antibodies, and phage are maintained by complex sets of forces such as hydrophobic and van der Waals bonds that can be formed or broken upon the change of pH, different washing

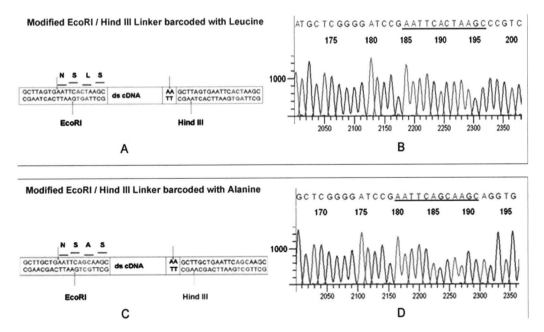

Fig. 1. Bar coded *EcoRI*/*Hind*III directional linkers used for the construction of T7 phage cDNA libraries. (**A**) The modified linker with the bar coding sequence obtained by adding triplet nucleotides in frame (color coded in pink and blue) and it resulted in the addition of amino acid "Leucine" in the linker region of the cDNA. (**B**) Partial sequence result representing the underlined linker sequence of the T7 phage clone obtained from T7 phage cDNA library constructed from OVC0156 ovarian tumor. (**C**) The modified linker with the bar coding sequence that resulted in the addition of amino acid "Alanine" in the linker region of the cDNA. (**D**) Partial sequence result representing the underlined linker sequence of the T7 phage clone obtained from T7 phage cDNA library constructed from OVCAR3 ovarian cancer cell line.

conditions, temperature of the reaction environment *(26, 27)*. Second, any noticeable divergence from a saturated-exponential shape of enrichment (**Fig. 2c**) such as a sudden increase in the titer between two consecutive cycles (magnitude more than 3–6 times) or early plateau of the titer curve might be indicative of an irregular distortion of the enrichment process and, hence, may dramatically diminish the diversity of the clones for a particular fraction. In an extreme situation, the recovered fraction contains a few or just a single clone that binds tightly to the antibodies on the beads which may be considered "overbiopanning." The process of enrichment proceeds at relatively slow degree in the beginning of biopanning (cycles 1 and 2) with rapid progression between cycles 3 and 5 (**Fig. 2a, c**). The extent of clonal diversity can be determined by PCR amplification of the cDNA inserts and comparing the sizes from a group of at least 20 phage clones from each biopanning (**Fig. 2b, d**).

Generally, after four cycles of biopanning, the immunoreactive phage clones are picked from multiple independent patients and are robotically printed on protein microarrays to identify

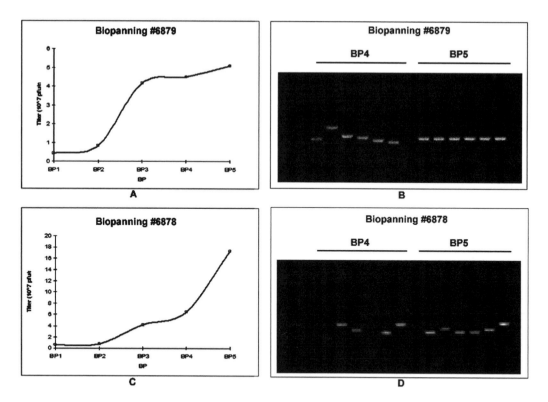

Fig. 2. Typical output eluant phage titers obtained after biopanning (cycles *1–5*) depicting variation in insert size. (**A**) Graphical representation (not the shape of an exponential function) of the output eluant phage titers as a function of biopanning. (**B**) Occurence of over-biopanning in fifth cycle (BP5) resulting in an unexpected jump in the titer value and corresponding lack of diversity of its clones as indicated by PCR amplification of phage clones picked up from biopanning 4 and 5 (BP4 & BP5). (**C**) Graphical representation (shape of an exponential function) of the output eluant phage titers resulting in the enrichment of immuno-reactive phage after the completion of each cycle of biopanning. (**D**) PCR amplification of the phage clones picked up from biopanning 4 and 5 (BP4 & BP5) showing retention of diversity in the pool of immuno-reactive phage as indicated by the range of insert sizes.

circulating serum antibodies produced by the cancer patient presumably to proteins from the cancer cells or tissue. Microarrays are processed with several sera obtained from cancer patients as well as healthy individuals. We previously used Cy3 (green fluorescent dye)-labeled T7 monoclonal antibody, directed against phage capsid protein, and Cy5 (red fluorescent dye)-labeled goat antihuman IgG that recognized the test subject's IgG bound to the antigens on the arrays for processing arrays *(24, 25)*. Recently we have introduced Alexa Fluor-labeled goat antimouse and goat antihuman secondary IgGs as secondary antibodies as described in **Subheading 3**. After processing, arrays are scanned and the ratio of antihuman IgG and anti-T7 capsid is determined by comparing the fluorescence intensities in the Cy5-Cy3 *(24, 25)* or Alexa Fluor-specific channels at each spot using standard image analysis programs. The microarray data are preprocessed and normalized using local background subtraction of the raw spot signals. The red over green channel intensity ratios are log-transformed and the data are normalized to the print-tip group median within each array. Mean of spot replicates (quadruplicate) is taken for further statistical analysis.

1.1.2. Validation of Biomarkers by Different Approaches

Bioinformatics approach. Initially, selection of clones for a second generation of protein microarray chips is performed by applying two-sided t-test or Bootstrapping ROC method *(28)* on the data set that comprised certain number of cancer patients, patients with benign or other diseases of the homologous tissue and healthy controls. These newly selected clones are printed on a second-generation antigen microarrays. These chips are processed with these and other samples that are now going to constitute the training set. Selection of clones and development of a model are conducted on this training set. For evaluation of the selected clones, validation is conducted on an independent test set that comprised other cancer patients, more healthy controls, and other benign and other diseases. All of the serum samples in these test sets cannot have been previously used in any phase of the study.

Biological Approaches

1. *Immunohistochemistry (IHC).* Statistical analysis of our microarray data revealed a panel of molecular markers (classifier) which showed highest reactivity with sera from epithelial ovarian cancer (EOC) patients and no reactivity with sera obtained from normal healthy individuals or from patients with benign or other gynecological diseases *(24)*. For the assessment of expression levels of these top-ranking biomarkers, like RCAS1, eIF5A, and Nibrin, paraffin-embedded formalin fixed tumor specimens were collected from ovarian cancer patients to test the protein level using immunohistochemical staining with commercially available antibodies to those biomarkers using a standard protocols *(24)*. We found that RCAS1 was highly expressed in 23 out of 30 early-stage and 27 out of 30 late-stage tumors. Likewise the antigen biomarker eIF5A (isolated twice) was also highly expressed in 13 out of 30 early-stage and 27 out of 30 late-stage tumors. The biomarker, p95 Nibrin, was positive in the sera of early- and late-stage EOC patients in our microarray analysis, but the immunohistochemistry showed that elevated expression was specific to late-stage cancers. This marker was expressed in only 1 out of 30 early-stage but 15 out of 30 late-stage tumors. The one early-stage patient who had a positive immunohistochemical reaction was a stage 1C patient who was never off therapy and died 2.5 years after diagnosis. All of these antibodies have no positive staining on normal ovaries or ovarian cysts. These data confirm our

hypothesis that these proteins are overexpressed in ovarian tumors, and it is likely that overexpression is the mechanism by which they become immunogenic. These data also indicate that our approach to identifying serum biomarkers may reveal tissue markers that are stage-specific at the immuno-histochemistry level *(24)*.

2. *Quantitative real-time PCR (Q-RT-PCR)*. The expression of immunoreactive antigens at the mRNA level could also be validated by performing Q-RT-PCR. Generally, a correlation between high protein expression (using IHC) as a result of high mRNA expression (using Q-RT-PCR) explains the underlying mechanism of generation of humoral immune response. In cases where high expression level of protein does not correlate with mRNA level, genetic mutation analysis should be pursued because mutations can lead to increased immunogenicity of an epitope thereby eliciting humoral immune response *(29)*.

Thus top-ranking antigens obtained from statistical and biological analyses are readily amenable to reformatting into an immunoassay as a diagnostic predictor of cancer as described earlier. The utilization of this diagnostic test in the clinic would be as a periodic, *in vitro* diagnostic screening immunoassay to detect the presence of cancer. The Epitomics approach has been adopted by others in the field of cancer antigen biomarkers *(30, 31)*. The strength of this approach is the developing of large panels of biomarkers from the antigen space within the human serum proteome that are less sensitive to interpatient variations in the population. This methodology is capable of accurate detection of antibodies in the sera of test subjects. The greater speed and simplicity of this serological approach may also be used for detection of autoantibodies in various autoimmune diseases and possibly even surrogate markers for disease for unknown etiology. A major advantage of our system is that we detect specific IgGs in serum. The IgG is the most stable, functional protein in serum having 5–10 times the half-life of other immunoglobulins as described earlier. To further verify the stability of serum IgGs, we have performed several tests with serum sample such as repeated freezing or left overnight at room temperature with little change in the results at the microarray analysis. Many serum analytes that are labile are generally subjected to interlaboratory variations due to differences in sample handling. In our approach, we identify biomarkers that are IgGs. We have found that leaving the blood overnight at 37°C also does not substantively alter the microarray results. However, the serum cannot be heated to 65°C or dried and rehydrated. Therefore, there should be little interanalyte stability variation among the biomarkers. We have successfully used sera from many other laboratories and serum banks. The only limitation is that the phage display technology cannot detect post-translational modification such as glycosylation. Therefore, the serum antibody repertoire that this technology utilizes for the detection of TAAs is directed toward amino acid epitopes of TAAs.

2. Materials

2.1. Preparation of Total RNA and mRNA from Fresh Tumor Specimen Obtained from Cancer Patient

1. *RNAlater®(Ambion, Austin, TX).* Used as stabilizing agent for tumor specimen (*see* **Note 1**).
2. *RNeasy Maxi Kit (Qiagen, Valentia, CA).* For extraction of total RNA from tumor tissues.
3. Absolutely mRNA Purification Kit (Stratagene, La Jolla, CA) for purification of mRNA from total RNA obtained from tumor tissues.

2.2. Northern Blotting for Quantitation and Quality Control of Tumor Poly(A)-Selected mRNA

1. Agarose (Sigma-Aldrich, St. Louis, MO).
2. Formaldehyde (Sigma-Aldrich, St. Louis, MO).
3. *10× MOPS (Sigma-Aldrich, St. Louis, MO).* 0.22 M MOPS, 0.030 M NaAc, 0.5 M EDTA. Adjust pH 6.6–7.8 with 5N NaOH.
4. Formamide (Sigma-Aldrich, St. Louis, MO).
5. RNA Marker (0.28–6.58 kb) (Promega Corporation, Madison, WI).
6. *Ethidium Bromide (Sigma-Aldrich, St. Louis, MO).* Dissolve at 10 mg/mL in water.
7. *20× SCC.* 3.0 M NaCl, 0.3 M sodium citrate. Adjust pH to 7.0 with concentrated HCl.
8. *NaAc/Methylene Blue for staining the RNA marker.* 0.5 M Sodium acetate, pH 5.0, 0.045% (w/v) Methylene Blue (Fisher Scientific, Pittsburgh, PA). Store at room temperature.
9. *RadPrime DNA Labeling Kit (Invitrogen Corporation, Carlsbad, CA).* Used for labeling cDNA probe for hybridization.
10. Gel blot paper (Schleicher & Schuell, Keene, N.H).
11. Nylon transfer Membrane (Hybond-N+) from GE Healthcare Biosciences Corp, Piscataway, NJ).
12. *Hybridization buffer.* 0.14 M Na_2HPO_4, 0.06 M NaH_2PO_4, 1 mM EDTA, 7% (w/v) SDS, 1% (w/v) BSA.
13. *Wash Buffer 1.* 2× SSC, 0.1% SDS.
14. *Wash Buffer 2.* 0.5× SSC, 0.1% SDS.

2.3 T7. Bacteriophage cDNA Library

1. *Eighty percent glycerol.* 80% (v/v) in water and autoclave.
2. *Fifty percent polyethylene glycol 8000 (PEG). Dissolve 100 g PEG in deionized water with stirring, autoclave, and bring the volume to 200 mL with sterile deionized water.*
3. *Tris-EDTA (TE). 10 mM Tris–HCl, pH 8.0, 1 mM EDTA.*
4. *62.5% CsCl.* (25 g CsCl + 15 mL deionized water).

2.4. Growth Media for Bacteriophage T7

1. *LB.* Add 10 g Bacto peptone (Fisher scientific, Pittsburgh, PA), 5 g Yeast extract (Fisher scientific, Pittsburgh, PA), 10 g NaCl (Fisher scientific, Pittsburgh, PA) per liter. Adjust pH to 7.5 with 1N NaOH. Autoclave for 20 min and store at room temperature.
2. 20× M9 salt solution (Fisher scientific, Pittsburgh, PA). Autoclave and store at room temperature.
3. Twenty percent glucose solution (Fisher scientific, Pittsburgh, PA). Autoclave and store at room temperature.
4. One molar $MgSO_4$ (Fisher scientific, Pittsburgh, PA). Autoclave and store at room temperature.
5. 50 mg/mL (w/v) Carbenicillin (Sigma-Aldrich, St. Louis, MO) (*see* **Note 2**).
6. 0.1 M Isopropyl-1-thio-β-D-galactopyranoside (IPTG) (Sigma-Aldrich, St. Louis, MO) (*see* **Note 2**).
7. 3.5 mg/mL (w/v) Phenylmethylsulfonylfluoride (PMSF) (Sigma-Aldrich, St. Louis, MO). This solution has to be freshly prepared before use.
8. Protease inhibitor cocktail (Sigma-Aldrich, St. Louis, MO).
9. Two percent (w/v) Gelatin (Sigma-Aldrich, St. Louis, MO). Autoclave and store at room temperature.

2.5. Biopanning of T7 cDNA Phage Displayed Libraries with Human Sera

1. 1× Phosphate-buffered saline (1× PBS) (Sigma-Aldrich, St. Louis, MO).
2. Protein G PLUS-agarose beads (Santa Cruz Biotechnology, Inc., Santa Cruz, CA).
3. 1% (w/v) Sodium dodecyl sulfate (SDS) (Sigma-Aldrich, St. Louis, MO) in water.

2.6. Agar Plates for Plaque Assay of Bacteriophage T7

1. 0.7% (w/v) agar in LB and autoclave (for performing plaque assay).
2. 1.5% (w/v) agar in LB and autoclave (for preparing plates).

2.7. Protein Microarrays

1. *1× Phosphate-buffered saline (1× PBS).* 0.136 M NaCl, 0.0026 M KCl, 0.0017 M KH_2PO_4, 0.01 M Na_2HPO_4. Adjust pH to 7.4. Filter PBS through 0.22-μm membrane (Fisher scientific, Pittsburgh, PA) using vacuum.

2. *PBS-T.* 0.1% Tween-20 (v/v) in PBS.
   Four percent milk solution. Add 4 g of powdered milk in 100 mL of 1× PBS. Mix with magnetic stirrer for 30–40 min. Centrifuge for 10 min at 9300 × g and decant the milk solution. Store it at 4°C until use.
3. T7 monoclonal antibody (EMB Chemical Inc., San Diego, CA), Alexa Fluor 532 goat antimouse IgG (H + L) and Alexa fluor 647 goat antihuman IgG (H + L) (Invitrogen Corporation, Carlsbad, CA).

3. Methods

This study describes a novel approach to clone and evaluate utility of tumor antigens in high throughput to detect serum antibodies on protein arrays. Multiple steps of selection of tumor antigens are used in this process. First, a differential biopanning technique is employed to screen a tumor-derived T7 phage display cDNA library so as to isolate cDNAs coding for antigenic proteins binding with antibodies present specifically in the sera of cancer patients but not with antibodies in the sera of healthy women. The selected phage clones are then robotically printed on protein microarrays and processed with several sera (from cancer patients and healthy individuals) and T7 mouse monoclonal antibody (directed toward phage capsid protein). We employ Alexa fluor 647 (red fluorescent dye)-labeled antihuman IgG to detect patient serum IgGs binding to clones on the microarrays. The red fluorescent intensity representing the binding of the test subject's IgG molecules on the same spot of phage proteins is compared with an Alexa flour 532 (green fluorescent dye)-labeled antimouse IgG to detect the T7 phage capsid protein. This latter reagent binds to every T7 phage clone and serves to normalize for variations in the amount of each antigen clone at each spot. We perform these microarray assays at a 1:300 dilution of each patient's serum. The digitized dye ratio data derived from the images are analyzed by IMAGENE™ software. Next, the processed chips are scanned using axon scanner, and the intensity of each spot is quantified using IMAGENE™ software (Biodiscovery). Statistical analyses are performed as described previously.

3.1. Serum Samples

1. Blood samples from cancer patients and healthy individuals are obtained from different institutions. Processing of blood to extract serum is performed in our laboratory. Briefly, blood samples are centrifuged at 150 × g at 4°C for 20 min and supernatants are stored at −80°C until use.

3.2. Isolation of Total RNA and mRNA from Fresh Tumor Specimen

1. *Isolation of mRNA from total RNA.* Total RNA is prepared from fresh tumor specimen (suspended in RNA*later*®) using RNeasy Maxi Kit following manufacturer's instructions.

2. Purification of Poly(A)+ mRNA is performed using Absolutely mRNA Purification Kit by following the instructions as suggested by the manufacturer. Poly(A)+ mRNA is quantitated by UV spectroscopy and the process of poly(A) selection is repeated. Twice poly(A) selected mRNA is stored at –80°C for use in library preparation. For quality control, northern blot is performed with the double poly(A)+ selected mRNA obtained from tumor tissues and comparing the hybridization signal for a GAPDH probe with that detection in 20 times more micrograms of total RNA (*see* **Note 3**).

3.3. Northern Blotting of Double Poly(A)+ mRNA

1. *Preparation of agarose gel.* 1.5% Agarose (w/v), 1× MOPS, 3% Formaldehyde (v/v). 10 μg of total RNA or 0.4 μg of mRNA are mixed separately with RNAase-free water to make the final volume to 5.5 μL. To each add 1.0 μL 10× MOPS, 3.5 μL Formaldehyde, 10 μL Formamide, and 2 μL of 6× loading dye.

2. The RNA samples together with RNA ladder (0.28–6.58 kb) are heated to 65°C for 15 min, chilled in ice and run at 100 V for 1 h.

3. The gel is stained with 0.5 μg/mL ethidium bromide and photograph is taken. The gel is then destained with distilled water and treated with 10× SSC for 15 min (two times).

4. A glass plate is placed on a plastic container containing 10× SSC. A wick (made from Gel blot paper) is placed on the glass plate with two ends touching the solution. Three Gel blot papers (soaked in 10× SSC) are placed on top of the wick. The gel is placed upside down on the wick. The nylon membrane is placed on top of the gel along with three presoaked Gel blot papers. A stack of paper towels are placed on top of the Gel blot papers. Another glass plate (with a heavy weight on top) is placed over the stack of paper towels. This completes the setup for the northern blotting and is kept overnight.

5. After 16–24 h, the setup is disassembled, and the nylon membrane is air-dried for 5–10 min, UV crosslinked on both sides.

6. The portion of the membrane containing the RNA marker is cut off and stained with NaAc/Methylene Blue. The marker is washed in distilled water until the bands become visible.

7. The membrane is prehybridized for 1–2 h in a sealed bag containing 10 mL hybridization buffer.

8. Next, the membrane is allowed to hybridize with the cDNA probe that has been labeled with (α-^{32}P) dCTP using RadPrime DNA Labeling kit (one million counts per mL).

9. After 16 h of hybridization, the membrane is washed with wash buffer 1 at room temp for 10 min (repeated two times).

10. Next, the membrane is washed with wash buffer 2 at 65°C (repeated two times).

11. After the second wash, the membrane is quickly wrapped up in saran wrap and is placed in an X-ray film cassette with film for a suitable exposure of time.

3.4. Construction of the OVCA T7 Phage cDNA Library

1. This is performed using Novagen's OrientExpress cDNA Synthesis (Random primer system) and Cloning system as per manufacturer's suggestions (EMB Chemical Inc., San Diego, CA: cDNA manual, TB247; T7Select System, TB178).

2. The OrientExpress Random Primer System is used to achieve orientation-specific cloning between *Eco*RI and *Hin*dIII sites. Briefly, first- and second-strand cDNA syntheses are sequentially carried out in the presence of 5-methyl dCTP. After second-strand synthesis, the cDNA is treated with T4 DNA polymerase to blunt the ends. Addition of *Eco*RI/*Hin*dIII Directional Linker d(GCTTGAATTCAAGC) at the d(A)n:d(T)n end created a *Hin*dIII site d(AAGCTT) in which the two underlined bases are derived from cDNA. The two dTs are provided on the 5′ end of each first strand by the *Hin*dIII random primer d(TTNNNNNN). In order to differentiate cDNAs from different sources we have introduced bar coding sequences as triplet nucleotide bases at two different locations of the directional *Eco*RI/*Hin*dIII linker as indicated in blue and pink colors without introducing stop signals (**Fig. 1a, c**). The translation start site is located on the T7 vector (not shown), and translation of the three nucleotides (in pink) in the linker region in the correct reading frame has resulted in the addition of an extra amino acid, for example, "L" and "A" as described in **Fig. 1a, c**. Three other nucleotide bases (in blue) are added to maintain the palindromic sequence of the linker. Thus, sequence result of the bar coded directional linkers present in each T7 phage clone (**Fig. 1b, d**) indicated the source of cDNAs used for the construction of T7 phage cDNA libraries. This approach permits pooling of libraries for each biopanning experiment. Excess linkers and small cDNAs (< 300 bp) are removed by a gel filtration step as described in Novagen's manual TB 247. Digestion of cDNAs with both *Hin*dIII and *Eco*RI thus yielded cDNA molecules ready for directional insertion into *Eco*RI/*Hin*dIII vector T7Select 10-3 arms. After vector ligation and packaging using T7 packaging extracts, the phages are plated to determine the library titer. About 50 phage

clones are randomly picked up and PCR is performed with T7 forward primer (TCTTCGCCCAGAAGC**TGCA**G) and T7 reverse primer (CCTCCTTTCAGCAAAAAACCCC), to determine the insert sizes. The insert size range is found to be between 300 bp and 1.5 kb.

3. *Amplification of packaged libraries by liquid culture method.* Ten milliliters of LB/carbenicillin medium is inoculated with a single colony of BLT5615 from a freshly streaked plate. The mixture is shaken at 37°C overnight. One milliliter of the overnight culture is added to 90 mL of LB/carbenicillin medium and is allowed to grow until OD_{600} reaches 0.4–0.5. IPTG (1 mM), M9 salts (1×), and glucose (0.4%) are added and the cells are allowed to grow for 20 min. An appropriate volume of culture is infected with phage library at MOI of 0.001–0.01 (100–1,000 cells for each pfu). The infected bacterial culture is incubated with shaking at 37°C for 1–2 h until lysis is observed. Glycerol (0.02%) and PMSF (0.02 M) are added to the cell lysate to block proteolysis of the capsid fusion proteins. The phage lysate is centrifuged at 8,000 × *g* for 10 min. The supernatant is collected and is stored at 4°C. The lysate is titered by plaque assay under standard conditions. The libraries are stored at –80°C after purification by polyethylene-glycol precipitation and ultracentrifugation through a stepwise CsCl gradient (please refer to T7Select System Manual TB178 for detail procedure).

3.5. Selection of T7 cDNA Phage Displayed Libraries with Human Sera

1. *Affinity selection with sera from normal individuals.* Twenty-five microliters of Protein G Plus-agarose beads (*see* **Note 4**) is taken in 0.6 µL Eppendorf tube and washed twice with 1× PBS. Washed beads are blocked with 1% BSA at 4°C for 1 h. The beads are then incubated at 4°C for 1 h with 250 µL of pooled sera at a dilution 1:20 from 20 healthy women. After 3 h of incubation, beads are washed three times with 1× PBS and then incubated with tumor-derived phage library (~10^{10} phage particles). After incubation, the mixture is centrifuged at 850 × g for 2 min to remove phage nonspecifically bound to the beads and the supernatant (phage library) is collected for biopanning.

2. *Biopanning of the selected phage mixture with serum from patient with ovarian cancer.* Protein G Plus agarose beads are placed into a 0.6-mL Eppendorf tube and washed two times with 1× PBS. Washed beads are blocked with 1% BSA at 4°C for 1 h. The beads are then incubated at 4°C for 3 h with 250 µL of serum from ovarian cancer patient at a dilution 1:20. After this incubation, the beads are washed three times with 1× PBS and are incubated with phage library supernatant mentioned earlier (termed as Biopanning 1, BP1) col-

lected for biopanning at 4°C for overnight (shorter times of incubation have not proven successful using model antibody systems). After incubation, the mixture is centrifuged at 3,000 rpm for 2 min and supernatant is discarded. Beads are washed three times with 1× PBS. To elute the bound phage 1% SDS is added to the washed beads and the mixture is incubated at room temperature for 10 min (*see* **Note 5**). The bound phage is removed from the beads by centrifugation at 8,000 rpm for 8 min. Eluted phage is transferred to liquid culture for amplification (50 µL elution to 5 mL bacterial culture). Four rounds of affinity selection and biopanning are carried out with amplified phage obtained after each biopanning. The number of biopanning cycles generally determines the extent of the enrichment for phage that binds to the sera of patient with ovarian cancer. This strategy allows for one cycle of biopanning to be performed in a single day. Two biopanning experiments are performed with the library of differentially selecting clones between control and cancer patient sera. The selection is to isolate phage antigen clones that did not bind to control sera pooled from 20 control women but did bind to a patient serum. This set of phage clones represent epitopes that are indicative of the presence of cancer as recognized by the host immune system.

3.6. Protein Microarrays

1. Phage clones are spotted in quintuplicate onto FAST™ slides (Schleicher & Schuell, Keene, N.H) by a robotic microarrayer, Prosys 5510TL (Cartesian, Inc.). The microarrays are blocked in 4% milk for 1 h at room temperature, rinsed in 1× PBS for two times, and incubated with human serum (preadsorbed with 120 µg of bacterial lysate, *see* **Note 6**) at a dilution of 1:300 and T7 antibody, at a concentration of 0.15 µg/mL at room temperature for 1 h. The microarray slides are washed three times in PBS-T three times 4 min each at room temperature and next incubated with Alexa fluor 532 goat antimouse IgG at a dilution of (1:40,000) and Alexa fluor 647 goat antihuman IgG at a dilution of (1:2,000) for 1 h in the dark. The microarrays are washed three times in PBS-T for 4 min each, then two times in PBS for 2 min each. The slides are centrifuged at $150 \times g$ for 3 min, dried with aerosol (pressurized air), and stored in the dark at room temperature.

2. The arrays were scanned in an Axon Laboratories 4100A scanner (Axon Laboratories, Palo Alto, CA) using 532-nm and 635-nm lasers. The ratio of anti-T7 capsid and antihuman IgG was determined by comparing the fluorescence intensities in the Alexa fluor 532 and Alexa fluor 647-specific channels at each spot using ImaGene™ software. (Biodiscovery, Inc., El Segundo, CA).

4. Notes

1. Fresh tumor specimens obtained from surgical resection should be cut into small pieces and suspended in RNAlater®. That way diffusion of RNAlater® into the tissue sections will be easier and it will help in the stabilization of tissues.

2. Carbenicillin and IPTG stock solutions are prepared in water and filter sterilized using 0.2-μm syringe filter. Both the solutions are aliquoted in 1.5-mL tubes and stored at –20°C.

3. There are two purposes for the northern blot analysis of the mRNA preparations. The first is to judge the integrity of the mRNA so that the bands revealed by the GAPDH probe are sharp and there is no hint of ribosomal RNA in the preparation. Secondly the intensity of the bands between the total 20 μg RNA and the 0.4 μg of poly(A) selected mRNA should be similar. If not then there is a problem with the quantitation of the mRNA using spectroscopy and the amount of mRNA used in the preparation of the cDNA library adjusted accordingly.

4. Protein G-PLUS agarose beads should be handled very carefully. The bead solution should never be vortexed. Only gentle mixing by hand is recommended.

5. One percent SDS should be prepared freshly just before use. Often, a variation in the concentration of SDS can interfere with the elution procedure and next round of amplification of the phage library (eluant) may not be successful.

6. Serum obtained from cancer patient also has circulating antibodies directed toward bacterial proteins that can nonspecifically interfere with the binding of other serum IgGs with their cognate antigens. Before processing protein microarrays, the patient's serum is preadsorbed with an optimal amount of bacterial extracts (as mentioned in **Subheading 3**) in order to sequester these antibodies. This results in the reduction of nonspecific binding of these bacterial antibodies on protein microarrays thereby improving the actual signal-to-noise ratio.

Acknowledgments

This work was supported by The Barbara and Fred Erb Endowed Chair in Cancer Genetics, The Gail Purtan Ovarian Cancer

Research Fund, The Sinai Guild, and grants from The Michigan Life Science Corridor Fund 085P300470, NIH grant CA100740, NIH grant U01 CA117478-01, and The Susan G. Komen Breast Cancer Foundation grant BCTR0504211 (M.A.Tainsky).

References

1. Anderson, K. S. and LaBaer, J. (2005) The sentinel within: exploiting the immune system for cancer biomarkers. *J. Proteome. Res.* 4, 1123–1133

2. Sahin, U., Tureci, O., Schmitt, H., Cochlovius, B., Johannes, T., Schmits, R., Stenner, F., Luo, G., Schobert, I., and Pfreundschuh, M. (1995) Human neoplasms elicit multiple specific immune responses in the autologous host. *Proc. Natl Acad. Sci. U S A* 92, 11810–11813

3. Disis, M. L., Calenoff, E., McLaughlin, G., Murphy, A. E., Chen, W., Groner, B., Jeschke, M., Lydon, N., McGlynn, E., Livingston, R. B., and Martin, A. C. (1994) Existent T-cell and antibody immunity to HER-2/neu protein in patients with breast cancer. *Cancer Res.* 54, 16–20

4. Disis, M. L., Pupa, S. M., Gralow, J. R., Dittadi, R., Menard, S., and Cheever, M. A. (1997) High-titer HER-2/neu protein-specific antibody can be detected in patients with early-stage breast cancer. *J. Clin. Oncol.* 15, 3363–3367

5. Gadducci, A., Ferdeghini, M., Buttitta, F., Cosio, S., Fanucchi, A., Annicchiarico, C., Gagetti, O., Bevilacqua, G., and Genazzani, A. R. (1999) Assessment of the prognostic relevance of serum anti-p53 antibodies in epithelial ovarian cancer. *Gynecol. Oncol.* 72, 76–81

6. Lechpammer, M., Lukac, J., Lechpammer, S., Kovacevic, D., Loda, M., and Kusic, Z. (2004) Humoral immune response to p53 correlates with clinical course in colorectal cancer patients during adjuvant chemotherapy. *Int. J. Colorectal Dis.* 19, 114–120

7. Conroy, S. E. and Latchman, D. S. (1996) Do heat shock proteins have a role in breast cancer? *Br. J. Cancer* 74, 717–721

8. Conroy, S. E., Sasieni, P. D., Fentiman, I., and Latchman, D. S. (1998) Autoantibodies to the 90kDa heat shock protein and poor survival in breast cancer patients. *Eur. J. Cancer* 34, 942–943

9. Sioud, M. and Hansen, M. H. (2001) Profiling the immune response in patients with breast cancer by phage-displayed cDNA libraries. *Eur. J. Immunol.* 31, 716–725

10. Nam, M. J., Madoz-Gurpide, J., Wang, H., Lescure, P., Schmalbach, C. E., Zhao, R., Misek, D. E., Kuick, R., Brenner, D. E., and Hanash, S. M. (2003) Molecular profiling of the immune response in colon cancer using protein microarrays: occurrence of autoantibodies to ubiquitin C-terminal hydrolase L3. *Proteomics* 3, 2108–2115

11. Brass, N., Racz, A., Bauer, C., Heckel, D., Sybrecht, G., and Meese, E. (1999) Role of amplified genes in the production of autoantibodies. *Blood* 93, 2158–2166

12. Naora, H., Yang, Y. Q., Montz, F. J., Seidman, J. D., Kurman, R. J., and Roden, R. B. (2001) A serologically identified tumor antigen encoded by a homeobox gene promotes growth of ovarian epithelial cells. *Proc. Natl Acad. Sci. U S A* 98, 4060–4065

13. Scanlan, M. J., Gout, I., Gordon, C. M., Williamson, B., Stockert, E., Gure, A. O., Jager, D., Chen, Y. T., Mackay, A., O'Hare, M. J., and Old, L. J. (2001) Humoral immunity to human breast cancer: antigen definition and quantitative analysis of mRNA expression. *Cancer Immun.* 1, 4

14. Chen, Y. T., Scanlan, M. J., Sahin, U., Tureci, O., Gure, A. O., Tsang, S., Williamson, B., Stockert, E., Pfreundschuh, M., and Old, L. J. (1997) A testicular antigen aberrantly expressed in human cancers detected by autologous antibody screening. *Proc. Natl Acad. Sci. U S A* 94, 1914–1918

15. Jager, D., Stockert, E., Gure, A. O., Scanlan, M. J., Karbach, J., Jager, E., Knuth, A., Old, L. J., and Chen, Y. T. (2001) Identification of a tissue-specific putative transcription factor in breast tissue by serological screening of a breast cancer library. *Cancer Res.* 61, 2055–2061

16. Jongeneel, V. (2001) Towards a cancer immunome database. *Cancer Immun.* 1, 3

17. Scanlan, M. J., Gure, A. O., Jungbluth, A. A., Old, L. J., and Chen, Y. T. (2002) Cancer/testis antigens: an expanding family of targets for cancer immunotherapy. *Immunol. Rev.* 188, 22–32

18. De, S. C., De, B. O., Faraoni, I., Lurquin, C., Brasseur, F., and Boon, T. (1996) The activation of human gene MAGE-1 in tumor cells is correlated with genome-wide demethylation. *Proc. Natl Acad. Sci. U S A* 93, 7149–7153

19. Stockert, E., Jager, E., Chen, Y. T., Scanlan, M. J., Gout, I., Karbach, J., Arand, M., Knuth, A., and Old, L. J. (1998) A survey of the humoral immune response of cancer patients to a panel of human tumor antigens. *J. Exp. Med.* 187, 1349–1354

20. Brass, N., Heckel, D., Sahin, U., Pfreundschuh, M., Sybrecht, G. W., and Meese, E. (1997) Translation initiation factor eIF-4gamma is encoded by an amplified gene and induces an immune response in squamous cell lung carcinoma. *Hum. Mol. Genet.* 6, 33–39

21. Stone, B., Schummer, M., Paley, P. J., Thompson, L., Stewart, J., Ford, M., Crawford, M., Urban, N., O'Briant, K., and Nelson, B. H. (2003) Serologic analysis of ovarian tumor antigens reveals a bias toward antigens encoded on 17q. *Int. J. Cancer* 104, 73–84

22. Jager, D., Jager, E., and Knuth, A. (2001) Immune responses to tumour antigens: implications for antigen specific immunotherapy of cancer. *J. Clin. Pathol.* 54, 669–674

23. Chen, Y. T., Gure, A. O., Tsang, S., Stockert, E., Jager, E., Knuth, A., and Old, L. J. (1998) Identification of multiple cancer/testis antigens by allogeneic antibody screening of a melanoma cell line library. *Proc. Natl Acad. Sci. U S A* 95, 6919–6923

24. Chatterjee, M., Mohapatra, S., Ionan, A., Bawa, G., Ali-Fehmi, R., Wang, X., Nowak, J., Ye, B., Nahhas, F. A., Lu, K., Witkin, S. S., Fishman, D., Munkarah, A., Morris, R., Levin, N. K., Shirley, N. N., Tromp, G., Abrams, J., Draghici, S., and Tainsky, M. A. (2006) Diagnostic markers of ovarian cancer by high-throughput antigen cloning and detection on arrays. *Cancer Res.* 66, 1181–1190

25. Draghici, S., Chatterjee, M., and Tainsky, M. A. (2005) Epitomics: serum screening for the early detection of cancer on microarrays using complex panels of tumor antigens. *Expert Rev. Mol. Diagn.* 5, 735–743

26. Carmen, S. and Jermutus, L. (2002) Concepts in antibody phage display. *Brief Funct. Genomic. Proteomic.* 1, 189–203

27. Smith, G. P. and Petrenko, V. A. (1997) Phage display. *Chem. Rev.* 97, 391–410

28. Pepe, M. S., Longton, G., Anderson, G. L., and Schummer, M. (2003) Selecting differentially expressed genes from microarray experiments. *Biometrics* 59, 133–142

29. Angelopoulou, K., Yu, H., Bharaj, B., Giai, M., and Diamandis, E. P. (2000) p53 gene mutation, tumor p53 protein overexpression, and serum p53 autoantibody generation in patients with breast cancer. *Clin. Biochem.* 33, 53–62

30. Wang, X., Yu, J., Sreekumar, A., Varambally, S., Shen, R., Giacherio, D., Mehra, R., Montie, J. E., Pienta, K. J., Sanda, M. G., Kantoff, P. W., Rubin, M. A., Wei, J. T., Ghosh, D., and Chinnaiyan, A. M. (2005) Autoantibody signatures in prostate cancer. *N. Engl. J. Med.* 353, 1224–1235

31. Zhong, L., Hidalgo, G. E., Stromberg, A. J., Khattar, N. H., Jett, J. R., and Hirschowitz, E. A. (2005) Using protein microarray as a diagnostic assay for non-small cell lung cancer. *Am. J. Respir. Crit Care Med.* 172, 1308–1314

Chapter 4

Analysis of Glycans on Serum Proteins Using Antibody Microarrays

Songming Chen and Brian B. Haab

Summary

Antibody arrays can be employed for the profiling glycan structures on proteins. Antibody arrays capture multiple, specific proteins directly from biological samples (such as serum), and lectin and glycan-binding antibodies probe the levels of specific glycans on the captured proteins. We use a practical method of partitioning microscope slides to enable the convenient processing of many detection reagents or samples. A critical first step in the procedure is the chemical derivatization of the glycans on the spotted capture antibodies, which prevents lectin binding to those glycans. We describe those methods along with the methods for preparing and treating serum samples, running the experiments, and designing and interpreting the experiments.

Key words: Antibody arrays, Glycan profiling, Lectin detection, Serum biomarkers.

1. Introduction

Antibody microarrays have proven to be very valuable for their ability to obtain high-sensitivity measurements of multiple proteins using low sample volumes *(1)*. This capability has been applied to many different research topics, particularly in cancer research *(2, 3)*. Recently we have further developed the antibody array method to enable the probing of carbohydrate modifications on proteins *(4)*. The ability to accurately measure the variation in specific carbohydrate structures on specific proteins in biological samples has many important applications. For example, the more careful characterization

Michael A. Tainsky, *Methods in Molecular Biology, Tumor Biomarker Discovery, Vol. 520*
© Humana Press, a part of Springer Science+Business Media, LLC 2009
DOI: 10.1007/978-1-60327-811-9_4

of glycan alterations associated with cancer could be used to determine the prevalence of particular structural alterations or the correlations with clinical factors. Conventional technologies for studying carbohydrates, such as separations-based methods or mass spectrometry, do not have the quantitative precision necessary to make comparisons between samples, nor do they have the throughput to look at population statistics. The method described here addresses those limitations.

The basic principle of the method is presented in **Fig. 1**. A biological sample, such as serum, is incubated on the surface of a microarray of immobilized antibodies. After proteins bind to the antibodies according to their specificities, the levels of specific glycan structures on the captured proteins are probed using lectins (proteins with glycan-binding activity) or antibodies targeting glycan epitopes. Different types of lectins and glycan-binding antibodies can be used to probe various glycan structures. An important first step in this procedure is a method to chemically derivatize the glycans on the immobilized antibodies. This step alters the glycans so that they are no longer recognized by the lectins or glycan-binding antibodies, ensuring that only the glycans on the captured proteins are probed. Each type of lectin recognizes its own, specific carbohydrate structure.

A description of the validation and optimization of the method was presented earlier *(4)*. The purpose of this chapter is to give detailed instructions on how to use the method in practice, along with the latest protocol enhancements. The description of this method will be presented in three sections (1) chemical derivatization of the glycans on the capture antibodies; (2) sample preparation; and (3) processing the microarrays.

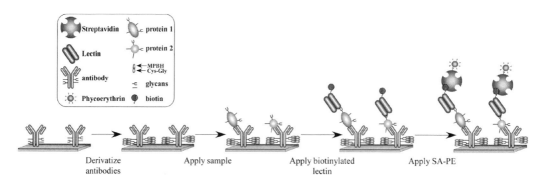

Fig. 1. The detection of glycans on proteins captured by antibody arrays. The drawing depicts antibodies immobilized on a planar surface. The glycans on the antibodies are derivatized to prevent lectin binding; a sample is incubated on the antibody array; proteins are captured by the antibodies; biotinylated lectins bind to the glycans on the captured proteins; and the level of bound lectin is determined by scanning for fluorescence from streptavidin-B-phycoerythrin.

2. Materials

2.1. Reagents

1. NaIO$_4$ (Pierce Biotechnology, Rockford, IL).

2. 4-(4-N-Maleimidophenyl) butyric acid hydrazide hydrochloride (MPBH) (Pierce Biotechnology, Rockford, IL).

3. Cysteine–Glycine (CysGly) dipeptide (Sigma-Aldrich, St. Louis, MO).

4. Streptavidin-B-Phycoerythrin (Invitrogen, Carlsbad, CA).

5. Neuraminidase (New England Biolabs, Ipswich, MA).

6. Protease Inhibitors (one tablet dissolved in 10 mL buffer) (Roche Applied Science, Indianapolis, IN).

7. Biotinylated lectins (Vector Labs, Burlingame, CA, and other suppliers).

8. Mouse, goat, sheep, and rabbit IgG antibodies, and chicken IgY antibodies (Jackson ImmunoResearch Labs, West Grove, PA).

9. Tween-20 (Sigma-Aldrich, St. Louis, MO).

10. Brij-35 (Sigma-Aldrich, St. Louis, MO).

2.2. Solutions

1. Coupling Buffer (0.04 M sodium acetate, pH 5.5).

2. Coupling Buffer + 0.1% Tween-20.

3. Phosphate-buffered saline (PBS), pH 7.4 (137 mM NaCl, 2.7 mM KCl, 4.3 mM Na$_2$HPO$_4$, 1.4 mM KH$_2$PO$_4$).

4. Tris-buffered saline (TBS).

5. *PBST0.1*. PBS + 0.1% Tween-20.

6. *PBST0.5*. PBS + 0.5% Tween-20.

7. PBST0.1 + 1 mM CysGly (prepare immediately before use).

8. Coupling Buffer + 200 mM NaIO4 (prepare immediately before use).

9. Coupling Buffer + 1 mM MPBH + 1 mM CysGly (prepare immediately before use).

10. PBST0.5 + 1% bovine serum albumin (BSA).

11. PBST0.5 + 0.1% (BSA) + 1 μg/mL Streptavidin-B-Phycoerythrin.

12. 10× Sample buffer (1% Tween-20 + 1% Brij-35 in 1× TBS).

13. *4× IgG/Y cocktail*. 400 μg/mL of goat, sheep, mouse, and chicken antibody, 800 μg/mL rabbit antibody, in TBS.

14. *20× protease inhibitor solution*. Dissolve one tablet of protease inhibitor into 0.5 mL of distilled water (prepare immediately before use).

2.3. Hardware and Instruments

1. Microscope slide staining chambers with slide racks (Shandon Lipshaw, Pittsburgh, PA, cat. No. 121).
2. Microscope slide boxes (several versions available).
3. Wafer-handling tweezers (Techni-Tool, Worcester, PA, cat. No. 758TW178, style 4WF).
4. Slide Imprinter, for printing wax partitions on slides (The Gel Company, San Francisco, CA).
5. Clinical centrifuge with flat swinging buckets for holding slide racks (Beckman Coulter, Fullerton, CA, among others).
6. Microarray scanner (several versions available).

3. Methods

This method described here assumes access to antibody microarrays. The selection and treatment of antibodies and the fabrication of antibody arrays are covered in previous publications *(3, 5, 6)*. Antibody microarrays can be stored in a vacuum-sealed slide box with desiccant in a refrigerator for months without loss of activity (*see* **Note 1**).

3.1. Chemically Derivatize the Glycans on the Capture Antibodies

Because antibodies are glycoproteins, the lectins used as the detection probes could bind to the capture antibodies on the arrays, which would interfere with the specific detection of the glycans on the proteins captured by the antibodies. A reliable method to prevent that interference is to chemically modify the glycans on the capture antibodies after they have been immobilized. The *cis*-hydroxyl groups of the glycans on the spotted antibodies are gently oxidized to convert to aldehyde groups, which are reacted with a hydrazide-maleimide bifunctional crosslinking reagent, which then reacts with a cysteine–glycine (CysGly) dipeptide. The CysGly dipeptide adds bulk to the derivatized carbohydrates to hinder lectin binding.

The chemically blocking procedure should be finished within a working day without interruption. All chemical solutions, such as $NaIO_4$, MPBH, and CysGly, should be prepared right before the reactions.

Some lectins or antibodies target glycan structures which are rare in antibodies, such as the Lewis blood group structures or O-linked *N*-acetyl-Glucosamine (*O*-GlcNAc), so these reagents do not bind to the capture antibodies. Therefore the chemical derivatization step is not necessary in those cases. A preliminary experiment to look at the level of lectin and antibody binding to capture antibodies would help determine if glycan derivatization is necessary. A slight loss in affinity may be evident after chemical derivatization *(4)*, so it may be important to make this determination. IgE antibodies seem to be particularly susceptible to affinity loss.

1. If the microarray slides are stored refrigerated in a vacuum-sealed pack, equilibrate the slides to room temperature for 30 min before opening vacuum seal. This equilibration will prevent condensation on the slides.

2. If using wax partitioning of the slides, print the desired pattern onto the slides using the SlideImprinter (*see* **Fig. 2** and **Subheading 3.3**) (*see* **Note 2**).

3. Briefly rinse all the slides with PBST0.1 followed by Coupling Buffer + 0.1% Tween-20, and wash the slides in Coupling Buffer + 0.1% Tween for 10 min at room temperature with gentle shaking (*see* **Note 3**). The slide washing steps can be performed by placing the slides in slide racks in a slide staining chamber.

4. Prepare 200 mM $NaIO_4$ in 1× Coupling Buffer (*see* **Note 4**).

5. Pour the $NaIO_4$ solution into a flat-bottom glass or plastic container to a depth sufficient to easily cover a microscope slide lying flat (about 5 mm) (*see* **Note 5**). Place the microarray slides in the bottom of the container facing up, submerging them, and cover the cassette with aluminum foil to keep the slides dark. Incubate the slides for 5 h with gentle shaking at 4°C (*see* **Note 6**). This step could be performed in a cold room.

6. Prepare the Coupling Buffer + 1 mM MPBH + 1 mM CysGly solution about 30 min before the end of the previous step (*see* **Note 7**).

7. Using the wafer-handling tweezers, remove the slides, briefly rinse them in Coupling Buffer + 0.1% Tween-20, and wash them for 3 min in the same buffer with gentle shaking at room temperature.

8. Pour the Coupling Buffer + 1 mM MPBH + 1 mM CysGly solution into a flat-bottom container as before, and place the slides in the bottom of the container facing up. Incubate at room temperature for 2 h with gentle shaking.

9. Prepare the PBST0.1 + CysGly solution about 30 min before the previous step finishes.

10. Wash the slides in PBST0.1 for 3 min.

11. Pour the CysGly solution into a cassette, place the slides on the bottom of the cassette facing up, and incubate at 4°C overnight with gentle shaking (*see* **Notes 8** and **9**).

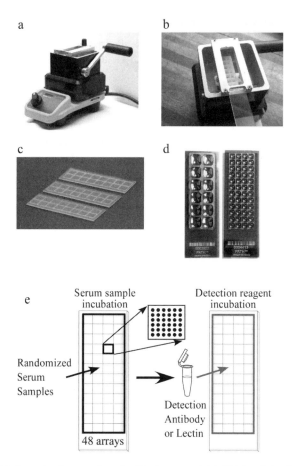

Fig. 2. High-throughput processing of antibody arrays. (**a**) A SlideImprinter device (The GelCompany, San Francisco, CA) is used to imprint wax patterns onto microscope slides. A bath of wax is melted on a hotplate, and (**b**) a slide is inserted upside-down into a holder above the bath. Pulling the level forward elevates a stamp out of the bath to contact the slide, (**c**) leaving a pattern of wax on the slide. (**d**) Various designs of stamps can be used, such as one that partitions 12 regions on a slide (*left*), or another that partitions 48 regions on a slide (*right*). The liquid loaded into each region remains segregated from the other regions. (**e**) Strategy for detecting a glycan structure on many samples. 48 different serum samples are randomized and incubated on 48 identical antibody arrays on a single microscope slide. Each array contains up to 144 spots. After the proteins bind to the antibodies, a glycan structure on the captured proteins is detected with a lectin or glycan-binding antibody.

3.2. Preparation of the Serum Samples

3.2.1. Serum Sample Dilution and Mixture

Low concentrations of detergents, such as Tween-20 and Brij-35, should be added to the serum samples to reduce nonspecific binding to the capture antibodies. We also recommend mixing in small amounts of nonspecific antibodies to compete for possible serum protein binding to the capture antibodies. The types of antibodies that are represented on the microarrays should be added to the serum samples. For example, if mouse IgG antibodies are used on the arrays, then normal mouse IgG antibodies (from nonimmunized mice) should be added to the sera. Tween-20 and Brij-35 are added to a final concentration of 0.1%, and the nonspecific antibodies also are added to 100 μg/mL, using 1× PBS as a carrier buffer. In addition, some serum proteases may be activated if serum samples are highly diluted. We recommend using a protease inhibitor cocktail in the diluent buffers.

The serum should be diluted so that the antigens of interest are in the linear-response range of detection. Low-abundance antigens, such as cytokines, are best detected using low dilution factors, such as 1.5–2×, and high-abundance antigens, such as serum transferrin, may require dilution factors of several thousand-fold. The optimal dilution factor can be determined experimentally. Serial dilutions of pooled sera should be analyzed on arrays (using the methods described later), and the signals should be plotted with respect to the dilution factors. The dilution factor for subsequent experiments should be set in the range that shows an approximately linear relationship between signal and dilution factor.

Another consideration in determining the appropriate dilution factor is that some detection lectins may show high backgrounds (high binding to the slide substrate) when using high concentrations (low dilution factors) of serum. The dilution factor may need to be increased in those cases to reduce backgrounds.

Here is an example of the preparation of 100 μL of a serum sample with a two-fold dilution factor:

1. 50 μL serum

2. 10 μL Sample buffer

3. 10 μL 10× TBS.

4. 25 μL of 4× IgG/Y cocktail

5. 5 μL of 20× protease inhibitor solution

3.2.2. Enzymatic Stepwise Removal of Terminal Glycans on the Serum Proteins

This optional step can be used in addition to the standard serum preparation method to provide more information about the glycan structures on the captured proteins. Some sugar groups are not accessible to lectin detection because they are masked by terminal glycan groups. Through the sequential, enzymatic removal of terminal glycan structures, the inner glycan groups can be made accessible to lectin detection. Certain enzymes, such as neuraminidase and galactosidase, can function without denaturing the target proteins, so that the proteins are still recognized by the capture antibodies. The following procedure describes the removal of terminal sialic acid groups using the enzyme neuraminidase. Some optimization may be required for other enzymes.

1. Add 4 µL of 10× reaction buffer (from the neuraminidase reaction kit) and 2 µL of the 20× protease inhibitor solution into 34 µL of serum sample.

2. Add 1 µL of neuraminidase into the mixture, and incubate at 37°C for 4 h.

3. Continue the serum sample preparation as described in **Subheading 3.2.1** (*see* **Note 10**).

3.3. Detection of Glycans on Captured Glycoproteins

This step describes the incubation of serum samples on the arrays and the probing of the captured proteins with glycan-binding reagents. We recommend partitioning the microscope slides so that multiple microarrays can be run on each slide, which saves on supply costs and makes it convenient to run many samples or detection reagents. A practical and versatile method to partition microscope slides is to imprint hydrophobic wax borders around each of the microarrays (**Fig. 2a–d**). These borders prevent liquid from leaking from one array to another, and they are thin enough to allow scanning using conventional microarray scanners. The borders can be applied using a commercially available instrument, and various patterns of borders can be applied to fit particular experimental needs. A design using 48 microarrays on a single slide is useful for probing many samples (**Fig. 2e**).

The detection lectins or glycan-binding antibodies should be chosen to target the particular glycan structures specific to the needs of each project. The specificities of some widely used lectins and antibodies for glycan detection are listed in **Table 1**, which contains information compiled from various sources *(7–11)*. Some lectins have broad specificities or bind more than one sugar type, such as *Lens culinaris Agglutinin* (LCA), which binds both α-Mannose and α-Fucose; other lectins recognize very specific sugar units, such as *Phaseolus vulgaris Leucoagglutinin* (L-PHA), which binds branched *N*-acetyl lactosamine (LacNAc). Antiglycan antibodies can be a good alternate detection reagent, but antibodies against common sugars are not available due to difficulties in their generation. A caveat in using antiglycan antibodies is that they may have higher crossreactivity than other antibodies, as suggested by a specificity study using carbohydrate microarrays *(12)*. Therefore, multiple lectins or antibodies may be used to obtain a reliable and a broader profile of the glycan structures present on the captured proteins. A good resource for searching glycan epitopes and their antibodies can be found in GlycoEpitope Database (http://www.glyco.is.ritsumei.ac.jp/epitope/) maintained by Kawasaki laboratory in Research Center for Glycobiotechnology, Ritsumeikan University.

1. If continuing from the chemical derivatization step (**Subheading 3.1**), wash the microarray slides in three baths of PBST0.5 for 3 min each.

Table 1

Glycans	GBPs	Lectin name or antibody clones	Lectin specificities or glycan structures
Fucose (Fuc)	AAL	*Aleuria aurantia* lectin	Fuc (preferably (α1-6)-linked Fuc)
	LCA	*Lens culinaris* Agglutinin	(α1-6)-linked Fuc
	PSA	*Pisum sativum* Agglutinin	(α1-6)-linked Fuc
	UEA I	*Ulex europaeus* Agglutinin I	Terminal or subterminal Fuc (α1-2) Gal
	LTL	*Lotus tetragonolobus* lectin	Fuc (α1-2) Gal (β1-4)[Fuc α1-3] Glc/GlcNAc), other difucosyl carbohydrates
	AAA	*Anguilla anguilla* Agglutinin	Fuc (α1-3) GlcNAc
α-linked galactose (αGal)	Antibody	2.10G, Gal-13, M86	Gal(α1-3)Gal(β1-4)GlcNAc-R
	GS IB4	GSL I-isolectin B4	Terminal aGal
	MOA	*Marasmius oreades* Agglutinin	Gal (α1-3)Gal(β1-4) GlcNAc/Glc
α-linked *N*-acetyl galactosamine (αGalNAc) (including Tn antigen (GalNAc α1 – Ser/Thr))	Antibody	B1.1, 5F4, 83D4, BRIC 111, Ca3256, Ca3268, Ca3638, CU-1, ETn1.01, FBT3, HBTn1, IE3, MLS128, NCC-LU-35, NCC-LU-81, Tn5,	GalNAc α-Thr/Ser (Tn antigen)
	HPA	*Helix pomatia* Agglutinin	Terminal αGalNAc
	HAA	*Helix aspersa* Agglutinin	α/βGalNAc
	VVL	*Vicia villosa* lectin	α/βGalNAc
	DBA	*Dolichos biflorus* Agglutinin	GalNAc (α1-3) GalNAc
	LBL	Lima Bean lectin (*Phaseolus lunatus*)	GalNAc (α1-3) Gal
	MPL	*Maclura pomifera* lectin	αGalNAc
	SBA	Soybean Agglutinin	αGalNAc
	WFA	*Wisteria floribunda* lectin	GalNAc (α/β1-6/3) Gal
β-linked galactose (βGal)	PNA	Peanut Agglutinin	Terminal βGal
	RCA120	*Ricinus communis* Agglutinin I	Terminal βGal as in Lactose/LacNAc
	ABA	*Agaricus bisporus* Agglutinin	βGal on T antigen
	ACA	*Amaranthus caudatus* lectin	βGal on T antigen

(continued)

Table 1
(continued)

Glycans	GBPs	Lectin name or antibody clones	Lectin specificities or glycan structures
β-linked *N*-acetyl galactosamine (βGalNAc)	SJA	*Sophora japonica* Agglutinin	βGal and βGalNAc
	PTL II	*Psophocarpus tetragonolobus* lectin II	βGal and βGalNAc
	SBA	Soybean Agglutinin	βGalNAc and αGalNAc
	WFA	*Wisteria floribunda* lectin	GalNAc (α/β1-6) Gal and Gal-NAc (α/β1-3) Gal
GalNAc(β1-3) Gal(β1-4)Glc-NAc	Antibody	TH2	GalNAc(β1-3)Gal(β1-4) GlcNAc-R
GalNAc(β1-4) [Fuc(α1-3)] Glc(β1-)	Antibody	AK97	Gal(β1-4)[Fuc(α1-3)]Glc(β1-)-R
GalNAc(β1-4) [Neu5Ac(α2-3)] Gal(β1-)	Antibody	2A3D2, 2D11E2, CT1, CT2, DMAb-1, DMAb-2, DMAb-3, DMAb-4, DMAb-5, KM531, YHD-06	GalNAc(β1-4)[Neu5Ac(α'-3)] Gal(β1-)-R
GalNAc(β1-4)Gal	Antibody	2D4	GalNAc(β1-4)Gal-R
T antigen (Gal-β1-3 GalNAc α1 – Ser/Thr)	Antibody	49H.24, 49H.8, 5A8, 8D8, A78-G, Ca3114, Ca3741, HB-T1, HH8, TF1, TF2, TF5	Gal (β1-3) GalNAc a-Thr/Ser (T antigen)
	BPL	*Bauhinia purpurea* lectin	Gal (β1-3) GalNAc or terminal αGalNAc
	PNA	Peanut Agglutinin	Terminal Gal (β1-3) GalNAc a-Thr/Ser (T antigen), terminal βGal
	Jacalin	Jacalin	Gal (β1-3) GalNAc α-Thr/Ser , GalNAc α-Thr/Ser(Tn)
	VVL	*Vicia villosa* lectin	Terminal Gal β1-3 GalNAc α-Thr/Ser or terminal αGal-NAc α-Thr/Ser
Sialyl T antigen	Antibody		Neu5Ac (α2-3)Gal(β1,3)Gal-NAc] α-Ser/Thr
Disialyl T antigen	Antibody	QSH2	Neu5Ac(α2-3)Gal(β1-3) [Neu5Ac(α2-6)]GalNAc(α1-) Ser/Thr

(continued)

**Table 1
(continued)**

Glycans	GBPs	Lectin name or antibody clones	Lectin specificities or glycan structures
Terminal Galactose 3-*O*-Sulfate	Antibody	M14-376, Sulph 1	HSO3(-3)Gal-R
Sialyl Tn antigen	antibody	B72.3, C1282, CC102, CC49, HB-STn1, 3C2, MLS132,	Neu5Ac (α2-3) GalNAc](α-)-Ser/Thr
Glucose (Glc)	VFA	*Vicia faba* Agglutinin	α-linked Glc and α-linked Man
	Con A	Concanavalin A	α-linked Glc and α-linked Man
N-acetyl-Glucose (GlcNAc)	GSL II	*Griffonia (βandeiraea) simplicifolia* lectin II	Terminal βGlcNAc or αGlcNAc
	PVL	*Psathyrella velutina* lectin	βGlcNAc
O-linked GlcNAc (*O*-GlcNAc)	Antibody	CTD110.6, HGAC39, HGAC85, RL2	GlcNAc(β1-)Ser/Thr
Chitobiose (GlcNAc (β1-4) GlcNAc)	WGA	Wheat germ Agglutinin	(GlcNAc (β1-4) GlcNAc)n repeats
	DSL	*Datura stramonium* lectin	GlcNAc oligomer
	LEL	*Lycopersicon esculentum* (tomato) lectin	GlcNAc oligomer
	STL	*Solanum tuberosum* (potato) lectin	GlcNAc oligomer
	UDA	*Urtica dioica* Agglutinin	GlcNAc oligomer
LacNAc (Gal (β1-4) GlcNAc)	Antibody	1B2 (to terminal LacNAc)	Terminal LacNAc
	ECL	*Erythrina cristagalli* lectin (ECL, ECA)	Terminal LacNAc
	RCA120	*Ricinus communis* Agglutinin I	LacNAc (binding inhibited by terminal sialic acid)
Branched (β1-6) LacNAc	PWM	Pokeweed mitogen lectin	Gal (β1-4) GlcNAc (β1-6)-R
	L-PHA	*Phaseolus vulgaris* leucoagglutinin	Gal (β1-4) GlcNAc (β1-6)-R
6-Sulfo LacNAc	Antibody	AG107, DD1, DD2, M-DC8	Gal(β1-4)[HSO$_3$(-6)]GlcNAc-R
6,6'-Sulfo LacNAc	Antibody	DD1, M-DC8	HSO$_3$(-6)Gal(β1-4)[HSO$_3$(-6)]GlcNAc(β1-)-R

(continued)

Table 1
(continued)

Glycans	GBPs	Lectin name or antibody clones	Lectin specificities or glycan structures
6,6,6'-Sulfo Lac-NAc	Antibody	DD1	HSO$_3$(-6)Gal(β1-4)[HSO$_3$(-6)] GlcNAc(β1-3)[HSO$_3$(-6)] Gal(β1-)-R
LDN (LacdiNAc)	Antibody	100-2H5-A, 114-2H12-C, 259-2A1, 273-3F2, 99-2A5-B, SMLDN1.1,	GalNAc(β1-4)GlcNAc-R
LDN-F	Antibody	204-6A1, 294-2A1, SMLDNF1	GalNAc(β1-4)[Fuc(α1-3)] GlcNAc-R
Acharan sulfate	Antibody	MW3G3	-{[HSO$_3$(-2)]IdoA(α1-4) GlcNAc(α1-4)}n-
Lewis a	Antibody	7LE, PR.5C5, PR 4D2, T174, B369, BC9-E5, CF4-C4 DG4-1	Gal(β1-3)[Fuc(α1-4)] GlcNAc(β1-)-R
Dimeric Lewis a	Antibody	NCC-ST-421	Gal(β1-3)[Fuc(α1-4)] GlcNAc(β1-3)Gal(β1-3) [Fuc(α1-4)]GlcNAc(β1-)-R
Disialyl Lewis a	Antibody	FH7	Neu5Ac(α2-3)Gal(β1-3) [Neu5Ac(α2-6)][Fuc(α1-4)] GlcNAc(β1-)-R
3'-Sulfo Lewis a	Antibody	F2, 91.9H	HSO$_3$(-3)Gal(β1-3)[Fuc(α1-4)] GlcNAc-R
Sialyl Lewis a (CA19-9)	Antibody	121SLE, CA199.02, 2M1, SPM110, 241, 192	Neu5Ac (α2-6))Gal(β1-3) [Fuc(α1-4)]GlcNAc-R
Lewis a- Lewis x Hybrid Antigen	Antibody	43-9F, NCC-ST-421	Gal(β1-3)[Fuc(α1-4)] GlcNAc(β1-3)Gal(β1-4) [Fuc(α1-3)]GlcNAc(β1-)-R
Lewis b	Antibody	2-25LE, T218, SPM194, 1116NS-10, YB-2	Fuc(α1-2)Gal(β1-3)[Fuc(α1-4)] GlcNAc(β1-)-R
Trifucosyl-Lewis b Antigen	Antibody	IMH2	Fuc(α1-2)Gal(β1-3)[Fuc(α1-4)] GlcNAc(β1-3)Gal(β1-3) [Fuc(α1-4)]GlcNAc(β1-)-R
Lewis c	Antibody	K21	Fuc(α1-2)Gal(β1-3)[Fuc(α1-4)] GlcNAc(β1-3)Gal(β1-3) [Fuc(α1-4)]GlcNAc(β1-)-R
Sialyl Lewis c	Antibody	C-50, DUPAN-2	Neu5Ac(α2-3)Gal(β1-3) GlcNAc(β1-)-R
Lewis x	Antibody	15C02, 28, ZC-18C, FR4A5, HI98, W6D3, P12, 1G10, 73-30, 80H5, FH2, LeuM1, MC-480, MMA, SH1, WGHS-29-1	Gal(β1-4)[Fuc(α1-3)] GlcNAc(β1-)-R

(continued)

Table 1
(continued)

Glycans	GBPs	Lectin name or antibody clones	Lectin specificities or glycan structures
Sialyl Lewis x	Antibody	CSLEX1	Neu5Ac (α2-6)Gal(β1-4) [Fuc(α1-3)]GlcNAc-R
Dimeric Lewis x	Antibody	FH4	Gal(β1-4)[Fuc(α1-3)] GlcNAc(β1-3)Gal(β1-4) [Fuc(α1-3)]GlcNAc(β1-)-R
3'-Sulfo Lewis x	Antibody	MIN/3/60, SU59	HSO$_3$(-3)Gal(β1-4)[Fuc(α1-3)] GlcNAc-R
6-Sulfo Lewis x	Antibody	AG107, AG273, AG97	Gal(β1-4)[Fuc(α1-3)][HSO3(-6)]GlcNAc(β1-)-R
Sialyl 6-Sulfo Lewis x	Antibody	2F3, 2H5, G162, G72, HECA-452	Neu5Ac(α2-3)Gal(β1-4) [Fuc(α1-3)][HSO$_3$(-6)] GlcNAc(β1-)-R
6'-Sulfo Sialyl Lewis x	Antibody	2F3, 2H5, CSLEX1 / CSLEX-1, HECA-452, SNH3 / SNH-3	Neu5Ac(α2-3)[HSO$_3$(-6)] Gal(β1-4)[Fuc(α1-3)] GlcNAc(β1-)-R
6,6'-Disulfo Sialyl Lewis x	Antibody	2F3, 2H5, G27011, G27037, G27039, G2706, HECA-452	Neu5Ac(α2-3)[HSO$_3$(-6)] Gal(β1-4)[Fuc(α1-3)][HSO$_3$(-6)]GlcNAc(β1-3)Gal(β1-)-R
Sialyl Lewis i-x (VIM-2)	Antibody	CF4, HE-10, VIM-2	Neu5Ac(α2-3)Gal(β1-4) GlcNAc(β1-3)Gal(β1-4) [Fuc(α1-3)]GlcNAc(β1-)-R
Sialyl Lewis x-i	Antibody	FH6	Neu5Ac(α2-3)Gal(β1-4) [Fuc(α1-3)]GlcNAc(β1-3) Gal(β1-4)GlcNAc(β1-3) Gal(β1-)-R
Cyclic Sialyl 6-Sulfo Lewis x	Antibody	G159	Cyclic Neu5Ac (α2-3) Gal(β1-4) [Fuc(α1-3)][HSO$_3$(-6)] GlcNAc-R
Lewis y	Antibody	BR55, F3, A70-C/C8, A63-D/B12, 3S193, AH6, BR96, H18A, YB-2	Fuc(α1-2)Gal(β1-4)[Fuc(α1-3)] GlcNAc- (β1-)-R
Trifucosyl-Lewis y	Antibody	KH1	Fuc(α1-2)Gal(β1-4)[Fuc(α1-3)] GlcNAc(β1-3)Gal(β1-4) [Fuc(α1-3)]GlcNAc(β1-)-R
Mannose (Man)	Con A	Concanavalin A	Terminal α-Man, branched tri-Man
	LCA	*Lens culinaris* Agglutinin	Terminal α-Man
	GNL	*Galanthus nivalis* lectin	Terminal Man (α1-2)Man, Manα(α1-6) Man
	BanLec	Banana lectin (*Musa acuminata*)	a-Man, 3-O-a-Man, branched tri-Man

(continued)

Table 1
(continued)

Glycans	GBPs	Lectin name or antibody clones	Lectin specificities or glycan structures
O-Mannosyl Glycan (Mammalian)	Antibody	IIH6	Neu5Ac(α2-3)Gal(β1-4) GlcNAc(β1-2)Man(α1-) Ser/Thr
Sialic acid (Neu5Ac)	SNA	*Sambucus nigra* lectin	α2-6 linked Neu5Ac
	MAL II	*Maackia amurensis* lectin II	Neu5Ac (α2-3) Gal
	SSA	*S. sieboldiana* Agglutinin	NeuAc(α2-6)Gal/GalNAc
	TJA-I	*Trichosanthes japonica* Agglutinin I	NeuA(α2- 6)Gal
	PSL	*Polyporus squamosus* lectin	Neu5Ac (α2-6)Gal(β1-4)Glc-NAc/Glc
	LPA	*Limulus polyphemus* Agglutinin	Neu5Ac
	LFA	*Limax flavus* Agglutinin	Neu5Ac
9-*O*-Acetyl Sialic Acid	Antibody	493D4, CH#-FcD	Neu5Ac9Ac(α2-)-R
Poly-*N*-Acetyl-neuraminic acid	Antibody	12E3, 1E6, 2-2B, 5A5, 735, H.46, OL28, S2-566	(Neu5Ac) n
KDN-Gal (KDN: 3-deoxy-D-glycero-D-alacto-nonulosonic acid)	Antibody	Kdn3G	KDN(α2-3)Gal(β1-)-R
Poly-KDN	Antibody	Kdn8kdn	(KDN)n
Neu5Ac(α2-3)Gal (Monosialogan-glioside)	Antibody	202	Neu5Ac(α2-3)Gal-R
Neu5Ac(α2-3) Gal(β1)	Antibody	FCM1	Neu5Ac(α2-3)Gal(β1-)-R
Neu5Ac(α2-3) Gal(β1-4)Glc	Antibody	M2590, MSG-1	Neu5Ac(α2-3)Gal(β1-4)Glc-R
Neu5Ac(α2-3) Gal(β1-4)Glc-NAc	Antibody	M2590, NS24, SPS-20	Neu5Ac(α2-3)Gal(β1-4) GlcNAc-R
Neu5Ac(α2-8) Neu5Ac(α2-3) Gal	Antibody	A1-245, A1-267, HJM1, R24	Neu5Ac(α2-8)Neu5Ac(α2-3) Gal-R
Neu5Ac(α2-8) Neu5Ac(α2-3) Gal(β1-4)Glc	Antibody	DMAb-19, DMAb-7, DMAb-8, DSG-1, GMB7	Neu5Ac(α2-8)Neu5Ac(α2-3) Gal(β1-4)Glc-R

(continued)

Table 1
(continued)

Glycans	GBPs	Lectin name or antibody clones	Lectin specificities or glycan structures
Blood Group A Trisaccharide	Antibody	3-3[a], AC1001, AC12, B2C114, CB, HB29-36, K7422, K7522, K7516, S10-11A6,	GalNAc(α1-3)[Fuc(α1-2)] Gal(β1-)-R
Blood Group A Type 1	Antibody	AH16, AH21, CB, CLH6, HB29-36, T36	GalNAc(α1-3)[Fuc(α1-2)] Gal(β1-3)GlcNAc(β1-)-R
Blood Group A Type 2	Antibody	11D4, 3A7, AH16, CB, HB29-36, T36	GalNAc(α1-3)[Fuc(α1-2)] Gal(β1-4)GlcNAc(β1-)-R
Blood Group A Type 3	Antibody	CB, HB29-36, K45aF3, M2, MRG-1	GalNAc(α1-3)[Fuc(α1-2)] Gal(β1-3)GalNAc(α1-)-R
Blood Group A Type 4	Antibody	CB, HB29-36, M2,	GalNAc(α1-3)[Fuc(α1-2)] Gal(β1-3)GalNAc(β1-)-R
Blood Group B Type 2	Antibody	3A7, CLCP-19B,	Gal(α1-3)[Fuc(α1-2)]Gal(β1-4) GlcNAc(β1-)-R
Blood Group H Disaccharide	Antibody	1E3, 3H1, B389	Fuc(α1-2)Gal(β1-)-R
Blood Group H Type 1	Antibody	0.BG.5, 17-206, 1E3, 1E5, 3H1, BE2, H1B4	Fuc(α1-2)Gal(α1-3)GlcNAc(β1-)-R
Blood Group H Type 2	Antibody	0.BG.5, 1E3, 1E5, 3A5, 3H1, 92 FR A2, B376, B389, B393, BE2, BRIC231, H1B4, YB02	Fuc(α1-2)Gal(β1-4)GlcNAc(β1-)-R
Blood Group H Type 3	Antibody	1E3, 3H1, MBr1	Fuc(α1-2)Gal(β1-3)GalNAc(α1-)-R
Blood Group H Type 4	Antibody	1E3, 3H1, MBr1	Fuc(α1-2)Gal(β1-3)GalNAc(β1-)-R
SSEA-1	Antibody	SSEA-1	Gal(β1-4)[Fuc(α1-3)] GlcNAc(β1-3)Gal(β1-4) GlcNAc(β1-3)Gal(β1-)-R
SSEA-3	Antibody	MC631, SSEA-3	Gal(β1-3)GalNAc(β1-3)Gal(α1-)-R
SSEA-4	Antibody	MC813-70	Neu5Ac(α2-3)Gal(β1-3) GalNAc(β1-3)Gal(α1-)-R
Heparan Sulfate	Antibody	10E4, AO4B08, HepSS1, HK249, HS3A8, HS3B7, HS4C3, HS4E4, J403, JM13, MW3G3, NAH46, RB4EA12,	-[{[$\pm$(HSO$_3$(-2))GlcA(β1-4)] or[$\pm$(HSO$_3$(-2))IdoA(α1-4)]} ($\pm$(HSO$_3$(-3))$\pm$[(HSO$_3$ or CH$_3$CO)(-2)]$\pm$(HSO$_3$(-6)) GlcN]n-
Delta-Heparan Sulfate	Antibody	3G10	Unsaturated HexA-R

(continued)

Table 1
(continued)

Glycans	GBPs	Lectin name or antibody clones	Lectin specificities or glycan structures
Keratan Sulfate	Antibody	5D4	-{HSO$_3$(-6)GlcNAc(β1-3)$\pm$[HSO$_3$(-6)]Gal(β1-4)}n-
P1 Antigen	Antibody	P001, Pk002	Gal(α1-4)Gal(β1-4)GlcNAc-R
Pk Antigen	Antibody	38.13, P001, Pk002, PK67	Gal(α1-4)Gal(β1-4)Glc-R
HNK-1	Antibody	334, 4F4, Elec39, HNK-1, L2, M6749, NC-1, NGR50, NSP-4, VC1.1	HSO$_3$(-3)GlcA(β1-3)Gal(β1-4)GlcNAc-R
I-Antigen	Antibody	Anti-I Ma, anti-I Woj, C6	Gal(β1-4)GlcNAc(β1-6) [Gal(β1-4)GlcNAc(β1-3)] Gal(β1-4)GlcNAc(β1-)-R

2. Incubate the slides in a blocking solution of PBST0.5 + 1% BSA for 1 h with gentle shaking (*see* **Note 11**).

3. Wash the slides in three baths of PBST0.5 for 3 min each.

4. Spin the slides at 1,000 × g for 1 min to dry the slides (*see* **Note 12**).

5. Place the slides in a slide chamber containing a moist paper towel at the bottom. The paper towel will humidify the chamber and prevent evaporation during the serum incubation.

6. Apply the serum solutions to their designated arrays and incubate at room temperature for 1 h with gentle shaking. The volume applied to each array depends on the size of the array. Using the 48-array/slide design shown in **Fig. 2e**, about 7 µL thoroughly covers the each array.

7. Prepare the glycan-binding detection reagents. Biotinylated lectins should be prepared in PBST0.1 with 0.1% BSA at a concentration of 10 µg/mL. The optimal concentration may be lower for certain high-affinity lectins; this value can be determined experimentally. Biotinylated antibodies (*see* **Note 13**) should be prepared at 1 µg/mL in the same buffer as the lectins.

8. Wash the slides in three baths of PBST0.1 for 3 min each.

9. Spin the slides at 1,000 × g for 1 min to dry the slides.

10. Apply the biotinylated lectin or antibody solutions onto each array, and incubate the slides in a humidified slide box at room temperature for 1 h with gentle shaking.

11. Prepare streptavidin-B-phycoerythrin in PBST0.1 + 0.1% BSA at a concentration of 1 μg/mL.

12. Wash the slides in three baths of PBST0.1 for 3 min each.

13. Spin the slides at $1,000 \times g$ for 1 min to dry the slides.

14. Apply streptavidin-B-phycoerythrin to each array, and incubate the slides in a humidified box at room temperature for 1 h with gentle shaking.

15. Wash the slides in three baths of PBST0.1 for 3 min each.

16. Spin the slides at $1,000 \times g$ for 1 min to dry the slides.

17. Scan the slides using a microarray scanner with appropriate resolution (10 μm or better) and emission and excitation settings. If the slides will not be scanned immediately, store them vacuum sealed with desiccant in the refrigerator.

3.4. Data Analysis and Interpretation

The lectin-binding levels on the arrays can be interpreted in light of the known binding specificities of the lectins. By using multiple lectins or glycan-binding antibodies, more information about the glycan structures can be gathered. When looking at changes in lectin-binding level between samples, it must be remembered that the underlying core protein concentrations might fluctuate along with the amount of a given glycan on the protein. We recommend running sandwich immunoassays to determine the core protein concentrations, which will allow a comparison between core protein changes and glycan changes. Sandwich immunoassays may be conveniently run using the same antibody microarrays as used for the assay described here, only detecting with antibodies against the core proteins rather than detecting with lectins or glycan-binding antibodies. Detailed descriptions of those types of experiments are found elsewhere (13–15).

The researcher should also be aware that lectin-binding levels can be affected by other factors besides the glycan level or the protein level. These factors include the number of the glycan repeats, the location of the glycan epitope in the overall carbohydrate structure, and the presence of outer glycan groups that block binding. For example, Ricinus Communis Agglutinin I (RCA_{120}) binding to LacNAc is inhibited by sialic acid groups at the terminus of glycan chains (4). Another consideration is that some lectins might bind more than one sugar group, so the relative contribution of the different sugar groups to the overall signal can be ambiguous. Therefore results must be interpreted with some caution. This method is ideal for high-throughput screening of the associations of glycan structures with disease or conditions, and complementary techniques can be used to further elucidate the glycan structures in selected samples.

4. Notes

1. Vacuum sealing helps to preserve the antibodies and proteins. Slide boxes can be vacuum sealed using a moderately priced vacuum packaging device such as the FoodSaver. Punch a hole in the slide box to ensure the air in the slide box is removed. Further removal of moisture can be achieved by placing a small desiccant pack in the slide box.

2. The wax partition should stay on throughout all procedures. However, if some thinning or weakening of the lines in observed, the wax can be reprinted at any step. Simply wash and dry the slides and reapply the wax. It may be most convenient to do that before the BSA blocking. Some surfaces, particularly hydrogel surfaces, may not hold wax well. To partition those surfaces, we recommend a gasket system available from several suppliers (The GelCompany, Grace-Biolabs).

3. Two forms of the Coupling Buffer are used here: with and without Tween-20. We have observed that the addition of the detergent prevented the slide coating from peeling off during the long incubation in the oxidation step when using the PATH slide from GenTel Biosciences (Madison, WI); other slide coatings may behave differently. The Coupling Buffer without Tween-20 should be used for the other reactions.

4. The concentration of $NaIO_4$ needed to oxidize the *cis*-hydroxyl groups varies somewhat between monosaccharides *(4)*. Sialic acid is the easiest to oxidize, while mannose seems to be the most difficult. When profiling many types of glycans, we suggest using around 200 mM $NaIO_4$, which will efficiently oxidize all types of glycans, but if the targets are only sialic acid or glucose, the $NaIO_4$ concentration can be 50 mM or less. The optimal conditions for *cis*-hydroxyl oxidation are pH < 4 and 4°C. Higher pH or temperature may decrease the reaction efficiency. At the concentration of 200 mM and 4°C, sodium paraperiodate may precipitate onto the slides, but it can be washed off without negative effect. We recommend storing the $NaIO_4$ in a vacuum-sealed package with desiccant at −20°C and preparing the solution immediately before use.

5. The lid of a pipette-tip box works well for this step. About 50 mL of solution is sufficient for a typical lid, and five slides can lie flat in the lid.

6. Shaking is necessary to ensure even access of the solution to all areas of the slides. Shaking can also help to avoid

precipitate formation. Push the slides to the bottom of the box so that they will not float on top of each other. To ensure the slides stay on the bottom of the container, a clip can be affixed to the side of the container to hold the edges of the slides down.

7. The optimum reaction pH for the maleimide groups on the MPBH is between 6.5 and 7.5. The purpose of the addition of CysGly at this step is to eliminate the possible reaction between the maleimide groups and the cysteine groups on antibodies, which could negatively affect the antibody activities.

8. The reaction between CysGly and the maleimide group of MPBH can be finished at room temperature in 2 h. The overnight incubation at 4°C is designed for a consecutive two-day protocol. If planning to store the slides after blocking, this step can be carried out at room temperature for 2 h, followed by washing, drying, and storage.

9. Since the effect of long-term storage of the blocked slide has not been tested, we suggest finishing the lectin detection immediately after the chemically blocking. The whole procedure will take two consecutive days.

10. It is not necessary to remove or denature the enzymes in the reaction mixture. Heat denaturation of the enzyme may denature the serum proteins and may not able to be captured by the capture antibodies. No negative result or increasing background was found when this reaction mixture was used in glycan detection assays.

11. Blocking reagents that contain glycans, such as milk, may result in high backgrounds and should be avoided.

12. Higher drying speeds may cause the coatings of certain slides, such as the PATH slide, to peel slightly at this step. This possibility can be minimized by slower spinning or drying the slides in a flat, facing-up position.

13. Many of the lectins can be obtained biotinylated, but some lectins and most antibodies will need to be biotinylated by the user. This process can be achieved using commercially available biotinylation reagents such as the NHS-biotin, Hydrazide-biotin, etc. from Pierce Biotech or other suppliers.

References

1. Kingsmore, S. F. (2006) Multiplexed protein measurement: technologies and applications of protein and antibody arrays. *Nat Rev Drug Discov* 5, 310–320

2. Haab, B. B. (2005) Antibody arrays in cancer research. *Mol Cell Proteomics* 4, 377–383

3. Haab, B. B. (2006) Applications of antibody array platforms. *Curr Opin Biotechnol* 17, 415–421

4. Chen, S., Laroche, T., Hamelinck, D., Bergsma, D., Brenner, D., Simeone, D., et-al. (2007) Multiplexed analysis of glycan

variation on native proteins captured by antibody microarrays. *Nat Methods* 4, 437–444

5. Haab, B. B. and Zhou, H. (2004) in *Protein Arrays*, ed. Fung, E. (Humana Press, Totowa, NJ), pp. 33–45

6. Orchekowski, R., Hamelinck, D., Li, L., Gliwa, E., vanBrocklin, M., Marrero, J. A., et-al. (2005) Antibody microarray profiling reveals individual and combined serum proteins associated with pancreatic cancer. *Cancer Res* 65, 11193–11202

7. Kelly, L. S., Kozak, M., Walker, T., Pierce, M., and Puett, D. (2005) Lectin immunoassays using antibody fragments to detect glycoforms of human chorionic gonadotropin secreted by choriocarcinoma cells. *Anal Biochem* 338, 253–262

8. Kuno, A., Uchiyama, N., Koseki-Kuno, S., Ebe, Y., Takashima, S., Yamada, M., et-al. (2005) Evanescent-field fluorescence-assisted lectin microarray: a new strategy for glycan profiling. *Nat Methods* 2, 851–856

9. Manimala, J. C., Roach, T. A., Li, Z., and Gildersleeve, J. C. (2006) High-throughput carbohydrate microarray analysis of 24 lectins. *Angew Chem Int Ed Engl* 45, 3607–3610

10. Wearne, K. A., Winter, H. C., and Goldstein, I. J. (2007) Temporal changes in the carbohydrates expressed on BF01 human embryonic stem cells during differentiation as embryoid bodies. *Glycoconjugate Journal* in press

11. Wearne, K. A., Winter, H. C., O'Shea, K., and Goldstein, I. J. (2006) Use of lectins for probing differentiated human embryonic stem cells for carbohydrates. *Glycobiology* 16, 981–990

12. Manimala, J. C., Roach, T. A., Li, Z., and Gildersleeve, J. C. (2007) High-throughput carbohydrate microarray profiling of 27 antibodies demonstrates widespread specificity problems. *Glycobiology* 17, 17C–23C

13. Chen, S. and Haab, B. B. (2007) in *Clinical Proteomics*, eds. Van Eyk, J. and Dunn, M. (Wiley, VCH, Weinheim, Germany)

14. Forrester, S., Kuick, R., Hung, K. E., Kucherlapati, R., and Haab, B. B. (2007) Low-volume, high-throughput sandwich immunoassays for profiling plasma proteins in mice: identification of early-stage systemic inflammation in a mouse model of intestinal cancer. *Molecular Oncology* in press

15. Nielsen, U. B. and Geierstanger, B. H. (2004) Multiplexed sandwich assays in microarray format. *J Immunol Methods* 290, 107–120

Chapter 5

Glycoproteomic Analysis by Two-Dimensional Electrophoresis

Mary Ann Comunale and Anand Mehta

Summary

Changes in N-linked glycosylation are known to occur during the development of cancer. For example, increased branching of oligosaccharides has been associated with metastasis and has been correlated to tumor progression in human cancers of the breast, colon, and melanomas. Increases in core fucosylation have also been associated with the development of hepatocellular carcinoma (HCC). To a large extent, the proteins to which these N-linked glycans are attached have been unknown. However, with the advent of sensitive glycan analysis and proteomic technologies, the ability to comprehensively identify all the fucosylated proteins in a given population is now a possibility. This method, generally referred to as targeted glycoproteomics, is shown as applied to the detection of proteins present in the fucosylated proteome of a liver cancer cell line but is generally enough to be applied in many other situations.

Key words: Hepatocellular carcinoma, Glycosylation, Hepatitis B virus, Proteomics, Glycomics.

1. Introduction

Changes in the glycosylation of glycoproteins are one of the many molecular changes that accompany transformations to neoplasia (1, 2). Increased branching of oligosaccharides associated with glycoproteins has been associated with metastasis (3) and has been correlated to tumor progression in human cancers of the breast, colon, and melanomas (4). Indeed, lectin staining for branched oligosaccharides in human colorectal carcinoma sections provides an independent prognostic marker for tumor recurrence and patient survival (5). In contrast, the addition of a bisecting N-acetylglucosamine residue prevents branching and suppresses lung metastasis of melanoma cells (6). However,

Michael A. Tainsky, *Methods in Molecular Biology, Tumor Biomarker Discovery, Vol. 520*
© Humana Press, a part of Springer Science+Business Media, LLC 2009
DOI: 10.1007/978-1-60327-811-9_5

mutations responsible for cancer initiation have not been found in genes of the protein glycosylation pathway. This indicates that changes in glycosylation may reflect or contribute to the malignant phenotype downstream of oncogenic events. Thus, it is becoming urgent to develop methodologies that can complement the genomic and proteomic approaches (for identifying differences in DNA or protein expression, respectively) with technologies that can evaluate changes in post-translational modifications such as glycosylation.

Changes in glycosylation have also been show to occur with the development of hepatocellular carcinoma (HCC). The most notable change is an increase in the level of fucosylation of AFP *(7, 8)* and is believed to be an accurate marker for HCC *(9–11)* (a biantennary N-linked glycan with core fucose is shown in **Fig. 1**). Although the molecular mechanism of increased fucosylation in HCC is not clear *(12, 13)*, it is known that the increase is not

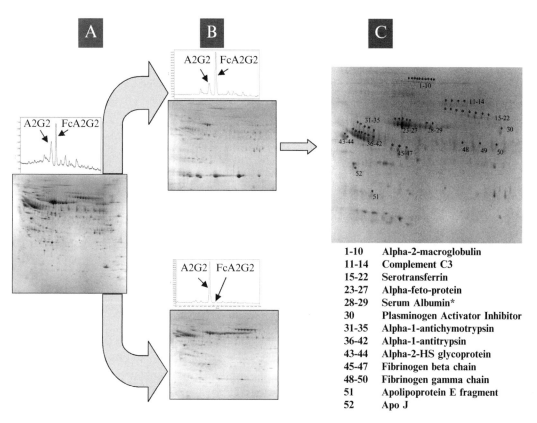

1-10	**Alpha-2-macroglobulin**
11-14	**Complement C3**
15-22	**Serotransferrin**
23-27	**Alpha-feto-protein**
28-29	**Serum Albumin***
30	**Plasminogen Activator Inhibitor**
31-35	**Alpha-1-antichymotrypsin**
36-42	**Alpha-1-antitrypsin**
43-44	**Alpha-2-HS glycoprotein**
45-47	**Fibrinogen beta chain**
48-50	**Fibrinogen gamma chain**
51	**Apolipoprotein E fragment**
52	**Apo J**

Fig. 1. Lectin extraction and glycan analysis of fractionated glycoproteins from Hep G2 cells. (**a**) Glycan analysis and 2DE of the total secreted Hep G2 proteins; (**b**) lectin fractionation of the secreted Hep G2 proteins showing the bound (fucosylated) and unbound nonfucosylated glycoproteins resolved via 2DE. The glycan profiles from each fraction is given above the 2DE and highlights the extraction efficiency (> 98%) (**c**) Identification of the lectin-bound glycoproteins from secreted Hep G2 cells. Features were identified by tryptic digestion and mass spectroscopy analysis. As these are glycoproteins, features may represent a single proteins family of glycoforms. Features are as indicated in the bottom list.

restricted to AFP *(14, 15)*. However, a comprehensive comparative analysis of all the fucosylated glycoproteins in HCC patients has not been performed. This type of study has been limited due to the absence of a suitable technology to allow the examination of large pools of unknown proteins. With the advent of sensitive glycan analysis and proteomic technologies, the ability to comprehensively identify all the fucosylated proteins in patients with HCC and to identify those proteins for the development of diagnostic markers is now a possibility.

2. Materials

1. Cell culture and collection of cell-secreted proteins.
2. RPMI 1640 media (Biowhittaker Cat. No. 12-702F).
3. Fetal bovine serum (Mediatech Inc. Cat. No. 35-011-CV).
4. Dulbecco's phosphate-buffered saline – DPBS (Mediatech Inc.Cat. No. 21-031-CV).
5. EDTA-free Protease Inhibitors (Roche Diagnostics Cat. No.04693132001).
6. Amicon Centriplus YM-10 (Waters Cat. No. 4421).
7. Tris (Hydroxymethyl Aminomethane)-buffered saline(10 m M Tris-HCL, 137 mM sodium chloride, pH 7.4).
8. Protein Assay Kit (Bio-Rad 500-0122).

2.1. Glycan Analysis

1. Spot picker for 2D gels, 3.0 mm (The Gel Company Cat No. P2D3.0).
2. 12% polyacrylamide gels.
3. Acetonitrile (Thermo Fisher Scientific Inc. Cat. No 51101).
4. 100 and 20 mM Ammonium Bicarbonate solution, pH 7.
5. 0.5 M DTT.
6. 0.5 M Iodoacetamide.
7. Fixing solution: 10% methanol, 7% acetic acid.
8. *N*-Glycanase plus (Prozyme Cat. No.GKE-5010B).
9. 5-mL luer lock syringes (BD Ref. No. 301603).
10. Millex-LCR syringe filter unite (Millipore #SLCR 013 NL).
11. 2-AB (2-aminobenzomide) glycan-labeling reagent (Prozyme Cat. No. GKKK-404).
12. Chromatography paper (Whatman Cat. No. 3030 700).
13. Amide-80 normal-phase column (Tosoh Bioscience Cat. No. K391-83H).

14. *50 mM aq. ammonium formate pH 4.4.* Prepare a stock solution of 2 M ammonium formate, pH 4.4. Place pH meter and balance in an empty fume hood. Weigh 92.06 g of formic acid (70 mL) into a beaker using a glass pipette. Place the beaker in an ice slurry with salt (−10°C). Add 500 mL Milli-Q water while stirring. Adjust pH of solution to 4.0 by adding ammonium solution (105.5 mL). Do not add in large quantities as it will produce a rapid and potentially dangerous increase in temperature. Remove solution from ice bath and adjust the pH to 4.4 (approximately 45.5 mL ammonium solution). Increase volume to 1 L in a volumetric flask. Dilute 50 mL of stock to 2 L with Milli-Q water prior to use.

15. Glucose homopolymer labeled with 2AB (Prozyme Cat. No. GKSB-503) for the glycan standard.

16. *Exoglycosidase buffer.* 0.2 mM Zinc Acetate, 0.15 M sodium chloride in a 0.5 M citrate/phosphate buffer, pH 4.5.

2.2. Lectin Extraction

1. *Lectin-binding buffer 10×.* 10 mM $MgCl$, 10 mM $MnCl$, and 10 mM $CaCl_2$ in 40 mM Tris-Buffered Saline, pH 7.4. (TBS may be stored, salts must be added fresh).

2. Agarose-bound *Lens culinaris* agglutinin, *Vicia fabia*, and *Pisum sativum* lectins for the extraction of core fucosylated proteins. Inhibiting/eluting Sugar: 200 mM α-methyl mannoside/200 mM α-methyl glucoside mixture.

3. Agarose-bound *Aleuria aurantia* lectin for the extraction of core and outer arm fucosylated proteins. Inhibiting/Eluting Sugar: 100 mM l-fucose.

4. Wide orifice pipette tips (Rainin Cat. No. HR-250WS).

5. 0.45-μm cellulose acetate spin-X centrifuge tube filters (Costar Cat. No. 8162).

6. Microcon centrifugal filter devices, 10,000 MWCO.

2.3. First-Dimension (IEF) Electrophoresis

1. Protean IEF system (Bio-Rad Laboratories Cat. No.165-4000).

2. *10 mL Solubilization buffer.* 7 M Urea, 2 M Thiourea, 4% Chaps, vortex and mix until in solution. You may warm to help solubilization, but keep water bath at or below 32°C. Add 0.4% ampholytes stock (2:1:1) pH 3–10, 2–4, and 9–11, (for 3–10NL IEF strips), 65 mM DTT, and 5 mM Tributylphosphine (Bio-Rad Cat. No. 163-2101) and bromophenol blue.

3. Cold (−20°C) acetone, acetone-compatible centrifuge tubes, centrifuge and rotor with 13,000 $\times g$ capability.

4. ReadyStrip IPG strips, pH 3–10, nonlinear, 17 cm (Bio-Rad Cat. No.163-2009).

5. *IEF strip-reducing buffer.* 6 M urea, 2% SDS, 1.5%DTT, 30% glycerol, and 50 mM Tris pH 6.8.

6. *IEF strip alkylation buffer.* Alkylated in 6 M urea, 2% SDS, 3% iodoacetamide, 30% glycerol, and 50 mM Tris pH 6.8.

2.4. Second-Dimension Electrophoresis

1. Protean IEF System (Bio-Rad Cat. No. 165-4000).

2. Protean II XL Ready Gel Precast Gel, Tris–HCl, 8–16%, 17-cm IPG well, 1.0- mm thick, 18.3 × 19.3 cm ($W \times L$) (Bio-Rad Cat. No. 161-1453).

3. Protean II xi cell (Bio-Rad)

4. Cooling tank.

5. CCD digital camera or Odyssey infrared imaging system (Li-Cor Biotechnology, Lincoln, Nebraska USA).

6. 2D gel imaging software such as nonlinear dynamics progenesis Workstation gel imaging software package (Nonlinear USA Inc., Durham, NC).

2.5. Mass Spectrometry, Maldi-TOF Analysis

1. Spot picker for 2D gels, 3.0 mm (The gel company Cat No. P2D3.0).

2. 50% Methanol/7% Acetic Acid 25 mM ammonium bicarbonate/5% acetonitrile, 25 mM ammonium bicarbonate/50% acetonitrile, and 100% acetonitrile.

3. 10 mM DTT.

4. 50 mM iodoacetamide.

5. Sequencing-grade modified trypsin (Promega Cat. No. V511).

6. 50mM ammonium carbonate buffer containing 5 mM $CaCl_2$.

7. *Extraction solution.* 50% acetonitrile/0.1%TFA.

8. Millipore Zip-TipC_{18} (MilliporeZTC18M960).

2.6. SDS Polyacrylamide Gel Electrophoresis/ Western Blot Analysis

1. *Reducing separating buffer (4×).* 0.25 M Tris, pH 6.8, 40% glycerol, 8% SDS, 40 mL Glycerol, 8% β-Mercapto-ethanol, and a little bromophenol blue. Once SDS and BB are dissolved, filter with a 0.2-μm syringe filter. Store aliquots in –20°C.

2. *Running buffer (5×).* 125 mM Tris, 0.96 M glycine, 0.5% (w/v) SDS. Store at room temperature.

3. Prestained molecular weight markers: (Invitrogen Cat. No. LC5925).

4. XCell-surelock (Invitrogen EI0001).

5. Precast 12% Tris–Glycine polyacrylamide gels (Invitrogen EC60085Box).

6. *25× Novex Tris–Glycine transfer buffer.* 12 mM Tris Base, 96 mM Glycine.

7. XCell II Blot Module (Invitrogen Cat. No. EW9051).

8. *Western blot transfer buffer.* 40 mL 25× Novex Transfer Buffer (Invitrogen Cat. No. LC3675), 200 mL methanol, and 760 mL Milli-Q water.

9. Chromatography paper (Whatman Cat. No. 3030 700).

10. PVDF membrane (Millipore Cat. No. IPF00010).

11. *Blocking buffer.* 1× TBS is (50 mM Tris–HCl, pH 7.6, 150 mM sodium chloride) containing 5% nonfat dried milk, and 0.1% Tween 20.

2.7. Lectin Fluorophore-Linked Immunosorbent Assay (FLISA)

1. 10 mM sodium periodate ($NaIO_4$) (Sigma Cat. No. 71859-25G).

2. Ethylene glycol.

3. Sodium Carbonate Buffer, pH 9.5.

4. Nunc-Immuno™ Modules for ELISA (Nunc Cat. No. 469949).

5. Phosphate-Buffered Saline (PBS) pH 7.2.

6. 3% Bovine serum albumin (Fisher Cat.No. BP1600-100) in PBS.

7. Scantibodies Heterophyllic Blocking Agent (Scantibodies Laboratory, Cat. No. 31X762).

8. Biotinylated Aleuria Aurantia Lectin (Vector Laboratories, Cat No. B-1395). Make a 4 µg/mL solution in PBS. This can be aliquoted and stored at −20°C.

9. Strepavidin-800 CW IR-Dye (Li-Cor Biosciences, Cat. No. 926-32230).

10. *Wash Buffer.* 1× TNT (10 mM Tris, pH 8.0; 0.15 M NaCl; 0.1% Tween-20).

11. Odyssey infrared imaging system (Li-Core Biotechnology, Lincoln, Nebraska USA) or some other imaging system.

3. Methods

To identify glycan modifications of interest and the N-linked glycosylated polypeptides that contain these modifications, a system of glycan profiling followed by polypeptide identification was developed. The basic design of our comparative approach is given in **Fig. 1**. Briefly, polypeptides from a sample are subjected to chemical or enzymatic treatment to release *N*-glycans. The *N*-glycan pools, representing contributions from all glycoproteins present in the sample, are resolved by neutral-phase HPLC. Specific glycoproteins are "extracted" using affinity reagents (such as Lectins) to target specific protein glycoforms. To control for extraction efficiency, glycan sequencing of the enriched fractions is performed.

The HPLC glycosequencing technology, employing fluorescent labeling of released oligosaccharides, permits the routine analysis of as little as 100 fmol of a particular glycan *(16)* and has allowed the detailed analysis of a variety of different glycoproteins present in minute amounts *(17)*. A fifth-order polynomial equation is generated from the glucose ladder standard and used to convert retention time of standards (both glucose oligomers and known reference oligosaccharides) into glucose units (Gu). All subsequent data are reported in Gu values. With this method of standardization all column conditions are normalized, and very slight variations in temperature or buffers, which would cause shifts in retention times, will not affect Gu values. Gu values have been determined for the major glycan structures and shown to be highly reproducible *(16–20)*. Arm-specific substitutions of multiantennary sugars and the linkage of fucose can be determined by the corresponding Gu value and/or exoglycosidase digestion. Gu values are generally unique to specific substitutions, for example an N-linked biantennary glycan with an alpha 1-3 linked fucose will elute at 7.89Gu, while the biantennary with an alpha 1-2 linked fucose will elute at 7.42Gu. However when two glycans coelute, identification is achieved through a series of exoglycosidase digestions. When the HPLC methodology is combined with exoglycosidase digestions and computational analyses to reference glycan structures, exact oligosaccharide structural information is obtained rapidly with extremely high precision and quantification *(17)*.

If a glycan peak appears to be specific to a sample set, such as serum samples from those with liver cancer or, affinity chromatography to "extract" glycoproteins containing the glycan structures of interest is performed, as indicated in **Fig. 1**. Lectins are the usual affinity reagent utilized for the extraction of specific glycoproteins. An aliquot of the sample that bound the affinity ligand (called "bound") is subjected to chemical or enzymatic methods to release *N*-glycans, followed by neutral-phase chromatography, to confirm that the affinity chromatography successfully recovered the glycan structures of interest (**Fig. 1c**). The balance of the sample from the affinity purification of the glycoproteins is resolved by 2DE (Fig. 1c), and polypeptides of interest are recovered and identified by biochemical and immunological methods.

The "unbound" sample is the component of the sample that did not bind to the affinity reagent and is resolved in parallel with the "bound" to permit determine the efficiency of recovery by the affinity reagent.

3.1. Cell Culture and Collection of Cell-Secreted Proteins

These instructions assume the cells used are HepG2, HepG2.215, or AD38 but may be adapted for other cell lines or serum. Serum analysis is described in **Subheading 3.2**. This protocol assumes the use of cell culture hoods, refrigerated centrifuge capable of $5,000 \times g$.

Cell culture. Cells are grown up in 15 mL completed media RPMI 1640 containing 10% v/v FBS. Media is changed every 2–3 days until cells are confluent, and then the completed media is removed and the cells are washed four times with 5 mL ice-cold DPBS Ca/Mg free, removing any trace of serum from the cultures. Add 10–15 mL of serum-free RPMI 1640 (No FBS added). The cells are cultured for a 24–48 h period (depending on specific cell line vitality).

Collecting and concentrating the secreted proteins. Remove the media and put into a 50-mL conical tube. Add one tablet of EDTA-Free Protease Inhibitors per 10 mL of media collected. Spin at 4000 g 10°C for 10–15 min, remove supernatant, and discard any cellular material. In our experience with Hep G2 and Hep G2.215 cell lines, the media needs to be concentrated 50-fold for the proteins to be within a reasonable working concentration (10 mg/mL or greater). The media is concentrated and buffer exchanged into TBS using Amicon Centriplus YM-10 centrifugal filter devices at 10°C. The media is protein assayed using a standard Bradford Protein Assay to enable loading controls onto gels and sufficient protein concentration for glycan analysis.

Glycan Analysis via Normal-Phase HPLC:

These instructions assume the use of a speed vac, fume hood, sonicator, heat block, HPLC, and an Amide-80 column.

Preparation of Gel Plugs: Gel plugs are pulled from 12% polyacrylamide gels using a 3.0-mm spot picker and placed into individual 1.5-mL polypropylene tubes. 200 µL Acetonitrile is added to each tube and the gel plug is dehydrated. The acetonitrile is removed and the plug is rehydrated in 20 mM ammonium bicarbonate. The plugs are dehydrated in acetonitrile a final time; then after removing the acetonitrile the plugs are dried in a speed vac. The plugs may be stored for a short period of time at –20°C. However, they will, in time, adsorb atmospheric moisture and may need to be redehydrated prior to use.

Incorporation of Sample into Gel Plugs: 5 µL of concentrated media or human serum, 0.75 µL 0.5 M DTT, and 1.25 µL 20 mM ammonium bicarbonate are added to the 1.5-mL tube with a prepared gel plug and spun down. The sample is allowed to adsorb into the gel plug on ice for 15 min. When the plug has visibly swelled, cover gel plug with 20 mM ammonium bicarbonate, heat to 100°C for 3 min, allow cooling, and then add 1 μL 0.5 M iodoacetamide. Spin down gel plug/IAA and incubate for 30 min in the dark. Fix the gel plug in fixing solution for 30 min.

In gel deglycosylation of proteins. Gel plugs are dehydrated in acetonitrile, rehydrated in 20 mM ammonium bicarbonate, dehydrated in Acetonitrile, and then dried in a speed vac as was done in the initial preparation of the plugs. 0.5 μL of PNGaseF (5 mU) and 7 μL of 20 mM ammonium bicarbonate are added to the dried plug, spun down, and the enzyme is allowed to adsorb. Cover the plug with roughly 10 μL of 20 ammonium bicarbonate buffer so that it does not dry out and incubate overnight at 37°C.

Glycan purification. Spin down digested gel plugs, collect supernatant into a fresh microfuge tube. Add an additional 25 μL of Milli-Q water to the gel plug and sonicate for 30 s. Spin down, remove supernatant, and add to previous tube. Repeat sonication step two more times pooling all samples. Bring the solution up to 0.5 mL with Milli-Q water. Filter the collected glycans using a 5-mL syringe and Millex-LCR syringe filter unit. Dry down the glycans in a speed vac to prepare for labeling.

Glycan labeling and clean-up. Prepare 2-AB dye according to manufacturer's directions. Add 5 μL to *completely* dry glycans, spin down, and incubate for 3 h at 65°C. To clean up glycans, cut a strip of chromatography paper and draw pencil circles the size of a penny approximately 1 in. from the bottom of a 6-in. high strip. Label the circles and spot the 5-μL sample inside. Add 10 μL MeCN to the sample tube, vortex, spin down, and spot on top of the sample. Perform chromatography in the dark in a fume hood using a mobile phase of 4:1:1 Butanol: Ethanol: Water. Run the mobile phase to the top of the paper to remove excess dye, remove from chromatography vessel, and allow complet*e* drying. Carefully cut out the circles and place into 5-mL syringe. Suck 1.0 mL of Milli-Q water into a 5-mL syringe and cap with a Millex-LCR syringe filter unit. Invert the syringe, place into a tube rack, and shake for 15 min. Filter and elute the glycans, then dry the glycans in a speed vac.

Normal-phase HPLC. HPLC equipped with an Amide-80 column is used for the glycan separations. Mobile phase A is aqueous 50 mM ammonium formate, pH 4.4, and the mobile phase B is 100% acetonitrile. The column is heated to 30°C. The gradient is set as described in (**Table 1**).

Sample loading. Labeled glycans (**step 5**) are resuspended in 100 μL Milli-Q water and vortexed. 5 μL of sample, 25 μL of Milli-Q, and 70 μL of acetonitrile are mixed and injected on the HPLC. Injection volumes into the HPLC may be adjusted or if needed the sample mixing may be modified to accommodate higher or lower glycan concentrations.

Table 1
Gradient conditions for HPLC

Time	Flow	%A	%B	Curve
	0.4	20	80	6
152	0.4	58	42	6
155	0.4	100	0	6
157	1.0	100	0	6
162	1.0	100	0	6
173	1.0	20	80	6
177	1.0	20	80	6
178	0.4	20	80	6
200	0.4	20	80	6
201	0.0	20	80	6

Creating a standard curve and calculating glucose unit (GU) values. A standard curve is created to convert elution times into GU (glucose units). A glucose homopolymer labeled with 2AB is run on the column, and the standard curve is created using the first ten peaks elution times and assigning each peak the corresponding GU 1 through GU 10. This is graphed in a program like EXCEL, and the line of fit is derived from a fifth-order polynomial equation (16). This equation is then used to convert the unknown peak elution times into glucose units. It is important to run standards frequently.

Peak identification: Initial peak identification is accomplished by converting peak elution times into GU values using the polynomial equation derived from the standard curve. The glycan structures that correspond to the resulting GU can be searched at Glyco Base (http://glycobase.ucd.ie/cgi-bin/public/glycobase.cgi), a database developed by Pauline Rudd's group at Oxford Glycobiology Institute, and are now located at NIBRT Ireland. This database contains the possible glycan structures as well as enzyme information for exoglycosidase digestions to determine the absolute peak identity.

Exoglycosidase digestion for peak identification. Sequential exoglycosidase digestions for peak identification may be applied to the entire sample or to individually collected peaks. The glycans may be split into several tubes for a sequential digestion or may be digested one enzyme at a time, the peak collected from the HPLC, dried down, and enzymatically digested again. The series of enzymes used will be determined by the probable structure for that particular GU value. The glycans are dried to completion and brought up in 4 µL of a 5× exoglycosidase buffer; the appropriate units of exoglycosidase needed are added and the solution brought to 20 µL with Milli-Q water. A common starting point for exoglycosidase digestion is cleaving the sialic acid residues using Sialidase. However, depending on which Sialidase you use, you will cleave different linkages. If linkage data are not sought, Sialidase A will cleave all sialic acids regardless of linkage. It is important the exoglycosidases are used in a proper order to accurately determine sugar structure and attention is paid to linkage specificity. Again, this information is available in detail in the Glyco Base database.

3.2. Extraction of Core Fucose and Outer Arm Fucosylated Proteins

Extraction of core fucosylated proteins. A fresh 10× lectin-binding buffer is made. Divalent cations such as calcium and manganese are required for sugar-binding activity. This is most easily accomplished by first preparing individual 1 M stock solutions. Prepare the lectin slurry, consisting of LcH, PSA, and VFA, by adding 50 µL of suspended beads from each agarose-bound lectin that has been gently resuspended by gentle mixing into 1.5-mL Eppendorf tubes. Spin down at 4000 g and remove the supernatant. Wash the beads a total of three times with 1 mL of a 1× lectin-binding buffer, spinning down and removing the wash each time. After beads are washed, dilute the sample (concentrated media or serum) to 100 µL with 10× and 1× lectin-binding buffer, (i.e., for a 20-µL sample add 2 µL 10× and 78 µL 1×). Allow sample to incubate overnight at 4°C with mixing. To transfer the beads to a 0.45-µm spin column use a wide orifice pipette tip. Spin down to elute the nonbound proteins, rinse the original tube with 100 µL lectin-binding buffer, and using same pipette tip add to the spin column for another column wash (this will also will rinse the beads stuck inside the tip). Repeat this wash several times until the original tube and pipette tip has been rinsed thoroughly. Three 100-µL washes will be sufficient. Pool all the supernatants and keep on ice. Remove the spin column insert and place into a clean tube. Elute the bound proteins with 2 × 100 µL 200 mM Methyl-∝-D-gluco-pyranoside 200 mM ∝-Methyl-D-manno-pyranoside with 5–10 min incubation with mixing each time. Samples are concentrated and buffer exchanged to a final volume of 100 µL in TBS using Microcon Centrifugal Filter Devices, 10,000 MWCO.

Extraction of core and outer arm fucosylated proteins. The technique will be the same as described in **Subheading 2.1**, **item 1**. Lectin slurry consisting of Aleuria Aurantia Lectin (AAL) will replace the three lectin (LcH, PSA, & VFA) mixture and the eluting sugar used is 100 mM l-Fucose.

3.3. Two-Dimensional Gel Electrophoresis

IEF Sample Preparation and Sample Running: Samples are acetone precipitated prior to first dimension. Add ice-cold acetone to 80% of total volume, vortex, and cool to –20°C for 1 h. Centrifuge (14,000 rpm for 20 min at 4°C) and remove supernatant (carefully so as not to disturb the pellet) and air dry for 30 min. Resuspend pellet in 360 µL solubilization buffer, vortex periodically for 1 h, and apply to a 17-cm first-dimension strip. Gel rehydration is carried out for 14 h at 50 V and focused using the Protean System using the following gradient: 100 V for 200 Vh, 500 V for 500 Vh, 1,000 V for 1,000 Vh, 8,000 V for 48,000 Vh. After focusing, first-dimension gel strips are placed into glass tubes (gel side up) and are reduced for 10 min and then alkylated for 10 min prior to running the second dimension.

Second-dimension gel electrophoresis. The second dimension is resolved with an 8–18% acrylamide gradient gel. Current is set to constant milliamps at 20 mA/gel for 20 min and 40 mA/gel for 4 h with gels cooled to 14°C. Gels are immediately fixed. Gel staining can be accomplished by colloidal coomassie, silver, Sypro Ruby, or any mass spec-compatible staining technique.

Gel imaging and analysis. Gels can be digitally imaged using a 16-bit cooled CCD camera or by the Odyssey Imaging System. TIFF files of the gel images are analyzed using gel imaging software.

Mass spectrometry, MALDI-TOF analysis. This protocol assumes the use of a MALDI-TOF mass spectrometer and may also be used for protein identification using a MALDI-TOF-TOF or LC/MS/MS.

Preparation of gel plugs for MS analysis. Gel spots are picked from the gel, placed into clean Eppendorf tubes, and labeled. Destain each spot in 500 µL coomassie destain of 25 mM ammonium bicarbonate/5% acetonitrile. Incubate for 30 min under agitation, then remove the buffer. Add 200 µL 100% acetonitrile and incubate for 10 min. Remove acetonitrile and dry spots under vacuum. Add 100 µL of 10 mM DTT, spin down, and allow incubating for 1 h at 56°C. Spin down, remove the DTT solution, and then alkylate by adding 200 µL of 50 mM iodoacetamide. Allow incubating at room temperature for 45 min in the dark. Remove the IAA, then wash the gel plug with 200 µL of 100 mM ammonium bicarbonate. Spin down, remove wash, and then dehydrate gel plug one final time with Acetonitrile. Dry the gel plug in a speed vac. Gel plugs that have been de-N-glycosylated for glycan analysis can be used for protein identification. If the plug has been treated as described in **Subheading 3.2**, **steps 1–4** they have already been reduced and alkylated and only need to be dehydrated one final time with acetonitrile, dried in a speed vac, and moved on to **Subheading 3.5**, **step 2**.

To prepare 20 µg Promega Modified Trypsin, add 1 mL ice-cold 50 mM Ammonium Carbonate buffer containing 5 mM $CaCl_2$. Add 5–10 µL trypsin to the dried gel plug and keep on ice during rehydration. When plug is rehydrated, spin down, and remove any unabsorbed solution, then cover the gel plug with 50 mM ammonium bicarbonate so the plug does not dry out. Incubate for a minimum of 3 h to overnight at 37°C. Remove the solution from tube and collect. Extract the peptides by adding 1 volume of extraction solution vortex and add to previous collection. Repeat extraction and combine supernatants. Samples must be dried and reconstituted in 0.1% Trifluoroacetic acid.

Zip-tip C_{18}– cleaning of samples. The zip-tip is wetted with 60% Acetonitrile, 0.1% TFA. The tip is equilibrated with 0.1% TFA by washing with the equilibration solution a minimum of three times. The sample is aspirated into the pipette tip at least seven times to maximize binding of the sample to the tip. Wash the tip and dispense to waste with a minimum of five cycles of wash solution. To elute the sample take up 10 µL of elution solution and dispense into a clean tube. Repeat two more times.

Spotting the MALDI target – Dried droplet method. Apply 0.5 µL of zip-tipped sample onto target. Add 0.5 µL of CHCA matrix, mix with pipette action, and allow to air dry. Check for a uniform crystallization. If the sample looks "clumpy" after drying, the sample may be redissolved with 50% Acetonitrile 0.1% TFA and recrystallized.

Peptide mass maps are obtained using a Voyager-DE Pro Mass Spectrometer (PE Biosystems, Foster City, CA) operated in positive ion reflector mode. Setting will vary from instrument to instrument and must be optimized by the operator. Proteins can be identified from the peptide mass maps using the MASCOT online database www.matrixscience.comto search the nonredundant protein database.

Confirmation of proteins with increased fucosylation by western blot. These instructions assume the use of an Invitrogen XCell II Blot Module, although other electrophoresis and blotting equipment may be substituted.

SDS-PAGE. Samples that have been lectin extracted, and buffer exchanged are resolved by SDS-PAGE on a 12% polyacrylamide gel. Samples should be in an equivalent volume of 100 µL (instructions to buffer exchange lectin-extracted samples into 100 µL of TBS) so that comparisons can be made. The volume of sample needed to obtain a good signal on the blot may need to be determined; it is suggested to start with 6 µL. The 6 µL of sample is combined with 5 µL of 2× reducing loading buffer and heated to 100°C for 5 min. Molecular weight markers are loaded at 3 µL per lane and the samples are loaded at 10 µL per lane. The gel is run at 40 mA constant until the dye front is at the bottom of the gel.

Western Blot. The proteins are transferred to a PVDF membrane by immunoblotting. The Whatman paper, membrane, and sponges must all be presoaked in transfer buffer prior to assembly. The PVDF membrane must first be soaked in 100% methanol, rinsed briefly in Milli-Q water, then quickly placed into transfer buffer. Assemble the gel/membrane sandwich by placing two presoaked sponges on the cathode core followed by a single sheet of Whatman filter paper. Place the gel carefully on the stack followed by the presoaked PVDF membrane. Place another sheet of presoaked Whatman filter followed by enough sponges to fill the inner chamber of the blotter. Close the unit with the anode side, and squeezing tightly place the chamber into the unit and snap into place. Add transfer buffer so that the level is just to the top of the blot. Fill the outside chamber with distilled water and run the blot at 40 mA constant overnight.

Detecting proteins on the blot: The membrane is blocked by incubating with blocking buffer for 1 h at room temperature, then incubated overnight with desired antibody and developed using the Li-Core Odyssey imaging system.

3.4. Conformation of Proteins via Lectin-FLISA

This protocol infers the use of the Odyssey Infrared Imaging System (Li-Core Biotechnology, Lincoln, Nebraska, USA). Multiple methods can be used here from simple alkaline phosphatase and horseradish peroxidase to ECL-based methods. What is described is our use of the Li-Core Odyssey Infrared Imaging System.

3.5. Oxidation of Capture Antibody and Plate Preparation

1. Prepare 100 mM $NaIO_4$ and dilute to 10 mM in the capture antibody of choice and incubate for 1 h at 37°C with mixing. Add sufficient ethylene glycol to stop the $NaIO_4$ oxidation; a 1:1 ratio to the $NaIO_4$ will be sufficient. Add sodium carbonate buffer of pH 9.5, so the final antibody concentration is 1 μg/100 μL. Pipette 100 μL into each well and incubate the plate overnight at 4°C with gentle shaking. Remove and block plate in three percent BSA/PBS for 3 h at room temperature of if preferred, overnight at 4°C.

2. Rinse the plates three times with rinse buffer and dry plates stored at –20°C.

3.6. Fluorophore-Linked Immunosorbent Assay

1. Add sample to well, bringing the final volume to 100 μL with PBS. Incubate for 2 h with shaking at 37°C. Wash the wells five times with washing buffer, and then add 100 μL of AAL-Biotin (4 μg/mL) into each well. Add 100 μL AAL (4 μg/mL) in PBS and incubate for 1 h with shaking at room temperature. Wash the plate five times with wash buffer and then add 100 μL of strepavidin-IRDye (1:5000). Incubate for 1 h with shaking in the dark at room temperature. Wash the plate five times with wash buffer, and leave a final wash in the plate so the plate is not dry.

2. Image using the appropriate Odyssey settings.

4. Notes

1. When collecting supernatants from cell cultures, it is important to reduce the amount of serum proteins present. Cell lines vary in their sensitivity to serum-free conditions and this must be tested empirically. In addition, care must be taken to fully wash cells with PBS before the addition of serum-free media.

2. When making the ammonium formate (**Subheading 2.2**) it is imperative that one adds in the ammonium solution slowly. Large additions of ammonium solution will produce a rapid and potentially dangerous increase in temperature.

3. When making the solubilization buffer (**Subheading 2.3**), it is often useful to slightly warm the buffer to aid solubilization, but keep water bath at or below 32°C.

4. The In-gel release of N-linked glycans is used to "fix" proteins in place to allow easy release and purification of glycans (**Subheading 3.2**). One concern in the handling of the gel-plugs is static electricity that can make working with the plug difficult. For that reason, it is best to spin the plug in a microfuge before use.

5. For glycan analysis, labeling dye must be added to completely dry glycans. An aqueous condition will result in poor labeling.

6. When performing lectin extraction (**Subheading 3.3**), equivalent protein concentrations must be used to compare different cell lines or different cell treatments. For analysis of serum, equivalent volumes are best used.

7. It is important to fully wash the tubes containing the agarose beads as they can "stick" to the microfuge tubes and pipette tips (**Subheading 3.3**).

8. When performing acetone precipitation, make sure solubilization buffer fully rinses the side of the tubes to collect all precipitated protein. This is best performed by mild vortexing.

9. When loading first-dimension strip, make sure the plastic backing of the strip is flush with the front glass plate and the entire length of the IEF strip is flush with the second dimension to prevent gel streaking (**Subheading 3.4**).

References

1. Hakomori S (1996) Tumor malignancy defined by aberrant glycosylation and sphingo(glyco) lipid metabolism. *Cancer Res.* 56(23): 5309–18

2. Kobata A (1998) A retrospective and prospective view of glycopathology. *Glycoconj J.* 15(4): 323–31

3. Dennis JW, Laferte S, Waghorne C, Breitman ML, Kerbel RS (1987) Beta 1–6 branching of Asn-linked oligosaccharides is directly associated with metastasis. *Science.* 236(4801): 582–5

4. Fernandes B, Sagman U, Auger M, Demetrio M, Denni JW (1991) Beta 1-6 branched

oligosaccharides as a marker of tumor progression in human breast and colon neoplasia [see comments]. *Cancer Res.* 51(2): 718–23

5. Seelentag WK, Li WP, Schmitz SF, Metzger U, Aeberhard P, Heitz PU, Roth J (1998) Prognostic value of beta1, 6-branched oligosaccharides in human colorectal carcinoma. *Cancer Res.* 58(23): 5559–64

6. Yoshimura, M, Nishikawa A, Ihara Y, Taniguchi S, Taniguchi N (1995) Suppression of lung metastasis of B16 mouse melanoma by *N*-acetylglucosaminyltransferase III gene transfection. *Proc Natl Acad Sci U S A.* 92(19): 8754–8

7. Breborowicz J, Mackiewicz A, Breborowicz D (1981) Microheterogeneity of alpha-fetoprotein in patient serum as demonstrated by lectin affino-electrophoresis. *Scand J Immunol.* 14(1): 15–20

8. Miyazaki J, Endo Y, Oda T (1981) Lectin affinities of alpha-fetoprotein in liver cirrhosis, hepatocellular carcinoma and metastatic liver tumor. *Acta Hepatol. Jpn.* 22: 1559–68

9. Taketa K, Ichikawa E, Taga H, Hirai H, (1985) Antibody-affinity blotting, a sensitive technique for the detection of alpha-fetoprotein separated by lectin affinity electrophoresis in agarose gels. *Electrophoresis.* 6: 492–97

10. Taketa K, Sekiya C, Namiki M, Akamatsu K, Ohta Y, Endo Y, Kosaka K (1990) Lectin-reactive profiles of alpha-fetoprotein characterizing hepatocellular carcinoma and related conditions. *Gastroenterology.* 99(2): 508–18

11. Shiraki K, Takase K, Tameda Y, Hamada M, Kosaka Y, Nakano T (1995) A clinical study of lectin-reactive alpha-fetoprotein as an early indicator of hepatocellular carcinoma in the follow-up of cirrhotic patients. *Hepatology.* 22(3): 802–7

12. Hutchinson WL, Du MQ, Johnson PJ, Williams R (1991) Fucosyltransferases: differential plasma and tissue alterations in hepatocellular carcinoma and cirrhosis. *Hepatology.* 13(4): 683–8

13. Miyoshi E, Noda K, Yamaguchi Y, Inoue S, Ikeda Y, Wang W, Ko JH, Uozumi N, Li W, Taniguchi N (1999) Altered glycosylation of serum transferrin of patients with hepatocellular carcinoma. *J Biol Chem.* 264(5): 2415–23

14. Yamashita K, Koide N, Endo T, Iwaki Y, Kobata A (1989) Altered glycosylation of serum transferrin of patients with hepatocellular carcinoma. *J Biol Chem.* 264(5): 2415–23

15. Naitoh A, Aoyagi Y, Asakura H (1999) Highly enhanced fucosylation of serum glycoproteins in patients with hepatocellular carcinoma. *J Gastroenterol Hepatol.* 5(1): 43–68

16. Guile, G. R., P.M. Rudd, D.R. Wing, S.B. Prime, and R.A. Dwek (1996) A rapid high-resolution high-performance liquid chromatographic method for separating glycan mixtures and analyzing oligosaccharide profiles. *Anal Biochem.* 240(2): 21017.

17. Rudd PM, Mattu TS, Zitzmann N, Mehta A, Colominas C, Hart E, Opdenakker G, DwekRA (1999) Glycoproteins: rapid sequencing technology for N-linked and GPI anchor glycans. *Biotechnol Genet Eng Rev.* 16: 1–21

18. Rudd PM, Mattu TS, Masure S, Bratt T, Van den Steen PE, Wormald MR, Kuster B, Harvey DJ, Borregaard N, Van Damme J, Dwek RA, Opdenakker G (1999) Glycosylation of natural human neutrophil gelatinase B and neutrophil gelatinase B-associated lipocalin. *Biochemistry.* 38(42): 13937–50

19. Mattu TS, Royle L, Langridge J, Wormald MR, Van den Steen PE, Van Damme J, Opdenakker G, Harvey DJ, Dwek RA, Rudd, PM(2000) "O-glycan analysis of natural human neutrophil gelatinase B using a combination of normal phase-HPLC and online tandem mass spectrometry: implications for the domain organization of the enzyme. *Biochemistry.* 39(51): 15695–704

20. Rudd PM, Colominas C, Royle L, Murphy N, Hart E, Merry AH, Hebestreit HF, Dwek RA (2001) A high-performance liquid chromatography based strategy for rapid, sensitive sequencing of N-linked oligosaccharide modifications to proteins in sodium dodecyl sulphate polyacrylamide electrophoresis gel bands. *Proteomics.* 1(2): 285–289

Chapter 6

All-Liquid Separations, Protein Microarrays, and Mass Spectrometry to Interrogate Serum Proteomes: An Application to Serum Glycoproteomics

Tasneem H. Patwa, Yinghua Qiu, Jia Zhao, Diane M. Simeone, and David M. Lubman

Summary

Disease-related changes in serum proteins are reasonable targets for early detection particularly due to the noninvasive approach in obtaining samples. Glycoproteins specifically have been implicated in a variety of disease types ranging from immune diseases to cancers. High-throughput screening methods that can assess glycosylation states of all serum proteins in normal and diseased sample groups can facilitate early detection as well as shed light on disease progression mechanisms. Outlined here is a combination of liquid separation, protein microarray, and mass spectrometry approach to highlight candidate proteins involved in diseases through glycosylation mechanisms.

Key words: Immunodepletion, Lectin enrichment, NPS-RP-HPLC, Glycoprotein microarray, Lectin blot, Deglycosylation, Glycopeptide mapping, Nano-LC-MS/MS.

1. Introduction

Serum proteins are of increasing interest in disease-related research due to easy collection in clinical settings unlike more invasive biopsy procedures. Furthermore disease markers in the blood would facilitate rapid patient screening in early detection scenarios. However the complexity of the serum proteome makes studying such a medium for biomarker discovery particularly challenging. Blood contains proteins over a dynamic range of close to 15 orders of magnitude *(1)*. Such a range is thought to cover over

Michael A. Tainsky, *Methods in Molecular Biology, Tumor Biomarker Discovery, Vol. 520*
© Humana Press, a part of Springer Science + Business Media, LLC 2009
DOI: 10.1007/978-1-60327-811-9_6

15,000 proteins, most of which are of low abundance. However high-abundance proteins such as albumin, which make up nearly 65% of the serum content, make proteomic analysis of the proteins of lower abundance almost impossible. A variety of methods have been developed to remove high-abundance proteins from plasma and serum. Such methods reduce the complexity of serum samples making it amenable to further separation techniques.

Glycoproteins and their glycoforms are present on many cell surfaces and are often secreted by cells. They play important roles in functions such as cell–cell interaction, recognition, and the immune response. Studies have shown that glycoprotein characteristics, particularly changing of the glycosylation site or the complexity of the glycan structure itself, correlate well with the development of diseases, an example of which is cancer (2–4).

Presented here is a protocol that combines an all-liquid phase separation technique with protein microarrays, multilectin detection, and mass spectrometry to study changes in glycoprotein patterns in serum/plasma samples. Serum proteins are first depleted of the 12 most highly abundant proteins. The remainder are enriched for glycoproteins and further resolved by nonporous reversed-phase HPLC separations followed by printing using noncontact printing mechanisms on nitrocellulose slides. The resulting arrays are probed with a range of biotinylated lectins and streptavidin conjugated to a fluorescent tag to detect distinct glycan structures on the proteins (5). Such a study on a large sample set is able to highlight key differences in glycan expression on specific glycoproteins as a function of disease (6). Key differences in lectin response which are observed based on the array data can then be further interrogated using mass spectrometry to determine glycoprotein identity as well as specific glycan structural changes.

2. Materials

2.1. Immunodepletion

1. ProteomeLab IgY-12 proteome partitioning kit (Beckman Coulter, Fullerton, CA).

2. Spin filters, 0.45 μm (Millipore, Billerica, MA).

3. *10× Dilution buffer composition.* Tris–HCl Buffered Saline: 100 mM Tris–HCl, pH 7.4, 1.5 M NaCl.

4. *10× Stripping buffer composition.* 1 M Glycine-HCl, pH 2.5.

5. *10× Neutralization buffer composition.* 1 M Tris–HCl, pH 8.0.

6. 15 mL, 5 kDa MWCO Amicon filters (Millipore).

2.2. Lectin Enrichment	1. Agarose-bound lectin, Wheat Germ Agglutinin, (WGA) and Agarose-bound Concanavalin A (Con A), (Vector Laboratories, Burlingame, CA) – If enrichment based on other glycan groups is desired, alternate agarose-bound lectins can be used.
	2. Empty spin columns (column capacity: 0.9 mL) (Pierce, Rockford, IL).
	3. *Binding buffer composition*. 0.15 M NaCl, 20 mM Tris–HCl, 1 mM $MnCl_2$, 1 mM $CaCl_2$, pH 7.4.
	4. *Elution buffer composition*. 0.3 M *N*-acetyl-glucosamine and 0.3 M Methyl-α-d- mannopyroside in 20 mM Tris–HCl and 0.5 M NaCl, pH 7.0.
2.3. Nonporous Reversed-Phase HPLC	1. *NPS-RP-HPLC column*. 33 × 4.6-mm Micra Platinum column, ODSII (recommended) (Eprogen).
	2. Column heater.
	3. Deionized water was purified using a Millipore RG system (Bedford, MA).
	4. *Solvent A*. Sonicated deionized water with 0.1% trifluoroacetic acid (TFA).
	5. *Solvent B*. Sonicated acetonitrile (ACN) with 0.08% TFA.
2.4. Array Printing	1. Nanoplotter 2.0 (GeSiM).
	2. Nitrocellulose slides (Whatman, Inc).
	3. *Printing buffer composition*. 62.5 mM Tris–HCl (pH 6.8), 1% w/v Sodium dodecyl sulfate (SDS), 5% w/v dithiothreitol (DTT), and 1% glycerol.
2.5. Hybridization of Slides	1. *Blocking buffer*. 1% bovine serum albumin (BSA) in PBS-T (phosphate-buffered saline with 0.1% Tween-20).
	2. *Primary incubation buffer*. 5 μg/mL biotinylated lectin in PBS-T. Any biotinylated lectin can be used, but we have found that SNA, MAL, AAL, and ConA cover a majority of glycan structures of interest (**Fig. 1**).
	3. *Secondary incubation buffer*. 1 μg/mL Alexafluor555-conjugated streptavidin in PBS-T and 0.5% BSA.
	4. *Washing buffer* 1× PBS-T (with 0.5% BSA if wash is after the secondary incubation).
2.6. SDS-page	1. *Running buffer*. 0.192 M glycine, 25 mM Tris–HCl, 0.1% w/v SDS.
	2. Prestained molecular weight markers.

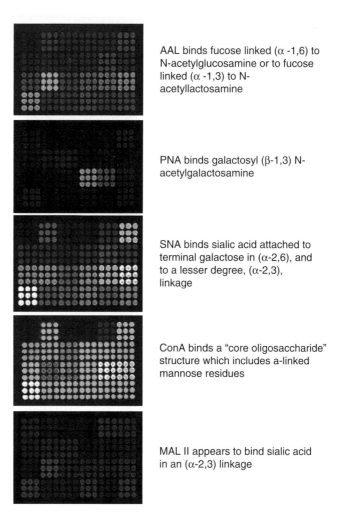

AAL binds fucose linked (α -1,6) to N-acetylglucosamine or to fucose linked (α -1,3) to N-acetyllactosamine

PNA binds galactosyl (β-1,3) N-acetylgalactosamine

SNA binds sialic acid attached to terminal galactose in (α-2,6), and to a lesser degree, (α-2,3), linkage

ConA binds a "core oligosaccharide" structure which includes a-linked mannose residues

MAL II appears to bind sialic acid in an (α-2,3) linkage

Fig. 1. Parts of array showing enriched glycoproteins from serum stained with five different lectins as indicated. All glycoproteins were printed in nine replicates to ensure reproducibility. Spots that appear white are in higher abundance and their signal is saturated. For quantitation purpose PMT gain of scanner would need to be reduced to ensure that spot intensities are not saturated.

2.7. Membrane Transfer and Lectin Blot

1. Filter paper (Whatman) and PVDF membrane is from BioRad.
2. *Transfer buffer.* 0.192 M glycine, 25 mM Tris–HCl, 1% Methanol.
3. *Blocking buffer.* 5% BSA in PBS-T.
4. *Primary incubation buffer.* 1 μg/mL biotinylated lectin in PBS-T containing 3% BSA.
5. *Secondary incubation buffer.* 100 ng/mL Alexaflor555-conjugated streptavidin in PBS-T containing 3% BSA.
6. *Wash buffer.* PBS-T

2.8. Glycopeptide Mapping	1. *Calibrant solution.* 2 μg/μL sodium iodide (NaI) and 0.05 μg/μL Cesium Iodide (CsI) in a 50:50 solution of isopropanol and water.

3. Methods

3.1. Sample Preparation

3.1.1. Serum Samples

1. Let samples sit at room temperature for a minimum of 30 min (and a maximum of 60 min) to allow the clot to form in the red-top tubes.

2. Centrifuge clotted sample at $1,300 \times g$ at 4°C for 20°min and transfer the serum into polypropylene-capped tube in 1 mL aliquots.

3. Freeze the sample at –80°C until further use.

3.1.2. Plasma Samples

1. Store patient plasma samples at –80°C until needed.

2. Before immunodepletion the samples need to be delipidated. Centrifuge the sample at $15,000 \times g$ for 15 min and pour out the lipid containing upper layer (*see* **Note 1**).

3.2. Immunodepletion

1. Thaw frozen sample on ice

2. Dilute 250 μL of thawed sample to a total volume of 625 μL with dilution buffer

3. Centrifuge the sample using a 0.45-μm spin filter for 1 min at $9,200 \times g$

4. Equilibrate the IgY-12 LC10 (*see* **Note 2**) column with 1× dilution buffer for 30 min. at a flow rate of 2.0 mL/min. at room temperature

5. Inject 625 μL of diluted sample and start the separation method which is as follows: 0.5 mL/min dilution buffer for 30 min; 2 mL/min dilution buffer for 5 min; 2 mL/min 1× stripping buffer for 20 min (*see* **Note 3**)

6. Collect the flow-through and eluted fractions. Add 1/10 volume of 10× neutralization buffer (1.6–1.8 mL) to eluted fraction (16–18 mL). Store depleted sample at –80°C if not used immediately

7. Concentrate the flow-through and bound protein samples to a volume compatible with the following step (500 μL to 2 mL) with an Amicon Ultra-15 centrifugal filter unit, 10,000 MW (*see* **Note 4**). **Figure 2a** shows a typical chromatogram observed during a depletion experiment when monitored at 280 nm

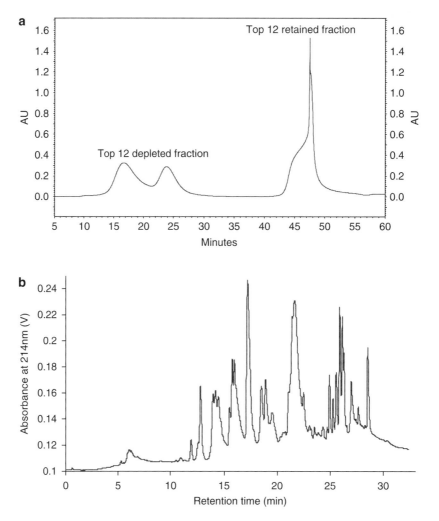

Fig. 2. Sample chromatogram from an (**a**) immunodepletion step and (**b**) Nonporous reversed-phase HPLC separation.

3.3. Lectin Enrichment

1. 1 mL of Agarose-bound lectin is packed into a disposable screw end-cap spin column with filters at both ends.

2. Prior to enrichment a solution of protease inhibitor cocktail is prepared and diluted in a ratio of 1:50 in all buffer that will be used. Depleted serum samples is buffer exchanged into 500 µL binding buffer using Amicon 5000 MWCO filter.

3. The column is first equilibrated with 500 µL of binding buffer.

4. Diluted sample is loaded on the column and incubated for 15 min at room temperature. The nonbinding fraction can be removed by centrifugation at 500 rpm for 2 min.

5. The column is washed with 600 μL of binding buffer to remove nonspecific binders. Bound glycoproteins are released and collected with 250 μL of elution buffer by centrifugation at 500 rpm for 2 min. The elution step is repeated twice to ensure good recovery of enriched glycoproteins.

3.4. Nonporous Reversed-Phase HPLC

1. Eluted, enriched glycoproteins are concentrated using a 10,000-MW centrifuge filter (Millipore) and reconstituted in deionized water.

2. The sample is loaded onto an ODS II (4.6 × 33 mm) column (Eprogen Inc.).

3. Proteins in sample are separated at a flow rate of 0.5 mL/min using the following gradient: 5–15% B in 1 min, 15–25% B in 2 min, 25–30% B in 3 min, 30–41% B in 15 min, 41–47% B in 4 min, 47–67% B in 5 min and 67–100% B in 2 min. Column temperature is maintained at 60°C and the separation process is monitored at 214 nm. Purified proteins are collected using a fraction collector. **Figure 2b** shows a typical NPS-RP-HPLC chromatogram seen with serum samples using the above gradient.

4. Separated proteins are stored at –80°C until further use.

3.5. Printing Arrays

1. All fractionated proteins are transferred to a 96-well print plate and dried down completely using a speedvac concentrator (Thermo).

2. The dried samples are resuspended in 15 μL of printing buffer and maintained on a shaker overnight at 4°C.

3. Microarrays are generated using a noncontact arrayer (GeSiM) that uses a piezo-electric mechanism to deposit droplets. The arrayer is programmed to deposit five droplets of 500 pL each per fraction spot and all spots are 600 μm apart.

4. At the completion of arraying, slides are left in arrayer overnight and then stored in a dessicator until further use.

3.6. Hybridization of Arrays

1. Dried slides are first blocked overnight using ~40 mL of blocking buffer per slide.

2. The slides are then hybridized in primary incubation buffer containing biotinylated lectin for 2 h at 4°C on a rotor. Hybridization is performed in plastic heat-sealable pouches that hold 4 mL of solution.

3. All slides are washed five times for 3 min each in PBS-T (*see* **Note 5a**).

4. Secondary incubation is accomplished in a secondary incubation buffer for 1 h at 4°C (again in heat-sealable pouches).

5. All slides are subsequently washed five times for 5 min each in PBS-T.

6. The slides are then spin-dried in a high-speed centrifuge for 15 min (*see* **Note 5b**).

3.7. Data Analysis (Genepix 6.0 and PCA + HC)

1. Processed slides are scanned on an Axon 4000A scanner with GenePix 6.0 software in the green channel.

2. PMT gain is typically maintained between ×400–700 on our instrument, depending on the lectin that is used to probe the array.

3. In cases where multiple samples are analyzed the GenePix 6.0 software facilitates spot intensity data integration so that all spot intensities can be further interrogated with principal component analysis (PCA) and hierarchical clustering (HC).

3.8. SDS-PAGE Gel Electrophoresis

In the case where multiple confident protein IDs are found by mass spectrometry it will be necessary to determine which protein in the mixture is causing a differential lectin response.

1. Fractions from the NPS-RP-HPLC separation that need to be interrogated further are dried and resuspended in 30 µl of Bio-Rad Laemmli sample buffer containing 350 mM DTT.

2. The sample is boiled in a water bath for 6–8 min.

3. A Bio-Rad ready gel (10% Tris–HCl) is loaded into a Mini-Protean cell (Bio-Rad, Hercules, CA).

4. Running buffer is introduced into the cell until it reaches close to the top. Make sure there are no leaks, otherwise current flow will be disrupted.

5. Load sample into the gel lanes (*see* **Note 6**).

6. The gel is run at 80 V until separation is achieved. Running times can range from 2 to 3 h. It is acceptable to make the low molecular materials run off the gel as this will facilitate improved separation of the higher molecular weight materials such as the glycoproteins of interest.

3.9. Membrane Transfer and Lectin Blot

1. Cut a PVDF membrane as well as a filter paper to the size of the gel (*see* **Note 7**).

2. Soak precut transfer membrane, filter paper and gel in transfer buffer for 5–10 min.

3. Wet the transfer apparatus (Amersham Biosciences) with transfer buffer.

4. Place two filter papers on bottom of transfer apparatus.

5. Place membrane on top of filter paper and remove any air bubbles using dry disposable pipettes by rolling it over the surface.

6. Transfer gel onto the membrane (Whatman) and remove air bubbles.

7. Place 2–3 filter papers on top of the gel and remove any air bubbles again.

8. Transfer for 3 h at 25 V. After transfer rehydrate the membrane in methanol

9. The membrane is blocked overnight at 4°C by immersing it in a solution of blocking buffer and leaving it on a shaker.

10. The following morning the membrane is incubated in primary incubation solution for 1 h at room temperature on a gel shaker.

11. The membrane is then washed six times for 15 min each using PBS-T.

12. After washing the membrane is incubated with secondary incubation solution for 1 h at room temperature on a gel shaker.

13. It is then washed four times for 15 min each with PBS-T.

14. The membrane is then immersed in an ECL analysis system (Pierce) by mixing the two components in a 1:1 ratio for 1 min.

15. The ECL-exposed membrane is placed between a plastic folder and in a transfer cartridge.

16. In a dark room a blue-sensitive autoradiographic film is placed on top of the membrane in the transfer cartridge and exposed for between 30 s and 1 min. At the end of the exposure the film is removed and checked to see if the exposure time is sufficient. Otherwise additional exposures are performed until an appropriate image is acquired (*see* **Note 8**).

3.10. Trypsin Digestion for Mass Spectrometry

1. Protein fractions from NPS-RP-HPLC are dried down to ~10 µL in a speedvac concentrator operating at 45°C.

2. The dried fractions are diluted with 40 µL of 100 mM ammonium bicarbonate (*see* **Note 9**) and 5 µL of 10 mM dithiothreitol (DTT).

3. 0.5 µL of TPCK modified sequencing grade porcine trypsin is added, and the samples are vortexed well and spun down.

4. The digestion mixture is incubated at 37°C overnight on an agitator.

5. Digestion is stopped by the addition of 0.5 µL of TFA to acidify mixture.

3.11. Protein Deglycosylation

1. 10 µL of 250 mM sodium phosphate, pH 7.5, and 2.5 µL 20× denaturation solution is added to dried digestion mixture. The solution is heated at 100°C for 5 min.

2. The heated solution is allowed to cool down and 2.5 µL of Triton-X is added to it.

3. 0.01 U (~2 µL) of PNGase F is added to deglycosylation mixture which is then left to incubate at 37°C overnight.

3.12. Protein Identification and Glycosylation Site Mapping by Mass Spectrometry

1. Before analysis by mass spectrometry, digested samples are completely dried down and reconstituted in HPLC-grade water to the volume required for injection.

2. The peptide mixtures are separated on a reversed-phase column attached to a Paradigm HPLC pump. A nanotrap platform is set up prior to the electrospray source. It includes a peptide nanotrap (0.15 × 50 mm) and a separation column (0.075 mm × 150 mm, C18). The peptide sample is first injected onto the trap column with 5% solvent B (0.3% formic acid in 98% ACN) at 50 µL/min for 5 min in order to desalt the sample.

3. The peptides are then eluted using the following gradient: 5–95% B at a flow rate of 0.25 µL/min over 45 min (*see* **Note 10**). Digested mixture can be used for protein identification purposes, but the deglycosylated sample should be analyzed if glycosylation site identification is desired.

4. A Finnigan LTQ mass spectrometer equipped with a nano-ESI source can be used to acquire spectra. A 75-µm metal spray tip is connected to the eluting end of the nanoseparation column and the spray voltage is set to 3 kV. The capillary temperature is 200°C, the spray voltage is 4.2 kV, and the capillary voltage is 30 V.

5. The instrument is operated in data-dependent mode with dynamic exclusion enabled. The MS/MS spectra on the five most abundant peptide ions in full MS scan are obtained. The high-abundance solvent or contamination peaks are placed in an exclusion list to avoid their selection for fragmentation and to maximize the useful tandem MS spectra. The normalized collision energy is set at 35% for MS/MS (*see* **Note 11**).

6. When searching the acquired spectra using the SEQUEST algorithm for matching identifications the following parameters are used: Threshold was set to 1,000, tolerances were set to 1.4 and 0.00 for precursor and fragment ions, respectively; modifications – Methionine oxidation (+18 Da), 0.984 on Asparagine (if deglycosylated sample is being searched), trypsin was indicated as a specific protease with two missed cleavages allowed. Positive protein identification was accepted for a peptide with X_{corr} of greater than or equal to 3.0 for triply, 2.5 for doubly, and 1.9 for singly charged ions (*see* **Note 12**).

3.13. Differential Glycopeptide Mapping

1. Digested peptide mixtures from target glycoproteins are separated by a capillary RP column (C18, 0.2 × 150 mm) (Michrom, Auburn, CA) on a capillary pump (Ultra-Plus II MD, Micro-Tech Scientific, Vista, CA).

2. The capillary column should be directly mounted onto a microinjector containing a 500-nL internal sample loop (Valco Instruments, Houston, TX).

3. Flow from the solvent delivery pump is split before it reaches the column in order to generate a flow rate of approximately 4 μL/min.

4. The gradient starts at 5% ACN, is ramped to 60% ACN in 25 min and finally ramped to 90% in another 5 min. Both solvents A (water) and B (ACN) contain 0.3% formic acid.

5. The separated peptides are detected by an ESI-TOF spectrometer (LCT premier, Micromass/Waters, Milford, MA). The following parameters are typically used: capillary voltage for electrospray at 3,200 V; sample cone at 45 V; desolvation temperature at 200°C; source temperature at 100°C; and the desolvation gas flow at 250 L/h.

6. The data are acquired in "V" mode and the TOF is externally calibrated using a Sodium Iodide and Cesium Iodide mixture.

7. The instrument is controlled by MassLynx 4.0 software. The experimental masses are matched with theoretical glycopeptide masses of target glycoproteins using GlyMod tool (http://www.expasy.ch/tools/glycomod/).

4. Notes

All solutions that require water should use MilliQ water with 18-MΩ resistance or DNA/RNAse-free water.

All buffers and solutions should be prepared fresh and should not be used for more than 1 week to ensure that they are clean. If solutions are stored then keep them away from light to prevent any growth of contaminants.

It is recommended to sonicate all solutions prior to use to ensure that air is eliminated. This minimizes air bubble problems during separations and also reduces streaking when probing slides and membranes.

1. Lipid layer will be viscous. Use a Pasteur pipette to remove layer carefully to prevent sample loss.

2. The immunodepletion column depletes the serum/plasma sample of the 12 most abundant proteins: albumin, IgG, α1-antitrypsin, IgA, IgM, transferrin, haptoglobin, α1-acid glycoprotein, α2-macroglobin, apolipoprotein A-I, apolipoprotein A-II, and fibrinogen so that they do not mask signal from lower-abundance proteins.

3. After depletion the column resin needs to be regenerated and stored appropriately. Detailed instructions about regeneration and storage can be found in the SOP manual of the kit. Essentially the column is first neutralized with neutralization buffer and then equilibrated in 1× dilution buffer containing 0.02% sodium azide and stored at 2–8°C in a refrigerator. Do not freeze this column. The Proteome Lab IgY-12 columns for different sample capacity (20 μL, 50 μL, 250 μL) are also available from Beckman–Coulter.

4. After enrichment a protein assay should be done to determine the protein content after depletion.

5a. Depending on the number of slides being processed it is a good idea to use a slide rack during the washing step. This will reduce the amount of time needed in transferring slides between solutions.

5b. Scanning immediately after hybridization ensures maximum signal. However if scanning will be accomplished later all slides should be stored in a clean, dark, and cool place to prevent photobleaching and increased background signal.

6. Make sure no air bubbles are introduced when loading gel lanes; otherwise, sample will disperse and overflow into other lanes contaminating sample.

7. Handle PVDF membrane with tongs and clean gloves in order to prevent introduction of contaminants onto membrane.

8. If exposure to ECL mixture is too long it may result in excessive background. This problem can be solved by allowing the membrane to chemiluminesce over time to reduce signal from background before exposing film to membrane, washing membrane for more time to lower background signal, or stripping all probing buffers off the membrane and rehybridizing it with all solutions.

9. Make sure that the pH of the digestion buffer is ~7.8 as adding DTT can lower pH slightly.

10. Gradient can be modified to ensure best separation depending on the sample of proteins being separated.

11. The capillary temperature should be optimized to ensure the best signal. The spray voltage needs to be increased when the spray tip is used over a longer time in order to

ensure a stable spray. It is also a good idea to enable dynamic exclusion in the run method as it will ensure maximum peptide coverage.

12. Tolerances should be used cautiously as they depend on the nature of the instrument that was used to acquire spectra. For example, peptide tolerance can be lower if a time-of-flight (TOF) instrument is used.

Acknowledgement

This work was supported by the National Institutions of Health under grants RO16M49500 and RO1CA106402.

References

1. Duggan, D.J., Bittner, M., Chen, Y., Meltzer, P., Trent, J.M., *Expression profiling using cDNA microarrays. Nat Genet*, 1999. 21(1 Suppl): p. 10–4.

2. Quackenbush, J., *Microarray analysis and tumor classification. N Engl J Med*, 2006. 354(23): p. 2463–72.

3. Hoheisel, J.D., *Microarray technology: beyond transcript profiling and genotype analysis. Nat Rev Genet*, 2006. 7(3): p. 200–10.

4. Anderson, L., Seilhamer, J., *A comparison of selected mRNA and protein abundances in human liver. Electrophoresis*, 1997. 18(3–4): p. 533–7.

5. Gygi, S.P., Rochon, Y., Franza, B.R., Aebersold, R., *Correlation between protein and mRNA abundance in yeast. Mol Cell Biol*, 1999. 19(3): p. 1720–30.

6. Chen, G., Gharib, T.G., Huang, C.C., Taylor, J.M., Misek, D.E., Kardia, S.L., Giordano, T.J., Iannettoni, M.D., Orringer, M.B., Hanash, S.M., Beer, D.G., *Discordant protein and mRNA expression in lung adenocarcinomas. Mol Cell Proteomic*, 2002. 1(4): p. 304–13.

Chapter 7

Reverse-Phase Protein Microarrays for Theranostics and Patient Tailored Therapy

Virginia Espina, Lance A. Liotta, and Emanuel F. Petricoin III

Summary

Analysis of the genome provides important information about the somatic genetic changes existing in the tissue; however, it is the proteins that do the work of the cell. Diseases such as cancer are caused by derangements in cellular protein molecular networks and cell signaling pathways. These pathways contain a large and growing collection drug targets, governing cellular survival, proliferation, invasion, and cell death. The clinical utility of reverse-phase protein microarrays (RPPA), a new technology invented in our laboratory, lies in its ability to generate a functional map of known cell signaling networks or pathways for an individual patient obtained directly from a biopsy specimen. Coupled with laser capture microdissection (LCM), the RPPA platform, the entire cellular proteome is immobilized on a substratum with subsequent immunodetection of the total levels and phosphorylated, or activated, state of cell signaling proteins. The results of which pathways are "in use" can then be correlated with biological and clinical information and serve as both a diagnostic and a therapeutic guide, thus providing a "theranostic" endpoint.

Key words: Cancer, Laser capture microdissection, Microarray, Molecular profiling, Protein, Proteomics, Tissue heterogeneity, Theranostics.

1. Introduction

Protein microarrays usually comprise immobilized protein spots on a solid surface substratum, which provides for the effective multiplexed analysis of many analytes at one time *(1–6)*. The individual protein spots may be heterogeneous or homogeneous in nature, and may consist of whole cell lysates, or phage lysates, an antibody, a nucleic acid, body fluid, drug or recombinant protein *(2, 3, 5–13)*. These immobilized bait molecules are detected

Michael A. Tainsky, *Methods in Molecular Biology, Tumor Biomarker Discovery, Vol. 520*
© Humana Press, a part of Springer Science + Business Media, LLC 2009
DOI: 10.1007/978-1-60327-811-9_7

using a signal-generating molecule such as a tagged antibody or a labeled ligand. The image can be generated from any number of colorimetric, flourimetric, radiometric, electrical, or evanescent means. If the analyte detection molecule is specific, the signal intensity of each spot is proportional to the quantity of applied tagged molecules bound to the bait molecule. The image is captured, analyzed, and correlated with biological information.

The focus of this topic is on reverse-phase protein microarrays (RPPA), a method that is different from forward-phase arrays, such as antibody microarrays (**Fig. 1**). Unlike a forward-phase approach, with the RPPA microarray format, what is immobilized is a cellular lysate, serum, or complex protein mixture, which is then queried with primary antibody against a specific analyte. Signal amplification is performed using highly sensitive third-generation tyramide amplification/precipitation chemistries (14–17).

Protein microarrays have broad applications for discovery and quantitative analysis, with applications in drug discovery, biomarker identification, and molecular profiling of cellular material. The overall utility of the RPPA lies in the ability to provide a portrait of the ongoing state of multiple in vivo kinase-driven signaling networks from a tissue biopsy, and to provide crucial information about protein posttranslational modifications, such as the phosphorylation states of these proteins (18–20). These analyses ultimately reflect the functional "activation" state of

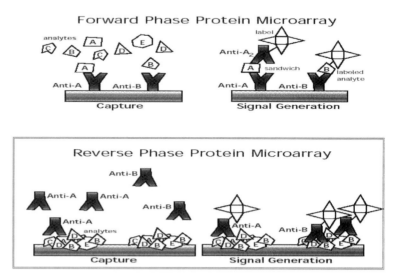

Fig. 1. Forward (*top*)- and Reverse (*bottom*)-phase protein microarrays. With the reverse-phase format, the printed zones comprise the analyte itself, usually in the form of a whole cell lysate or body fluid. An important attribute of the reverse-phase array is the requirement for only one antibody instead of a sandwich assay, which greatly expands the number of analytes that can be measured at one time.

cell signaling pathways and networks, which cannot be measured by gene expression microarrays. Indeed, "gene networks" is a misnomer since genes do not form functional networks per se – it is the proteins that form the networks. Identification of critical signaling disruptions within these networks can be a critical starting point for the discovery and use of diagnostic biomarkers that are also the therapeutic targets themselves: the beginning steps toward individualized therapy *(18, 21–23)* and theranostic applications. Characterization and analysis of protein cell signaling pathways in tissue serve two critical purposes: (1) stratifying patients for therapy and (2) discovery of predictive and prognostic markers for clinical implementation. The methods described encompass (1) preparation of a whole cell lysate from either cell culture or tissue samples, (2) protein lysate microarray printing, (3) immunostaining, and (4) microarray spot analysis.

2. Materials

2.1. Cellular Lysates

1. Cell culture, human or animal tissue sample. Satisfactory tissue samples for protein analysis are (1) frozen tissue sections, (2) ethanol-fixed, paraffin-embedded tissue, (3) formalin-fixed paraffin-embedded (FFPE) tissue, or laser capture microdissected (LCM) cell populations from the aforementioned tissues (*see* **Note 1**).

2. Microdissected samples on LCM caps with Safe-Lock Eppendorf Tubes, 0.5 mL (Brinkmann, Westbury, NY; catalog #22 36 361-1) or MicroAmp™ 500 mL Thin-walled Reaction Tubes (Perkin-Elmer Applied Biosystems, Foster City, CA; catalog #N801-0611).

3. Cell lysis buffer:

   T-PER™ (Tissue Protein Extraction Reagent, Pierce, Rockford, IL)
   2× Tris–glycine SDS loading buffer (Invitrogen, Carlsbad, CA)
   2-Mercaptoethanol (Sigma Aldrich, St. Louis, MO)
   5 M NaCl (300 mM final conc.).

4. Protease inhibitors for cell culture samples:

   200 mM PEFABLOC (AEBSF 4-(2-aminoethyl)-benzenesulfonyl fluoride hydrochloride) (Roche Applied Science, Indianapolis, IN; catalog #1 585 916)
   1 mg/mL Aprotinin (5 µg/mL final conc.), Roche #1583794

5 mg/mL Pepstatin A (5 µg/mL final conc.), Roche #1524488

5 mg/mL Leupeptin (5 µg/mL final conc.), Roche #1529048

5. Protease inhibitors for tissue samples:

Protease Inhibitor Cocktail (catalog #P2714 Sigma Aldrich, St. Louis, MO). Use 10 µL of protease inhibitor cocktail/mL of lysis buffer.

6. Phosphatase inhibitors:

1 mM orthovanadate (Sigma Aldrich) – please make this fresh every time
Sodium molybdate QC to 1 mM final
Sodium fluoride QC to 1 mM final
B-glycerophosphate QC to 75 mM final.

2.2. Printing Reverse-Phase Protein Microarrays

1. Nitrocellulose-coated glass slides (FAST slides, Whatman Schleicher & Schuell Biosciences, Keene, NH).

2. Microarray printing device (Aushon Biosystems 2470 Protein Arrayer, Burlington, MA).

3. Cellular lysate sample (minimum volume 30 µL).

4. 96-well or 384-well polypropylene microtiter plate.

5. Purified water (Type I reagent grade water).

6. 70% Ethanol.

7. Desiccant (Drierite anhydrous calcium sulfate, W.A. Hammond Drierite Co. Xenia, OH).

8. Ziplock-style plastic bags.

2.3. Immunostaining Microarrays

2.3.1 Microarray Pretreatment and Blocking

1. Reblot™ Mild Antigen Stripping solution 10× (Chemicon, Temecula, CA) (*see* **Note 2**).

2. Phosphate-Buffered Saline (PBS) without calcium or magnesium.

3. I-Block™ Protein-Blocking Solution (Applied Biosystems, Foster City, CA).

4. Tween 20 (DakoCytomation, Carpinteria, CA).

2.3.2.. Dakocytomation Autostainer Immunostaining

Immunostaining may be performed manually if an Autostainer is not available.

1. Validated primary antibody of choice (*see* **Note 3**).

2. Biotinylated, species-specific secondary antibody.

3. DakoCytomation Autostainer (DakoCytomation, Carpinteria, CA).

4. Catalyzed Signal Amplification (CSA) kit (DakoCytomation, Carpinteria, CA).

5. Biotin-blocking system (DakoCytomation, Carpinteria, CA).

6. Antibody diluent with background reducing components (DakoCytomation, Carpinteria, CA).

7. Tris-Buffered Saline with Tween (DakoCytomation, Carpinteria, CA).

8. Liquid DAB+ (Diaminobenzidene) (DakoCytomation, Carpinteria, CA).

2.3.3. Total Protein Blot Stain for Microarrays

1. Sypro Ruby Protein Blot stain (catalog #S-11791 Invitrogen/ Molecular Probes, Carlsbad, CA).

2. Fixative solution – 7% acetic acid, 10% methanol in dH_2O. (Acetic acid, glacial catalog #V193, Mallinckrodt; Methanol, absolute catalog #17-5 Sigma Diagnostics).

3. Standard UV transilluminator or a laser scanner (FluorChem 8800, Alpha Innotech Imager, San Leandro, CA) (*see* **Note 4**).

4. Sypro Red/Texas Red filter (490-nm longpass filter) or a 600-nm bandpass filter.

2.4. Microarray Spot Analysis

1. Spot analysis software of choice. Examples are ImageQuant® (Amersham Biosciences), MicroVigene™ (Vigene Tech, Billerica, MA), or P-SCAN (Peak quantitation with Statistical Comparative Analysis (http://abs.cit.nih.gov)).

2. High-resolution flatbed scanner (Epson® Perfection Scanner series 1640, Long Beach, CA or UMAX PowerLook 1120, Dallas, TX).

3. Adobe® Photoshop software.

3. Methods

The protocols describe: (1) protein lysate preparation, (2) protein (tissue) lysate microarray printing, (3) immunostaining, and (4) spot analysis. These protocols are uniquely designed for quantitative analysis of protein phosphorylation events in cellular lysates, with the concomitant analysis of the corresponding total (phosphorylated and nonphosphorylated) protein.

3.1. Protein Lysate Preparation

1. Samples may be cell culture lysates, microdissected tissue lysates, or other cellular lysates. Prepare lysates within one week of microarray printing. Long-term storage (>6 months) of protein lysates may result in protein degradation or diminished protein yield. If needed, store protein lysates at –80°C or in the vapor phase of liquid nitrogen.

2. Prepare cell culture lysis buffer:
   Cell Culture Lysis Buffer (per mL)

   915 mL TPER™

   60 mL 5 M NaCl (300 mM final conc.)

   10 mL 100 mM orthovanadate (1 mM final conc.) (boil vanadate 10 min in H2O to solubilize), Sodium Molybdate QC to1 mM final, Sodium Floride QC to 1 mM final, and B-glycerophosphate QC to 75 mM final

   10 mL 200 mM PEFABLOC (AEBSF)

   5 mL 1 mg/mL Aprotinin (5 µg/mL final conc.)

   1 mL 5 mg/mL Pepstatin A (5 µg/mL final conc.)

   1 mL 5 mg/mL Leupeptin (5 µg/mL final conc.)

   Note: final conc. of NaCl is 450 mM because TPER™ reagent contains 150 mM NaCl.

3. Spin at approximately $900 \times g$ for 10 min in refrigerated (4°C) centrifuge and remove any excess liquid from cell pellet. If cells were stored in DMSO, wash cell pellet twice with PBS without calcium or magnesium. Wash in approximately 15 mL of PBS without calcium or magnesium, spin at approximately $900 \times g$ for 10 min. Decant supernatant and repeat wash step with an additional 15 mL of PBS without calcium or magnesium. Thoroughly decant supernatant.

4. Suspend cell pellet in appropriate volume of lysis buffer, vortex 15 s, spin briefly, and incubate on ice for 20 min. Volume of lysis buffer: 1×10^6 cells/100 µL of extraction buffer or, for lymphocytes, 1×10^6 cells/µL of extraction buffer. Spin at approximately $3,000 \times g$, for 5 min and transfer supernatant to clean tube. If the proteins of interest are phosphorylated, phosphatase inhibitors should be added to the T-PER extraction buffer solution. If T-PER alone is used for preparation of cellular lysate, for example, if a Bradford-based protein assay is desired, then NaCl should be added to the T-PER reagent qc to 300 mM.

5. Perform protein assay of choice to determine protein concentration.

6. Dilute sample with 2× Tris–glycine SDS Sample Buffer (Invitrogen) + 2.5% 2-mercaptoethanol to 2 mg/mL based on the results of the protein assay. Store lysate at –80°C if needed (*see* **Note 5**).

3.1.1. Preparation of Tissue Lysate

1. The limited volume of the total cellular material from biopsy samples makes it necessary to use a slight modification of the lysis buffer recipe as compared to the cell culture lysis buffer. The following protocol describes a method for preparing whole cell lysates from laser capture microdissected (LCM) cells. The limited biopsy sample generally precludes

the use of total protein assays prior to microarray printing. To compensate for this, one microarray slide is stained for total protein using a Sypro Ruby Protein blot stain (*see* **Subheading 3.3.3**).

2. Prepare extraction buffer. Prepare a 4% solution of 2-mercaptoethanol (BME) using the 2× Tris–Glycine SDS Sample Buffer. For example: Add 40 μL of BME to 960 μL of SDS sample buffer. Using this 4% BME–SDS buffer, prepare a 1:1 solution of T-PER by adding equal parts of both. Example: Add 1 mL of BME–SDS buffer solution to 1 mL of TPER.

3. Pipette the desired quantity of the final extraction buffer onto the bottom of a clean 500-μl Eppendorf tube. Note: If the buffer is placed on or near the lip of the tube, wicking and loss of the sample will possibly take place during incubation of the samples.

4. Place the CapSure Transfer Film cap containing cells captured by LCM securely onto the tube. Invert and, using a slinging motion, deposit the buffer onto the surface of the cap. Vortex. Place the inverted tube with the extraction buffer resting on the surface of the cap into a 70°C ± 5 oven for 30 min to 2 h. At the end of the incubation, vortex the inverted tube again, and repeat **step 4** one more time. Place the tube into a microcentrifuge and spin the sample to the bottom of the tube. Remove supernatant to a clean, labeled Eppendorf tube if cell debris is present at the bottom of the tube. Discard the LCM cap and cap with the top of the Eppendorf. Store the lysate at –20°C until time to run the downstream assay.

5. It is not necessary to extract proteins immediately after microdissection. The caps of microdissected cells can be stored on a clean Eppendorf tube at –80°C until all samples have been collected.

6. Protease and phosphatase inhibitors should be added to the H&E-staining baths for tissue processing prior to LCM.

7. As a rule of thumb, use 15 μL of lysis buffer to solubilize 15,000 cells for microdissected tissue. More than one LCM cap may be used with a given volume of lysis buffer to concentrate the amount of protein in a given volume of lysis buffer (*see* **Note 6**).

8. Pipette the desired volume of lysis buffer in the bottom of the 0.5-mL microcentrifuge tube. Take care to avoid leaving droplets of lysis buffer near the lip of the tube. Place the LCM cap snugly on the tube. Invert the tube and mix well. Do not vortex. Place the tube, cap side down, in an oven or heat block at 70 ± 2°C for 15 min. Mix well after 15 min. Place back in oven for an additional 15 min. Mix well again. Spin tube at approximately 3,000 × g for 1–2 min. Remove and discard LCM cap (*see* **Note 7**). Transfer extracted protein

sample to a clean, labeled screw cap tube. Boil samples for 5–10 min before storing/printing microarrays. Store at –80°C if necessary.

3.2. Protein Tissue Lysate Microarray Printing

1. Each microarray comprises multiple samples, printed in dilution curves (usually a series of serial 1:2 dilutions), on a single slide. This format allows the comparison of multiple samples across an array for a given antibody (**Fig. 2**). Additionally, the dilution curve allows each antibody affinity to be matched with its optimal sample concentration and ensures that every analyte is analyzed and compared in its linear dynamic range. Nitrocellulose cannot be effectively stripped and reprobed; therefore, each slide is probed with a different antibody, generating a set of microarray slides for each set of antibody probes.

2. Quality control and comparison of microarrays across platforms and time require the use of control lysates and calibrators that are printed on each array (**Fig. 2**). These samples may be test

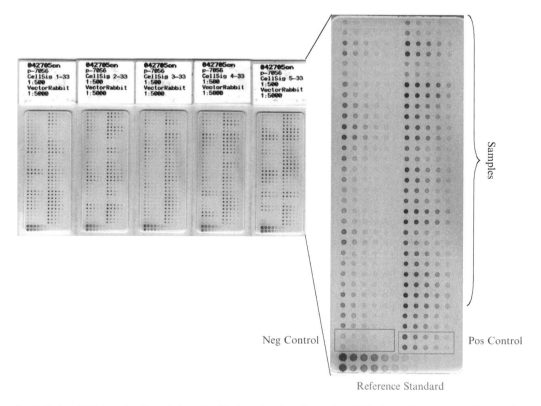

Fig. 2. Typical RPPA layout with controls and calibrators. A series of experimental test samples are arrayed in a series of five 1:2 dilutions (from *left* to *right*). Each sample is printed in duplicate, and the last spot in each series is a buffer alone control. On the bottom of every slide, a positive and negative control is printed as well as a reference standard calibrator.

samples, commercial cell lysates, peptides, phosphorylated peptide, or peptide mixtures. Ideally, the control lysate should contain the proteins(s) of interest that are being investigated in the test samples in a limited series of overall concentrations. For example, a series of controls could be an analyte at three predetermined concentrations of low, medium, and high levels. Control samples should be diluted in the same manner as the test samples, and the same control lysate should be printed on each array. Calibrators, such as a phosphopeptide, are arranged in a longer dilution curve such that the dynamic range of the assay is represented within the curve, providing a facile means of determining the level of any analyte in any experimental sample on the slide. The controls and calibrators allow for effective bridging of a given analyte across time and arrays and to calibrate the assay.

3. A minimum volume of 30 μL of lysate is required for printing microarrays in a dilution format from a 384-well microtiter plate. 15 μL of neat sample is used to prepare serial 1:2 dilutions of the lysate. An additional 15 μL of lysate is required for the neat sample. A minimum volume of 50μL of lysate is required for printing microarrays in a dilution format from a 96-well plate (25 μL of lysate to prepare the dilutions and 25 μL for the neat lysate).

4. Prepare additional lysis buffer for diluting the samples in a microtiter plate: 50 μL 2-mercaptoethanol, 950 μL 2× Tris–glycine SDS loading buffer, and 1 mL TPER™. Mix well. Prepare daily. Store at room temp. It is not necessary to add additional protease or phosphatase inhibitors.

5. Boil whole cell lysate: place screw cap tube containing the thawed lysate sample in a boiling water bath or heat block at 100°C for 5 min. Remove tubes from heat and allow tubes to cool to room temp. Spin briefly in a microcentrifuge.

6. Dilute samples to be printed on the array in appropriate dilutions in a microtiter plate. Typical dilutions are 1:2 serial dilutions with the final dilution lysis buffer only (neat, 1:2, 1:4, 1:8, 1:16, buffer only). The buffer only serves as a negative control spot (**Fig. 2**).

7. Set up the Aushon 2470 arrayer:

   (a) Select microtiter plate –96 well or 384 well.

   (b) Select number of microtiter plates.

   (c) Select number of hits per spot. Five hits/spot is recommended with a 384-well plate. Ten hits/spot is recommended with a 96-well plate (*see* **Note 8 and 9**).

   (d) Position nitrocellulose slides on printing platen. Load microtiter plate. Turn on humidifier if desired to achieve 30–70% humidity.

(e) Program appropriate dot spacing based on number of samples, replicate spots, and size of nitrocellulose pad (*see* **Note 10**).

(f) Print microarrays. Store printed slides in a slide box, inside a ziplock-style plastic bag. Add desiccant to the plastic bag prior to freezing. Store printed microarrays at –20°C.

3.3. Immunostaining

3.3.1. Microarray Slide Pretreatment and Blocking

1. Comparison of multiple phosphoproteomic endpoints for a group of samples on the array permits evaluation of the interconnected cell signaling proteins in the sample populations. Each microarray is probed with a single primary antibody directed against the protein of interest. Microarray slides used for immunostaining should be blocked prior to staining. Microarray slides used for Sypro Ruby protein staining *do not* require blocking, and *should not* be blocked.

2. Remove microarray slide(s) from freezer, and leave at room temperature for approximately 5–10 min. Prepare a 1× solution of Reblot™ mild solution in deionized water. Wash microarray slides with gentle rocking in 1× Reblot™ mild solution for 15 min. (*see* **Note 11**). Discard Reblot™ solution. Wash slides in PBS without calcium or magnesium twice, for 5 min each.

3. Block slides in I-block™ solution for a minimum of one hour at room temperature (*see* **Note 12**). Preparation of I-block™:Pour 500 mL of 1× PBS without calcium and magnesium into a 1,000-mL beaker and add a magnetic stir bar. Add 1 g of I-Block™ powder. Place beaker on hot plate with magnetic stirrer. Heat gently with stirring until solution becomes clearer (approximately 5–15 min). Do not boil. Allow I-Block™ solution to cool to room temp. Add 500 μL of Tween20. Store at 2–4°C for up to 7 days.

3.3.2. Microarray Immunostaining

1. Immunostaining requires the use of control slides for determining background staining due to secondary antibody alone. Each species-specific secondary antibody should be used to stain an individual microarray. Therefore, for any immunostaining run, one slide must be used as a negative (secondary antibody alone) control slide. The total number of slides to be stained is determined by the number and species of primary antibodies. For example, if three antirabbit primary antibodies and one mouse primary antibody are selected, a total of 6 microarray slides will be needed (4 antibodies + 2 controls).

2. Select primary antibodies of choice.

3. Select species-specific, biotinylated secondary antibodies.

4. Prepare CSA reagents following manufacturer's directions (*see* **Note 13**).

5. Prepare 1× TBST buffer per manufacturer's directions. Fill water reservoir with deionized water. Empty waste container if appropriate.

6. Load reagents and microarray slides on the Autostainer (*see* **Note 14**). Prime water. Prime buffer. Start run. Remove slides promptly at end of Autostainer run. Do not allow the Autostainer to add TBST to the slides after staining is complete (*see* **Note 15**). Allow slides to air dry away from direct light. Covering the slides lightly with a paper towel is adequate to reduce exposure to direct light. Label slides as to which antibody was used for immunostaining. Scan slides and store the stained slides in the dark at room temp.

3.3.3. Sypro Ruby Total Protein Staining of Microarray

1. The limited sample material from microdissected biopsy lysates precludes the use of spectrophotometric analysis of total protein prior to microarray printing. A microarray slide stained for total protein serves as a tool for normalizing spot intensity between samples (*see* **Note 16**).

2. Remove microarray slide(s) from freezer, and leave at room temperature for approximately 5–10 min (*see* **Note 17**).

3. Prepare fixative solution: 5.0 mL methanol, 3.5 mL acetic acid, and 41.5 mL dH$_2$O (final concentrations: 10% Methanol, 7% Acetic Acid). Mix well and store tightly sealed. Wash slide in dH$_2$O 2× for 5 min each with continuous agitation or rocking.

4. Fix slides by immersing in fixative solution (volume sufficient to cover slides) for 15 min. Place on orbital shaker or rocker. Wash in dH$_2$O 4× for 5 min each with continuous agitation or rocking. Immerse slides in Sypro Ruby Red stain (volume sufficient to cover slides) for 30 min at room temperature, in the dark. Cover container with aluminum foil to prevent photobleaching of the stain. Place on orbital shaker or rocker. Wash in dH$_2$O 4× for 1 min each, in the dark, with continuous agitation or rocking. Air dry slides at room temperature in the dark. Scan slides with a standard UV transilluminator or a laser scanner. Refer to http://probes.invitrogen.com/media/pis/x11791.pdf for a list of compatible scanning platforms.

3.4. Scanning and Data Analysis

1. The chromogenic detection system described allows the microarrays to be scanned on any high-resolution scanner (1,200 dpi) with software capable of a 14- or 16-bit scanning option for grayscale. Electronic images may be imported into a variety of spot analysis software programs, such as PSCAN (http://abs.cit.nih.gov), MicroVigene™ (Vigene Tech), or ImageQuant® (Amersham Biosciences).

2. Each array is scanned, regional and local background subtracted, the spot intensity analyzed, data are normalized to

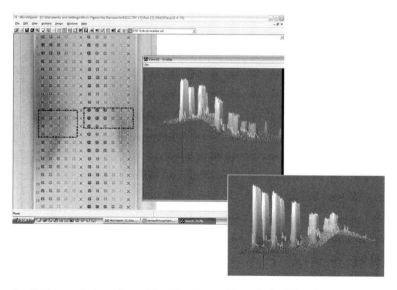

Fig. 3. Data analysis performed by MicroVigene (VigeneTech, MA) software program. Spot finding, regional and local background subtraction, and linear dynamic range finding are performed by the software program. Combined with the calibrator, this method provides for a reproducible and quantifiable value for every sample (*See Color Plates*).

total protein, and a standardized, single data value is generated for each microarray sample (**Fig. 3**). The data may be used to generate histograms, dendograms based on hierarchical clustering algorithms or Bayesian clustering analysis for generation of cell signaling network profiles.

3.4.1 Scanner Settings

(a) Place the microarray slides on the scanner.

(b) Scan at 600–1,200 dpi. Convert the image to grayscale. Save image as a 14- or 16-bit grayscale image.

(c) Save the image as a tiff file, compatible with the spot analysis software.

4. Notes

1. Analysis of protein from formalin-fixed tissues can be done using commercially available lysing solutions (e.g., Proteo SOL™ Tissue Extraction System, KPL Laboratories, Inc) or using three consecutive treatments of the LCM material with boiling TPER/SDS extraction buffer for 5 min each using 10–15 µL of lysate each time. Pool the lysates. Protein yield will be less than that from frozen tissue: approximately 40–50% as much. Extraction of high yield, quality protein from formalin-fixed tissue is generally difficult due to

the extensive crosslinks formed in formalin-fixed samples. Currently, the optimal tissue specimen for use with protein lysate microarrays is fresh tissue, immediately embedded in a cyroprotectant solution and frozen or snap frozen tissue.

2. Reblot™ solution is manufactured in two strengths: mild and strong. It is imperative that the mild solution be used with nitrocellulose-coated slides. The Reblot™ strong solution may cause the nitrocellulose to detach from the glass slide.

3. The primary antibody should be validated by Western Blot prior to use on a microarray. A validated antibody should show a single band at the specified molecular weight. Primary antibodies should be unconjugated and may be any species, with the only caveat being the biotinylated secondary antibody should be species matched with the primary antibody. Primary and secondary antibody concentration should be optimized for use on a microarray prior to use with patient samples. Typically primary antibody dilutions of 1:250, 1:500, and 1:1,000 are used to immunostain a set of microarrays. The secondary antibody concentration is held constant. Comparison of signal-to-noise ratio is used to determine the optimal concentration to use on the microarray. Secondary antibodies are optimized in a similar manner. A set of microarrays is immunostained with secondary antibody alone at a variety of concentrations and antibody diluent is used as the primary antibody. In general, the secondary antibody dilution that shows minimal staining is the optimal dilution. Verification of the optimal secondary antibody concentration may be performed by staining a microarray with an optimized primary antibody and the secondary antibody dilution of choice and accessing the signal to noise ratio.

4. Sypro Ruby blot stain is a ruthenium complex, exhibiting luminescence upon excitation with either UV-B or blue light. The luminescence may be visualized with UV epi-illumination sources, UV or blue-light transilluminators, or laser scanning instruments with excitation light at 450, 473, 488, or 532 nm. The emission peak of the ruthenium complex is approximately 618 nm *(24)*.

5. The binding capacity of the nitrocellulose is 9 µg/mm^3 with a 0.2-µm pore membrane *(25)*. Samples with protein concentrations greater than 2 mg/mL may saturate the nitrocellulose with concomitant loss of the dilution series in the printed diluted spots.

6. A common issue with microdissected tissue is minimal cell number on any given LCM cap. To effectively increase the cell number and protein concentration for a volume of lysis

buffer, it may be necessary to solubilize 2–3 LCM caps in one volume of lysis buffer. This is done by sequentially solubilizing the cells on LCM caps in the same volume of lysis buffer. To illustrate the process, one LCM cap is solubilized in lysis buffer. This first cap is discarded and a fresh LCM cap containing microdissected material is placed on a tube containing the lysis buffer used previously to solubilize the first LCM cap. The cells on this second cap are solubilized in the lysis buffer, effectively increasing the protein concentration in a given volume of buffer.

7. After solubilizing cells from an LCM cap, the efficiency of extraction may be determined by examining the cap surface with the aid of a microscope. Place the cap, polymer side down, on a clean glass microscope slide. Observe the surface of the polymer with a standard light microscope. Cellular material should not be visible on the polymer surface. If cells are still present, place the cap on the tube containing lysis buffer and continue heating the cap at 70°C for an additional 15 min. Repeat the process until the cells are solubilized.

8. Dot spacing on the microarray is a critical factor for ensuring successful spot intensity analysis. Careful planning of the array configuration prior to printing is essential. Spots placed too closely prevent discrimination of background areas from spot area with most spot analysis software programs. The 384-well format results in 12 horizontal spots, in two dilution curves for two different samples.

9. The Aushon arrayer can effectively print multiple aliquots on the same spot, effectively increasing the protein concentration/spot. Printing 5–10 hits/spot maximizes the protein binding capacity of nitrocellulose without saturating the nitrocellulose. The recommendation to print 10 hits/spot from a 96-well plate and 5 hits from a 384-well plate is based on dot-spacing restrictions in the x and y-axes from the different microtiter plate formats.

10. Typical microarrays with human samples are printed in triplicate for quality control and statistical analysis. Dot spacing is a function of pin diameter – dot spacing must be a minimum of 1.5× the pin diameter. FAST™ slides are manufactured in a variety of formats, with a 20 × 50 mm nitrocellulose pad being compatible with reverse-phase microarray format and the DakoCytomation Autostainer.

11. Wash time is critical with the Reblot™ mild solution. Extended wash times may cause the nitrocellulose to detach from the glass.

12. Microarrays may be blocked overnight at 4°C. The minimum blocking time is one hour.

13. The Autostainer grid layout is a modification of the CSA grid provided by the manufacturer. Additional TBST rinse steps have been added to ensure adequate rinsing of the microarray slides. 450 μL of reagent is added to the slide in each of the three drop zones.

14. Do not let the microarray slides dry while loading and prior to starting the Autostainer run. If necessary, pour I-block or 1× TBST on the slides. If the ambient humidity is low, a shallow tray of water may be placed inside the Autostainer during the staining run. Operate the Autostainer with the lid closed.

15. The DakoCytomation Autostainer is designed primarily for immunohistochemistry. In these procedures, the slides are kept moist with periodic rinses of TBST. The high salt content causes crystal formation on the nitrocellulose if the TBST is allowed to dry on the microarray slide. If crystal formation inadvertently happens, it may be possible to dissolve the crystals by washing the microarrays with PBS + 0.2% Tween20 for 1 h and then washing with PBS only. A final rinse in water is usually sufficient to remove the crystals. Additionally, the Autostainer may be programmed to include a final water step. Adding an "auxiliary" reagent step to the end of the program allows the Autostainer to run in an "overnight" mode. This auxiliary reagent is deionized water and the time is 840 min (14 h). The microarray slides will be rinsed with water following the DAB detection step. The Autostainer will remain in idle, waiting to dispense water in 840 min, allowing the operator to return in 14 h.

16. Syrpo Ruby staining is a permanent protein stain, detected by fluorescence with an excitation wavelength of 300 or 480 nm and an emission wavelength of 618 nm. The stain is photostable, allowing long emission lifetime and the ability to measure fluorescence over a longer time frame, minimizing background fluorescence.

17. Do not block (with I-block) the microarray slide used for total protein staining. Due to slight changes in the protein concentration per spot from the first slide printed to the last slide printed, an average protein concentration per spot for all slides printed within a run may be determined from one slide. Typically a slide representing the median slide of the printing run is selected for total protein staining. For example, if 25 slides were printed in a run, slide 13 would be selected for total protein staining.

18. Reblot™ is used to completely denature and keep denatured the protein analytes associated with the nitrocellulose substratum because the binding of the proteins to the nitrocel-

lulose, even in an SDS detergent background, can be weak, and indeed, the protein can begin to refold after spotting. The Reblot™ is used to fully denature the proteins for the reverse-phase array.

References

1. Liotta L. A., Espina V., Mehta A. I.et al., (2003) Protein microarrays: Meeting analytical challenges for clinical applications. *Cancer Cell* 3(4), 317–25.

2. Haab B. B., Dunham M. J., and Brown P. O. (2001) Protein microarrays for highly parallel detection and quantitation of specific proteins and antibodies in complex solutions. *Genome Biol* 2(2), RESEARCH0004.

3. Macbeath G. and Schreiber S. L. (2000) Printing proteins as microarrays for high-throughput function determination. *Science* 289(5485), 1760–3.

4. Macbeath G. (2002) Protein microarrays and proteomics. *Nat Genet* 32, 526–32.

5. Paweletz C. P., Charboneau L., Bichsel V. E., et al. (2001) Reverse phase protein microarrays which capture disease progression show activation of pro-survival pathways at the cancer invasion front. *Oncogene* 20(16), 1981–9.

6. Zhu H. and Snyder M. (2003) Protein chip technology. *Curr Opin Chem Biol* 7(1), 55–63.

7. Wilson D. S. and Nock S. (2003) Recent developments in protein microarray technology. *Angew Chem Int Ed Engl* 42(5), 494–500.

8. Templin M. F., Stoll D., Schrenk M.et al. (2002) Protein microarray technology. *Trends Biotechnol* 20(4), 160–6.

9. Schaeferling M., Schiller S., Paul H., et al. (2002) Application of self-assembly techniques in the design of biocompatible protein microarray surfaces. *Electrophoresis* 23(18), 3097–105.

10. Weng S., Gu K., Hammond P. W.et al.. (2002) Generating addressable protein microarrays with PROfusion covalent mRNA-protein fusion technology. *Proteomics* 2(1), 48–57.

11. Petach H. and Gold L. (2002) Dimensionality is the issue: use of photoaptamers in protein microarrays. *Curr Opin Biotechnol* 13(309–314.

12. Lal S. P., Christopherson R. I., and Dos Remedios C. G. (2002) Antibody arrays: an embryonic but rapidly growing technology. *Drug Discov Today* 7(18 Suppl), S143–9.

13. Humphery-Smith I., Wischerhoff E., and Hashimoto R. (2002) Protein arrays for assessment of target selectivity. *Drug Discov World* 4(1), 17–27.

14. Bobrow M. N., Harris T. D., Shaughnessy K. J., and Litt G. J. (1989) Catalyzed reporter deposition, a novel method of signal amplification. Application to immunoassays. *J Immunol Methods* 125(1–2), 279–85.

15. Bobrow M. N., Shaughnessy K. J., and Litt G. J. (1991) Catalyzed reporter deposition, a novel method of signal amplification. II. Application to membrane immunoassays. *J Immunol Methods* 137(1), 103–12.

16. Hunyady B., Krempels K., Harta G., and Mezey E. (1996) Immunohistochemical signal amplification by catalyzed reporter deposition and its application in double immunostaining. *J Histochem Cytochem* 44(12), 1353–62.

17. King G., Payne S., Walker F., and Murray G. I. (1997) A highly sensitive detection method for immunohistochemistry using biotinylated tyramine. *J Pathol* 183(2), 237–41.

18. Petricoin E., Wulfkuhle J., Espina V., and Liotta L. A. (2004) Clinical proteomics: revolutionizing disease detection and patient tailoring therapy. *J Proteome Res* 3(2), 209–17.

19. Grubb R. L., Calvert V. S., Wulkuhle J. D., et al. (2003) Signal pathway profiling of prostate cancer using reverse phase protein arrays. *Proteomics* 3(11), 2142–6.

20. Wulfkuhle J. D., Aquino J. A., Calvert V. S., et al. (2003) Signal pathway profiling of ovarian cancer from human tissue specimens using reverse-phase protein microarrays. *Proteomics* 3(11), 2085–90.

21. Liotta L. A., Kohn E. C., and Petricoin E. F. (2001) Clinical proteomics: personalized molecular medicine. *JAMA* 286(18), 2211–4.

22. Petricoin E. F., Zoon K. C., Kohn E. C., Barrett J. C., and Liotta L. A. (2002) Clinical proteomics: translating benchside promise into bedside reality. *Nat Rev Drug Discov* 1(9), 683–95.

23. Wulfkuhle J. D., Edmiston K. H., Liotta L. A., and Petricoin E. F. (2006) Technology Insight:

pharmacoproteomics for cancer-promises of patient-tailored medicine using protein microarrays. *Nat Clin Pract Oncol* 3(5):256–68.

24. Berggren K., Steinberg T. H., Lauber W. M., et al. (1999) A luminescent ruthenium complex for ultrasensitive detection of proteins immobilized on membrane supports. *Anal Biochem* 276(2), 129–43.

25. Tonkinson J. L. and Stillman B. A. (2002) Nitrocellulose: a tried and true polymer finds utility as a post-genomic substrate. *Front Biosci* 7, c1–12.

Chapter 8

Serum Proteomics Using Mass Spectrometry

Brian L. Hood, David E. Malehorn, Thomas P. Conrads, and William L. Bigbee

Summary

The identification and eventual application of tumor markers in cancer screening, early detection, diagnosis, and prognosis is a continuing focus of significant translational cancer research. While many new candidate markers have been discovered and at least partly characterized, very few have found widespread clinical application limited presently to the use of CA-125 in ovarian cancer, CEA, primarily in colon cancer, and PSA in prostate cancer screening and patient monitoring. The rapidly emerging field of cancer genomics and proteomics, and their clinical translation as "molecular diagnosis" and "molecular medicine" are already beginning to transform the field, and the accelerating growth of information and technology in this research area will undoubtedly transform the field of tumor markers and their application in the near future leading to improved molecular tools for cancer diagnosis, prognosis, and treatment and ultimately, to the emergence of novel and more effective cancer therapies, including improved approaches for immunotherapy and cancer prevention strategies. Toward this goal, herein are described detailed methods and workflows for mass spectrometry-based biomarker discovery in serum/plasma utilizing two complementary approaches – matrix-assisted laser desorption ionization time of flight (MALDI-TOF) and nanoflow reversed-phase liquid chromatography (RPLC)-tandem mass spectrometry (MS/MS). These discovery workflows incorporate both abundant protein depletion and sample fractionation upstream of analytical mass spectrometry to optimize the identification and quantitation of lower abundant species.

Key words: Serum proteomics, MALDI-TOF-MS, Nanoflow RPLC-MS/MS, Abundant protein depletion.

1. Introduction

Cancer biomarkers are broadly defined as molecular species detectable in biological specimens that represent alterations in normal cellular and tissue function associated with the malignant process. These tumor marker molecular species, most often proteins or glycoproteins but also phospholipids, DNA and epigenomically

Michael A. Tainsky, *Methods in Molecular Biology, Tumor Biomarker Discovery, Vol. 520*
© Humana Press, a part of Springer Science+Business Media, LLC 2009
DOI: 10.1007/978-1-60327-811-9_8

altered DNA, or RNA, and low molecular weight metabolites, may be produced directly by the tumor or by the body in response to the presence of the tumor. The detection and monitoring of these genetic, epigenetic, or biochemical changes, evaluated in the tissue or interest and/or in surrogate fluid biospecimens, are potentially useful markers for a variety of clinical applications.

Tumor markers can be discovered and studied directly in tumor tissue/cells, in exfoliated or distributed tumor cells, e.g., circulating tumor cells, or, in the case of circulating soluble tumor markers, in peripheral blood plasma or serum or other surrogate biospecimens including urine, saliva, sputum, cerebrospinal fluid, and tumor ascites' fluid or effusions. Although the characteristics of an ideal tumor marker depend to some degree on the category and clinical application of the marker, the general properties of an ideal tumor marker include (1) produced specifically by premalignant or malignant tissue early in the progression of the tumor; (2) produced at detectable levels in all patients with a specific malignancy; (3) expressed in an organ site-specific manner; (4) measurable in body fluids obtained noninvasively or in easily accessible tissue; (5) level is quantitatively related to tumor volume, biological behavior, or tumor progression; (6) relatively short lived, reflecting temporal changes in tumor burden or response to therapy; and (7) a standardized, reproducible, and validated quantitative assay exists. For screening and early detection markers to be applied in large clinically asymptomatic populations additional requisite characteristics include: (1) the utilization of surrogate biological specimens that can be obtained safely and noninvasively, e.g., blood or urine; (2) application of low cost/high throughput, validated, and standardized assays; and (3) relatively high sensitivity and very high disease specificity, i.e., to yield a very low false-positive rate (FPR) and a reasonable low false-negative rate (FNR).

Since the circulating peripheral blood compartment continuously perfuses all tissues of the body, including sites of emerging tumors, this constant biochemical flux permits the release and/or active secretion of protein species into the serum resulting in a rich biological milieu for potential tumor marker discovery and clinical application. These complex serum proteomic patterns and multianalyte profiles therefore contain biological information reporting the molecular etiology of tumor initiation and progression, and therefore can be evaluated for diagnostic features applicable to the discovery and characterization of all of the categories or tumor markers described. This rich spectrum of biomarkers, reflecting complex tumor-host cell interactions sampled in serum, provide biologically complementary information which, when used together in marker panels, can potentially provide improved diagnostic accuracy over that provided by traditional single tumor markers.

2. Materials

2.1. Maldi-TOF-MS-Based Discovery

2.1.1 Reagents

1. Enchant™ Life Sciences Multi-Protein Affinity Separation Kit (Pall Corporation).

2. Glycine buffer, 250 mM, pH 3.

3. Q Ceramic ᴴʸᵖᵉʳᴰ®ᶠ Ion Exchange Sorbent (Pall Corporation).

4. Anion exchange fractionation buffers:

   (a) *U9 denaturation buffer.* 9 M urea, 2% CHAPS, 50 mM Tris–HCl, pH 9; and dilutions in PBS to 1:4 and 1:9 (i.e., U2.3 and U1 buffers).

   (b) Resin Rehydration buffer, (50 mM Tris–HCl, pH 9).

   (c) *Wash buffer 1.* 50 mM HEPES with 0.1% n-octyl β-D-glucopyranoside (OGP), pH 7.

   (d) *Wash buffer 2.* 100 mM NaAcetate with 0.1% OGP, pH 5.

   (e) *Wash buffer 3.* 100 mM NaAcetate with 0.1% OGP, pH 4.

   (f) *Wash buffer 4.* 50 mM NaCitrate with 0.1% OGP, pH 3.

   (g) *Wash buffer 5.* 33.3% isopropanol/16.7% acetonitrile/0.1% trifluoroacetic acid.

5. *Calibration standards (Bruker).* Peptide Calibration Standard II and Protein Calibration Standard I).

6. α-cyano-4-hydroxycinnamic acid (CHCA; Bio-Rad), reconstituted as half-saturated according to manufacturer's directions, in 50% MeCN with 0.1% trifluoroacetic acid (TFA; Pierce Biochemicals).

7. Sinapinic acid (SPA; Bio-Rad), reconstituted as per manufacturer's directions, in 50% MeCN/0.5% TFA.

8. HPLC-grade water (ThermoFisher Scientific).

9. Magnetic bead purification kits (Bruker Daltonics) including derivatized superparamagnetic beads (e.g., IMAC-Cu, weak cation exchange WCX, hydrophobic interaction HIC-8) as well as binding, washing, and eluting buffers.

2.1.2. Supplies, Equipment, and Instrumentation

1. Blood collection containers (Becton-Dickinson).

2. Cryovials (ThermoFisher Scientific).

3. PCR adhesive tape.

4. Aluminum block (ThermoFisher Scientific).

5. Acroprep™ filtration plate (Pall Corporation, 1-mL wells, 0.45 μ GHP).

6. Deep-well MTP (ThermoFisher Scientific).

7. Nonbinding surface 96-well microplate (Corning).

8. Microplate shaker (DPC MicroMix5).

9. Swinging bucket centrifuge, MTP adapters (Sorvall).

10. Microcon YM-3 centrifugal concentrator (Millipore).

11. Microcentrifuge.

12. Polished steel MALDI target, 384 feature (Bruker Daltonics).

13. Gold ProteinChip™ array (Bio-Rad).

14. ClinProt™ robot pipettor tips (Bruker Daltonics).

15. ClinProt™ 96-well tube plates (BioZym, Bruker Daltonics).

16. ClinProt™ 96-well skirted plate (Greiner).

17. 0.2 mL 8-tube strips.

18. Aluminum plate-sealing tape.

19. Multichannel pipettors.

2.1.3. Specialized Equipment

1. MALDI-TOF mass spectrometer (*ultraflexII* TOF/TOF, Bruker Daltonics).

2. PBSIIc ChipReader™ (Bio-Rad) with AutoLoader™.

3. ClinProt™ liquid-handling robotic workstation, and operating software.

4. Biomek2000™ liquid-handling robotic workstation, and operating software.

2.2. Nanoflow RPLC-MS/MS-Based Discovery

2.2.1. Reagents

1. Phenylmethylsulfonyl fluoride, 100 mM in 100% ethanol.

2. Ammonium bicarbonate, 50 mM, pH 8.2, and 1 M.

3. Ammonium acetate, 1 M (for SCX dilutions).

4. Dithiothreitol, 1 M.

5. Iodoacetimide, 150 mM.

6. Sequencing-Grade Modified Trypsin (Promega).

7. Acetonitrile, Optima/HPLC Grade (ThermoFisher Scientific).

8. Water, HPLC Grade (ThermoFisher Scientific).

9. Formic Acid, HPLC Grade (Sigma-Aldrich).

10. Trifluoroacetic Acid, HPLC Grade (Sigma-Aldrich).

2.2.2. Supplies, Equipment, and Instrumentation

1. Agilent MARS High Abundant Protein Depletion Spin Columns (or alternate depletion kit) (Agilent Technologies).

2. BCA Protein Assay Kit (or comparable assay reagent) (Pierce).

3. PepClean™ C-18 Spin Columns (Pierce).

2.2.3. Specialized Equipment

1. Ultimate 3000 HPLC System (or comparable) (Dionex Corporation).

2. LTQ Linear Ion-Trap Mass Spectrometer (or comparable) (ThermoFisher Scientific).

3. Methods

3.1. Maldi-TOF-MS-Based Discovery

3.1.1 Serum Denaturation

Significant attention and great care is required to assure that serum samples are not compromised by variations in their collection and storage (*see* **Note 1**).

1. Distribute 40-µL serum samples (thawed, spun) in randomized layout into low-binding microplate on ice, e.g., atop an aluminum block in an ice bath.

2. With the multichannel pipettor, add 50 µL U9 buffer to all wells, and cover plate with PCR tape.

3. Incubate the plate with shaking 30 min at 4°C on a microplate mixer. (During this step, immunodepletion resin is pretreated and equilibrated – see later).

4. Add 110 µL of MPAS kit binding/washing buffer, or a physiologically isotonic and buffered solution such as TBS or PBS.

5. Store plate on ice until the depletion resin has been pretreated and re-equilibrated as described later.

3.1.2. Serum Depletion Using MPAS Depletion Kit

Samples are processed as two parallel aliquots, and under denaturing conditions (*see* **Note 2**). A resin pretreatment step is absolutely essential (*see* **Note 3**).

1. Combine the contents of MPAS Depletion Kit resin bottles; ~20 mL total volume will contain ~6.5 mL of settled resin, which is roughly two-third α-HSA and one-third α-IgG. This will process 32 serum aliquots of 40 µL each. The following instructions can be scaled to fit any part or all of a 96-well layout, with multiple kits required for more than 32 samples.

2. Centrifuge at low speed (1 min at 500 rpm) to settle the resin. Remove and discard the supernatant fluid.

3. Add PBS to bring volume to ~13 mL and resuspend the resin mixture.

4. Ensuring adequate resuspension throughout the process, use a multichannel pipet to deliver two 200 µL aliquots to four columns of a deep-well MTP filtration plate, positioned over, and locked onto an MTP receiver plate.

5. Uncover and spin the filter/receiver plate assembly in an MTP-adapter, swinging bucket rotor (1 min at 1,000 rpm) and discard the filtrate.

6. Repeat with a second aliquot of 200 µL resin suspension per well.

7. Aliquot 200 µL of U2.3 buffer to all wells. Cover the plate, and shake on the microplate mixer 5 min at room temperature. Agitation should be sufficient to visibly resuspend the resin.

8. Uncover and spin the filter/receiver plate assembly 1 min at 1,000 rpm and discard the filtrate.

9. Aliquot 200 μL of MPAS kit binding/washing buffer to all wells. Cover the plate, and shake on the microplate mixer 5 min at room temperature.

10. The plate can wait at this stage for some time to allow completion of serum denaturation, but not indefinitely, as some wells may drain by capillarity/gravity, possibly drying the resin.

11. When ready to receive the denatured serum samples, uncover and spin the filter/receiver plate assembly 1 min at 1,000 rpm and discard the filtrate.

12. Transfer denatured, diluted serum samples into their corresponding locations in the depletion MTP filter plate. Cover the plate, and shake on a microplate mixer 15 min at room temperature.

13. Uncover and spin the filter/receiver plate assembly 1 min at 1,000 rpm; save, cover and refrigerate the receiver plate with filtrates, as these represent the "depleted samples."

14. Attach a new receiver plate to the MTP filter; add 100 μL MPAS kit "binding/washing buffer" to each well. Cover the plate, and shake on the microplate mixer 5 min at room temperature.

15. Uncover and spin the filter/receiver plate assembly 1 min at 1,000 rpm; save, cover, and refrigerate the receiver plate with filtrates, which represent the "depletion column Rinse samples," first aliquot.

16. Repeat **steps 13–15**; combine the filtrate with that of the first rinsing step; if applicable, also combine the filtrates from the two replicate processing wells of each patient sample. At this point we routinely transfer the combined filtrates (~400 μL per patient sample) to a deep-well MTP, cover, and flash freeze for storage until a later concomitant processing of all samples in ensuing steps of concentration and profiling.

17. Attach a new receiver plate to the MTP filter; add 100 μL acidic glycine solution to each well. Cover the plate, and shake on the microplate mixer 5 min at room temperature.

18. Uncover and spin the filter/receiver plate assembly 1 min at 1,000 rpm; save, cover, and refrigerate the receiver plate with filtrates, which represent the "depletion column Strip samples," first aliquot.

19. Repeat **steps 17–18**; combine the filtrate with that of the first stripping step; if applicable also combine the filtrates from the two replicate wells of each sample. Neutralize and adjust the "Strip" fractions to > 50 mM Tris, pH 8 with 1 M Tris, checking pH of representative wells by spotting on pH paper. Neutralized filtrates can be transferred to deep-well MTP for flash freezing and storage as described earlier.

20. If continuing with processing, "Rinse" and "Strip" fractions are concentrated by microcentrifugation in an ultrafiltration unit, such as Millipore Microcon-YM3. Samples are concentrated > 20–30-fold 2–3 times, with discard of the filtrate, and retentate is serially diluted with 10 mM Tris, pH 8.

21. After concentration, retentates (~30–40 µL) are transferred into a 96-well skirted MTP, which can be flash-frozen and stored pending subsequent comparative profiling by magnetic bead purification, as described later.

22. Process consistency throughout this protocol can be monitored with simple "neat spotting" and spectrometry on a low-resolution PBSIIc instrument (*see* **Note 4**). For neat-spotting check by mass spectrometry, 1 µL SPA matrix solution is mixed with 1 µL of each sample, spotted [at least in duplicate] immediately on gold ProteinChip™ target, and air dried for ~1 h.

23. High-throughput matrix mixing and target spotting can be achieved on 12-chip arrays of the gold Proteinchips using the Biomek™ liquid-handling workstation. Automated spectrometry in the PBSIIc Chipreader™ with Autoloader™ is conducted as described later.

3.1.3. Anion Exchange Fractionation

The output of the depletion process is suitable for direct input into the AE fractionation protocol, being already urea denatured and pH adjusted. Fractionation ideally is performed immediately after depletion, with no protracted storage or intervening freeze-thaw cycle.

1. Assuming processing of two 40-µL serum aliquots from a given sample, the two depletions are combined (~400 µL) and adjusted to 600 µL with U2.3 buffer. This amount becomes distributed across 4 wells, in randomized layout, containing Q Ceramic HyperD®F resin (75 µL settled volume each), which is pretreated as described later.

2. Resin is resuspended and dispensed into a 50-mL conical centrifuge tube for bulk equilibration. The resin is allowed to settle (low-speed centrifugation may be helpful) and the ethanolic storage buffer is changed for 50 mM Tris–HCl, pH 9. After 5 min mixing (rotating mixer) the resin is again settled by gravity or centrifugation.

3. Repeat the buffer change twice.

4. After the last buffer change, the resin is resuspended, and sufficient slurry to comprise 75 µL settled resin volume is dispensed into each well in the MTP filtration plate, attached firmly to a low-binding MTP receiver plate.

5. The filter/receiver plate assembly is spun 5 min at 2,000 rpm to drain; the filtrate is discarded.

6. Aliquot 150 µL of U2.3 buffer into each well, cover the filter/receiver plate assembly, and shake 5 min vigorously

(Micromix Form 18, Amplitude 7) to thoroughly resuspend the resin.

7. The filter/receiver plate assembly is uncovered and spun 5 min at 2,000 rpm to drain; the filtrate is discarded.

8. At this point the diluted serum depletions are apportioned into 4 wells (150 μL each) in appropriately randomized locations. The filter/receiver plate assembly is covered and shaken 30 min at 4°C. At regular intervals the receiver plate is checked, and if any well has drained by gravity, the filtrate is returned to the well to remix with the resin.

9. The filter/receiver plate assembly is uncovered and spun 5 min at 2,000 rpm to drain; the receiver plate containing the filtrate is detached and refrigerated.

10. Attach a new receiver plate and aliquot 100 μL of U2.3 buffer into each well, cover, and mix the filter/receiver plate briefly (1 min).

11. Uncover and recentrifuge the filter/receiver plate assembly to collect the rinse; combine with the previous plate to constitute the unbound flow-through fraction.

12. Successive steps are performed comparably: two sequential 100-μL aliquots of buffer (Buffers 1–5, pH 7/5/4/3/organic) are added at each step, with 5-min shaking at 4°C, and centrifugation to collect filtrates, which are combined at each step.

13. The product of all replicates of each sample is combined for each elution step (~800 μL) and transferred to a deep-well MTP and flash-frozen for storage, pending concentration/buffer change.

14. Fractions are concentrated by microcentrifugation (Microcon-YM3) ~20-fold, twice serially, using 10 mM Tris, pH 8, and discarding the filtrate.

15. After concentration, retentates are brought to 30 μL volume with 10 mM Tris, pH 8, and transferred into a 96-well skirted MTP, which can be flash-frozen and stored pending subsequent comparative profiling by magnetic bead purification, as described later.

16. For process monitoring or for profiling without magnetic bead purification, samples are neat spotted with SPA matrix for spectrometry as described later.

3.1.4. Magnetic Bead Purification

Magnetic bead purification is performed on a liquid-handling robotic workstation (ClinProt™ Robot, Bruker Daltonics) with preprogrammed routines configured for optimized volumes and ratios of biofluid and ClinProt™ magnetic bead suspensions. Whereas these programs were initially developed for application to whole serum, their application to depleted, fractionated serum samples still results in robust profile generation from a variety of bead affinity types for the majority of these fractions. However, relative quantitation of a specific ion's intensity between different AE fractions may not be meaningful in light of the application of variable amounts of total protein, and in different analyte admixtures, in the purification reaction.

1. Prior to performing a purification run, sample-related information may be compiled with up to seven columns of columnar data in Excel, then exported as .csv format for input into the ClinProt™ robot operational software; this should include identifiers of sample groups targeted for subsequent classification model development. This information remains associated with samples processed in the system and is ultimately evinced in the structure of data files created during mass spectrometry.

2. Software directs the creation of a session-specific "method" file through selection of a preconfigured purification routine, based on magnetic bead type, and ratio of beads to sample volume, as well as (if desired) the number of matrix types and spotting replicates to be performed contemporaneously with purification.

3. The method file is automatically associated with the file name and location for the spectra to be created, as well as the AutoXecute method to be applied during ensuing spectrometry. This information is tracked in the system through the MALDI target unique identifier.

4. Activate the "Identify Plate" command to launch a new status window visualization, which provides graphical depiction of the work deck, as well as the current usage status for certain consumables positions. Reset current usage values for "workplate" and disposables (tips) if necessary.

5. The reagent rack illustration automatically calculates required volumes and positions of solutions (e.g., bead suspension, binding buffer, washing buffer, elution, and stabilization solutions) to provide for the method chosen and for the number of samples to process. Place adhesive aluminum foil over these containers (8-tube strips, or reservoirs) and securely attach the rack cover.

6. If performing target spotting coordinately with purification, install a cleaned target into the appropriate position on the work deck

7. Validate command sequence with "Checkmark" command to initiate a preview of the method; the "Undo" command must be selected in order to activate the "Start Processing" option

8. MTP plates with depleted/fractionated samples are typically introduced into the robot just prior to their use in the routine (pausing the robot), after which they are returned to refrigerated storage.

9. Occasional monitoring during processing runs is advisable to guard against jams (*see* **Note 5**).

10. For larger profiling projects, we terminate purification prior to target spotting in order to accrue purifications from multiple runs and perform contemporaneous matrix spotting. In this case the purification routine terminates with elution, and the workplate is transferred out of the robot into a magnetic separation plate. The eluates are carefully decanted and transferred to a fresh MTP for flash freezing and storage prior to matrix spotting.

3.1.5. Matrix Spotting and MALDI-TOF-MS

There is considerable flexibility of options, but also need for optimization in establishing conditions for spectrometry (*see* **Note 6**)

1. Clean MALDI targets thoroughly including rinses with matrix solvent (50% MeCN/0.25% TFA), sonication in 50% methanol bath, and rinses with acetone and ethanol. Attach target to a target frame adaptor and place onto the left rear of robot work deck.

2. Create a date- and target-specific method, and import sample-related annotation, as described earlier.

3. Select a pre-existing or customized "Targetprep" method for the performance of sample mixing with matrix, and target spotting.

4. Provide a 96-well skirted microplate, or "Matrix Plate" at the indicated position on the work deck. Provide the required volume of matrix solution (CHCA, half-saturated in 50% MeCN/0.25% TFA) as indicated, in the proper location in the reagent rack, covered with adhesive foil tape.

5. Validate command sequence with "Checkmark" command to initiate a preview of the method; the "Undo" command must be selected in order to activate the "Start Processing" option.

6. Visual observation during target preparation is advisable to assure effective mixture and consistent deposition, especially when small volumes are used to conserve samples. It may be necessary to adjust target placement, or to use "Reteaching" modules in the software, to ensure optimal alignment of deposited droplets within the center of the target features.

7. Peptide and/or protein calibrant mixtures can be added manually to interstitial locations within sentinel grid locations (e.g., at the corners and center of the target). The use of a single external calibration applied to all spectra of a larger experiment has been recommended as the most useful starting point for subsequent spectral alignment *(1)*.

8. The locations of deposited spots, as well as the imported sample annotation information, are embedded in the "AutoXecute" xml file which is created by the software and deposited in the

"AutoXecute Sequences" folder of the mass spectro-meter computer.

9. Mass spectrometry is being performed on the Bruker *ultraflex*II ToF instrument in linear mode, with gridless ion optics, using pulsed ion extraction of 120 ns, IS2 voltage 23.5 kV, lens 6 kV, matrix suppression by gating up to 800 Da, linear detector 1,650 V, mass range to 23 kDa, 1 GS/s sampling, 100 mV electronic gain. No high-energy prewarming shots are employed, given the relatively thin sample application over a larger area (relative to that achieved by Bruker AnchorChip™ targets).

10. Spectra collection is performed using the "AutoXMethod" with constant laser power (nominally 118 µJ, attenuated to roughly 30%) without the application of "Fuzzy" controller, which is a feature by which transients with insufficient intensity are rejected, and laser power increased.

11. Automated spectrometry conditions are designed to collect from a substantial number of locations (50 shots at 25 Hz, at 30 locations) within a feature to minimize any impact of surface irregularity or "sweet spots." Geometry of the raster is a small spiral beginning at the center of the feature, to avoid collection near the sometimes-irregular edges of dried droplets; target-specific teaching can be employed to ensure accurate alignment at the center of features.

12. For process monitoring and profiling by high mass range spectrometry on the PBSIIc instrument, samples are spotted with SPA matrix solution and spotted on gold ProteinChips. These are interrogated by an automated spot protocol which collects 192 transients from 16 different positions across the width of the feature, operating at relatively high laser power (225) with 20 kV source volts, 2,900 V detector, pulse 3 kV lag time 900 ns, mass deflection at 1,000 Da, and mass range extending to 160 kDa m/z.

3.1.6. Data Export and Analysis

These brief details concern options for spectral preprocessing and analysis algorithms which are resident in the Ciphergen and Bruker profiling software. There is a wide range of issues to consider when undertaking the analysis of profiling spectral datasets (*see* **Note** 7)

1. Spectra generated on the PBSIIc are compiled to a single "experiment" .xpt file, batch processed by:

    (a) Single external calibration, 7-in-1 peptide mix 1–7 kDa (Bio-Rad)

    (b) Spot-to-spot correction applied

    (c) Default smoothing by 25 pts; baseline subtraction by 8× expected peak width, average filtering at 0.2× EPW, noise definition over 1,500 Da

    (d) Total ion current normalization (> 1,500 Da) but only within AE fraction type; spectral rejection for normalization factor > 2 SD from mean N.F.

    (e) Peak clustering and analysis for sample group distinction using Biomarker Wizard™ software module. Note the Mann-Whitney U-test and Kruskal-Wallis H-test *p*-value calculations do not take sample replication into account.

    (f) Export to Ciphergen Express™ server, or else export/import as .xml files with all pertaining sample annotation and preprocessing information

2. Further processing and alternate analysis is available through Ciphergen Express™:

    (a) Overall spectral alignment, via recalibration to internal shared peaks

    (b) PCA and correlation/clustering analysis

    (c) Corrected calculations for putative biomarker significance

    (d) Export of peak cluster data to spreadsheet (.csv file)

3. Peak intensity data imports into Biomarker Pattern Software™ (BPS; v. 5) for recursive development of classification and regression tree (CART) models, which are optimized for minimum crossvalidation error.

4. Raw spectral files (.csv mz/intensity format) are exported for alternate spectral preprocessing, and statistical evaluation in parallel, using a Proteomics Data Analysis Package (PDAP) which has been developed at the University of Pittsburgh, using MATLAB™, and applied to several SELDI-TOF profiling studies *(2, 3)*.

5. MALDI-TOF spectral data generated from AutoXecute sequences, flowing from ClinProt™ robot preparation, are automatically structured for subsequent analysis by ClinProTools™ software (v.2)

    (a) The basic workflow "Peak Statistic Calculation" can be used to quickly calculate peak statistics using ClinProTools™ default settings. This workflow includes spectra recalibration and average spectra calculation, peak picking and area calculation, as well as peak statistic calculation.

    (b) The basic workflow "Model Generation" can be used to quickly calculate models using ClinProTools™ defaults settings. This workflow includes spectra recalibration and average spectra calculation, peak calculation and model generation based on the selected classification algorithm.

    (c) After running peak calculation, the peak intensity and peak list can be exported from ClinProTools™ to XML or ASCII (*.dat) format. Peak intensity data in ASCII format data can be imported into BPS software for development of classification and regression tree (CART) model or MATLAB™-based classification applications.

(d) MALDI-TOF raw spectral files (.dat mz/intensity format with tab delimiter) can be exported individually through the "Export" menu in flexAnalysis or batch process through a user-defined script, which need to be named with "FAMSMethod" extension.

3.2. Nanoflow RPLC-MS/MS-Based Discovery

3.2.1 High Abundant Protein Depletion from Serum

This procedure can be performed using a variety of commercially available depletion technologies (antibody- or chemistry-based) or by other noncommercial strategies (low-abundant proteome enrichment *(4)*) to remove high abundant protein(s) from serum. The method described later will highlight a procedure based on the Multiple Affinity Removal System (MARS, Agilent Technologies) with which we have had extensive and successful experience (*see* **Note 8**).

1. Dilute 15-µL serum with 185-µL sample loading buffer (Buffer A) for every replicate of serum to be depleted. Fifteen µL of serum corresponds to roughly 900 µg of total protein in serum (~60 mg/mL) with an expected binding capacity of 1 mg for each MARS column. Assuming an 85–90% depletion of the high abundant proteins, each replicate should yield ~90–130 µg per column. Using two MARS columns for balancing, this usually consists of four replicates (two runs through each column) for a sufficient recovery of total protein for downstream analysis.

2. Filter the entire diluted serum sample through a 0.2-µm spin filter (multiple spins) to remove particulates.

3. Following the manufacturer's protocol, deplete each serum sample as follows:

(a) Using the Leur-Lok syringe, wash spin column with 4 mL of Buffer A. Discard any solution in the sample collection tube.

(b) In a new sample collection tube, add 200 µL of diluted, filtered sample and spin at $100 \times g$ for 1 min. Let sample/column rest at ambient temperature for 5 min to allow for complete binding of high abundant proteins. Do not discard the flow-through.

(c) Add 400 µL Buffer A to MARS spin column and centrifuge at $100 \times g$ for 2.5 min. Collect the sample flow-through in the same tube as b (sample "F1").

(d) Transfer column to a new collection tube, add 400 µL Buffer A to the column and centrifuge at $100 \times g$ for 2.5 min (sample "F2"). Place both sample collection tubes on ice.

(e) Using the Leur-Lok syringe, elute the high abundant proteins bound to the column with 2 mL of Buffer B. Collect in a 15-mL falcon tube (sample "E2").

(f) Repeat **steps a–e** for the number of replicates to yield the desired amount of depleted serum.

4. Protein Desalting: Prerinse 5 kDa molecular weight cut-off (MWCO) centrifugal concentrators (one for each different serum sample) with 2 mL Buffer A by centrifuging at $2,000 \times g$ until volume is reduced to approximately 500 µL. Bring to 2 mL with Buffer A and repeat. Discard all residual buffer from the centrifugal concentrator. Pool all depleted serum samples (all "F1" and "F2" samples) and concentrate to approximately 500 µL as described earlier, continuing to add depleted serum until all has been concentrated to ~500 µL. Bring to 2 mL with 50 mM ammonium bicarbonate, pH 8.2, and concentrate again. Repeat twice more and transfer to a clean microcentrifuge tube.

5. Determine protein concentration of all samples (e.g., by a Bradford or BCA assay) and normalize all sample concentrations (i.e., 1 mg/mL) using 50 mM ammonium bicarbonate, pH 8.2.

6. Protein digestion: Samples are boiled for 5–10 min, cooled to ambient temperature, brought to 10 mM DTT, and incubated at 37°C for 30 min. Optional step: Cysteine residues can be alkylated by addition of concentrated iodoacetamide solution to a final concentration of 15 mM and incubated in the dark at 37°C for 1 h. Add trypsin at a 1:50 enzyme-to-protein ratio and incubate overnight at 37°C. The protein digest should be stored at −80°C

3.2.2. Sample Desalting

Desalting of samples prior to analysis must be carried out prior to liquid chromatography-mass spectrometry analyses. A recommended procedure is described using the C-18 desalting columns (Pierce PepClean™ C-18 Spin Columns).

1. Equivalent aliquots (~30 or 60 µg of total protein) of each serum protein digest are removed and brought to an equivalent volume with 50 mM ammonium bicarbonate. A one-third volume equivalent of concentrated loading buffer (20% acetonitrile/2% trifluoroacetic acid) is added to bring the sample to 5% ACN, 0.5% TFA. Sample is desalted on a single column (30 µg) or two columns (60 µg).

2. *Activation.* Add 200 µL of activation solution (50% acetonitrile) and centrifuge at $1,500 \times g$ for 1 min and discard flow-through. Repeat.

3. *Equilibration.* Add 200 µL equilibration solution (5% ACN, 0.5% TFA) and centrifuge at $1,500 \times g$ for 1 min and discard flow-through. Repeat.

4. *Sample Binding*. Load sample (in 200 μL aliquots) to column and centrifuge at $1,500 \times g$ for 1 min. Do not discard flow-through! Repeat as many times as is necessary to load all sample onto the column. Repeat with all flow-through to ensure complete sample binding. Retain flow-through for evaluation (if necessary).

5. *Wash*. Add 200 μL equilibration solution and centrifuge at $1,500 \times g$ for 1 min. Repeat twice more, retaining all flow-through for evaluation (if necessary).

6. *Elution*. Add 20 μL elution solution (70% ACN, 0.5% TFA) and centrifuge at $1,500 \times g$ for 1 min. Repeat and collect flow-through in the same tube.

7. Lyophilize all samples to dryness to remove organic solvent for downstream analysis and store at $-80°C$

3.2.3. Multidimensional Fractionation and LC-MS/MS Analysis

This method describes the use of a combined strong cation exchange (SCX)-reversed-phase liquid chromatography (RPLC) resolution of peptides first described by Yates *(5)*. In the present analysis, a multidimensional nanoflow LC (Dionex Ultimate 3000) is coupled online with a linear ion trap MS (ThermoFisher LTQ) for peptide identification. Peptides can be resolved prior to and decoupled from MS analysis using a variety of separation/fractionation techniques (ion exchange or reversed-phase chromatography, capillary electrophoresis, etc.) and can be analyzed using a variety of mass spectrometers with varying instrument parameters.

1. Lyophilized peptides are resuspended in 15 μL of 0.1% TFA (or an appropriate volume based on the size of the LC autosampler sample loop and syringe volumes) and transferred to an autosampler vial.

2. Following appropriate setup protocols for the LC instrumentation, sample is injected followed by a number of chromatographic resolution steps which are each subsequently analyzed by the mass spectrometer, described later for the SCX-RP-LC/MS/MS analysis methodology:

   (a) After injection, the sample is permitted to load onto the SCX column for 30 min at a flow rate of 3 μL/min in solvent A (2% ACN in water, 0.1% formic acid). (Note: The flow rate is based on the pressure limitations of the column). LC system capillary tubing should be plumbed so that peptides that do not bind to the SCX column continue along and bind to the reversed-phase column with the solvent going to waste.

   (b) Peptides are eluted from the reversed-phase column by switching the solvent flow to the reversed-phase column by a valve switching and introducing a linear gradient of

0.3% solvent B (100% ACN, 0.1% formic acid) over 140 min at a flow rate of 0.2 µL/min. This is followed by increasing the solvent composition to 95% solvent B in 15 min and a column "washing" step of 95% solvent B for 20–30 min.

(c) Solvent composition is reduced to 100% solvent A over 3–5 min and the reversed-phase column is re-equilibrated in 100% solvent A for 20–30 min at a flow rate of 0.5 µL/min prior to the next injection.

(d) The entire procedure is repeated using bolus 15 µL injections of increasing ammonium acetate salt concentrations (i.e., 20, 40, 60, 75, 100, and 500 mM in 0.1% TFA) to elute peptides from the SCX column to then bind to the reversed-phase column for subsequent analysis. A final 15 µL injection of a 50-mM ammonium bicarbonate, 50% ACN solution is used to recondition the system for the next full sample analysis.

(e) All "salt concentration," reversed-phase MS analyses are triggered at the beginning of the introduction of the gradient by a contact closure mechanism (between the LC and the MS), and data collection continues through the beginning of the wash phase of column (160 min). The mass spectrometer operates in a data-dependent manner where it first collects a broad m/z (350–1,800) scan event from which it subsequently selects the top seven most abundant molecular ions for tandem MS to obtain peptide sequence information. A variety of parameters are set for basic MS data collection and also to avoid redundant selection of ions that have been previously sequenced by the MS (dynamic exclusion) *see* **Note 9**.

3.2.4. Bioinformatic Analysis and Protein Identification

This method describes the use of the SEQUEST algorithm, contained in the Bioworks Software Suite (ThermoFisher Scientific) to search the raw data generated from the LC-MS/MS analysis described earlier. A variety of other search engines/data analysis tools may be used to analyze the data and are publicly accessible (Mascot, XTandem, PEAKS, etc.). In addition, acquisition and formatting an appropriate protein sequence database (such as the EMBL-EBI Integr8 web portal) is described later. A variety of database types and formats can be downloaded from the Internet for searching mass spectral data (NCBI, IPI)

1. *Database Setup*. Open a web browser and direct the home page to http://www.ebi.ac.uk/integr8/EBI-Integr8-HomePage.do.Browse the appropriate species and then go to the downloaded page. Save the FASTA formatted complete UniProtKB proteome database. Unzip and save as an appropriate name and date of download to track version changes/updates.

Within the database, the "|" character must be replaced with a "space" and the database must be saved as a .FASTA file.

2. *Searching.* Raw files are searched against the appropriate database using the appropriate criteria (source database, mass ranges and tolerances, enzyme specificity, modifications, etc. – saved as a .PARAMS file). SEQUEST will generate data files (.dta) and then result files (.out) following the search of the raw data against the database. Once searched, the results can be loaded in the Bioworks browser and filtered with the appropriate criteria (selected in the "Filter" tab), and the data can be exported as a SequestPeptide Microsoft Excel format. We typically export data with lower-than-desired filtering criteria and then further refine the dataset with more stringent criteria downstream.

3. *Bioinformatics – Data Combining:* Peptide exports as mentioned earlier can be imported into database software (in this case Microsoft Access) and then combined for each sample to generate a single, complete peptide list for each sample. Using the query function in Microsoft Access, we further reduce the data to contain only those peptide identifications that match our selection criteria (crosscorrelation and delta correlation scoring) and that are also unique to a single protein entry in the database (in SEQUEST this is represented by a empty "Count" field in the peptide export file). What will remain at this point for each sample is a culled list of all unique peptide identifications from a single analysis of several LC-MS/MS runs.

4. *Spectral Count Data Analysis.* From these individual sample data, a query can be generated to compare the total peptide identifications for each protein (in the case of the UniProt database, a unique Accession number) across all samples analyzed. This "spectral count," or total number of peptides identified per protein, method allows relative estimation of a protein's abundance within a given sample. Based on the experimental design, using equivalent amounts of total protein, processing all samples similarly, and injection of equivalent amounts for analysis, the assumption can be made that, all things being equal, the more the number of peptides identified for a given protein, the higher the likelihood that it is present in greater abundance.

4. Notes

1. Serum samples typically have experienced no more than two rounds of freeze thawing; many anecdotal reports *(e.g., 6, 7)* and recent systematic examination *(8)* discourage more than

this, and strongly indicate that rigorously consistent processing and storage history must be maintained and documented for all experimental and control samples involved. In our laboratory the second freeze (flash freezing in dry ice) occurs on the occasion of aliquotting thawed original patient samples into multiple small single-use aliquots. For serum processing, we thaw serum aliquots quickly in very cold water (4°C), then maintain tubes in an ice-cooled aluminum block during handling. Before distribution into low-protein binding polypropylene or polystyrene microtiter plate (MTP), the serum aliquots are centrifuged briefly (e.g., $13,000 \times g$ at 4°C) to sediment any insolubles and separated lipids.

2. We currently employ a split-and-combine strategy to minimize the impact of well-to-well variability in high-throughput immunodepletion and anion exchange fractionation processes. The depletion replicates are combined and split for AE fractionation, which likewise is done in two parallel reactions and ultimately combined. We employ such replication in light of a recent report that "batch of processing" is a significant contributor to variance observed in profiling spectra generated after AE fractionation (9). If the total number of samples processed necessitates the performance of multiple fractionation runs separated in time or employing different reagent batches, sample groups/types should be distributed across all runs to avoid biasing effects of inter-run variability.

3. The resins for affinity depletion *must* be pretreated to minimize the leaching of ligand components into serum samples. Prior to first use, a sample of buffer only should be processed, to expose the column resin to denaturing and stripping conditions, and then re-equilibration prior to binding with serum samples. Like others (10), we find the use of reuseable immunodepletion spin columns involves processing inconsistency due to incomplete cap sealing and attendant bead loss, as well as impracticability for very large sample sets. Similarly, we also have observed insufficient stripping of reuseable immunodepletion spin columns: this can require between 10 and 15 successive strippings to reduce eluted protein to levels undetectable by mass spectrometry (data not shown). Imperfect stripping/regeneration diminishes column capacity and lifetime, but also entails possible crosscontamination of column "Strip" fractions, increasingly being advocated for separate interrogation by profiling (10).

4. The PBSIIc instrument provides reasonably sensitive detection of larger molecular weight analytes by this method and can serve as a useful process control for monitoring the partitioning of serum analytes such as HSA and Ig. Neat-spotted MALDI as qualitative process control can require optimization

of the ratios and dilutions of matrix to maximize signal from dilute samples; very concentrated samples may form a glass. Variable composition and concentration between fractions may preclude quantitative assessment of analyte partitioning between fractions. Within fraction type, however, this can provide an early indication of processing stability between individual subject samples, and among their processing replicates. After depletion, this method reveals a primary high molecular weight signal at 79 kDa, presumed to represent transferrin *(11)*.

5. Problematic tip attachment or ejection can in turn result in impeded motion or jamming of the robot arm. We have modified a number of methods to introduce a considerably larger air gap, intended to minimize leakage of water from the needles into the top of those tips which are reracked and reused at multiple pipetting steps for shared reagents. Jams or interruptions can be cleared by rehoming the robot and relaunching the routine with the jump editor to the last successfully completed program line.

6. There have been recommendations to perform spectral generation only within a specific time window after spotting *(12, 13)*, but we are not able to accommodate this precise control logistically during larger profiling runs and given our protracted profiling times. However, all samples, in randomized layout within AE fraction, generally are accorded comparable time between spotting and spectrometry. Our present matrix-spotting conditions are formulated around the use of polished steel MTP targets; the deposition of 1–2 μL droplets to cover the majority of the area of these features; the desire to conserve samples yet provide adequate technical replication; balanced against the volatility of the matrix solution and attendant inconsistencies in its handling in small volumes. Recent communication illustrates the need, during projects of significant duration (weeks to months), to accurately standardize and routinely monitor laser energy output and calibrate laser attenuation *(8)*.

7. MALDI profiling data analysis issues

   (a) Sources of variability in mass spectrometric profiling have been increasingly reported *(6, 8, 14)* since an early indication of a possible ovarian cancer SELDI "signature" was subsequently associated with a date-of-run bias inadvertently applied to one sample group *(3, 15)*. Day-to-day purification variance has been documented *(9)*, and variance from mechanical sources attributed to causes from the sporadic, such as a source or detector failure *(16)* to the systematic, such as gradual decline in laser energy *(8)* or physical deviation in field strength due to target movement in the source (hence spot-to-spot correction in ProteinChip™

software). In the absence of the means by which to control all recognized (and even suspected) sources of artifactual distinction, diligent effort must be made to ensure that no one source is preferentially exerted against only one sample class.

(b) Spectra generated on the PBSIIc from neat spotting can be analyzed within ProteinChip™ software (v3.2.1) which is a well-developed suite of spectral preprocessing and viewing options, with multiple parameters for spectral noise reduction, baseline subtraction, and normalization. Historically, normalization in SELDI-TOF experiments was based on baseline-subtracted total ion current (TIC) beyond low-mass noise (i.e., >1,500 Da m/z). This was originally espoused as a possible means by which run-specific variations could be accommodated in large groups of spectra generated across multiple profiling sessions. We find this does not remove strong distinction associated with date of run, and this must necessarily be addressed in experimental layout through the randomized distribution of all sample groups across all processing and spectrometry sessions. Normalization would not be expected to be applied across spectra from distinct AE fractions, which are observed to have different protein concentrations and compositions, and thus inherently different patterns and intensities of signals.

(c) ClinProTools™ uses a standard data preparation workflow and supports grouping of spectra from multiple measurements. The standard workflow can be supplemented by applying additional filters to modify spectra, reduce data, and exclude spectra of lower quality from further processing. The result of data preparation is a collection of (normalized) peak areas for each spectrum. For all spectra, areas of the same peaks are calculated so that, for each spectrum, the same number of peak areas is obtained. Peak areas are used, which have a smaller variation between spectra than intensities of single points. For nearly all of these steps there are parameters, which can be chosen to adapt to the kind of spectra used and to control the number of peaks taken into account. The data preparation parameters can be set using the "Settings Spectra Preparation" and "Settings Peak Calculation" commands from the "Data Preparation" menu.

(d) A recent exemplary report (17) gives extensive details of an integrated workflow for the export, preprocessing and analysis of serum proteomic profile data. Specific recommendations are given for spectral preprocessing routines and classification algorithms, and even custom-written software made available, as "best practice" methods for adoption. However, there is little move toward consensus in the field, as the platforms for data generation, the sample types being analyzed, and even the desired practical endpoint in these studies vary widely. These fundamental differences underpin the very assumptions on which these analytical frameworks are established, developed, optimized, and validated. Another recent excellent report *(18)* shows the merit of the evaluative approach, in which a variety of analytical methods are applied to a common dataset, and the relative performances are all reported and compared. Reporting the result of only the method that appears to provide the best unvalidated performance constitutes a form of "model overfit," compromising generalizability. Based on a consistent performance endpoint or sufficiently broad range of studies, this evaluative approach may eventually result in consensus about critical questions such as modes of spectral alignment ("SpecAlign" *(19)* has many advocates for example) or classification [support vector machine (SVM) *(8, 18, 20)* has many advocates]. Our own analysis efforts are similarly highly comparative, where ultimate determination about the merits of spectral preprocessing or classification methods is judged on the robust and reproducible detection of features, and the stability (and crossvalidation, or external validation) of the classification models constructed therefrom, and not simply on the feasibility of feature isolation and identification *(17)*, although such practical concerns weigh heavily in planning for follow-on or validation studies.

8. All buffers and samples are to be kept on ice throughout the depletion protocol. Fifty mL aliquots of the column buffers should be supplemented immediately before use with protease inhibitor (0.1 mM PMSF final concentration). Each MARS spin column should be carried through the complete depletion protocol using only Buffer A as a blank sample to precondition the column before each day's use. Columns should be stored in Buffer A at the end of each day's use and stored at $4°C$.

9. It may be prudent to utilize a file-naming system to maintain the unique sample name/identifier at the end of the data file name when setting up the analyses to facilitate downstream bioinformatics, e.g., a file name such as ProjectName_Date_SaltConc_SampleID.raw. This will assist in combining the multiple analyses from a single sample downstream using standard database software using tables and queries.

References

1. Hauskrecht, M., Pelikan, R., Malehorn, D.E., Bigbee, W.L., Lotze, M.T., et-al. (2005) Feature selection for classification of SELDI-TOF-MS proteomic profiles. *Appl. Bioinformatics* 4, 227–246.

2. Pelikan, R., Bigbee, W.L., Malehorn, D.E., Lyons-Weiler, J., and Hauskrecht, M. (2007) Intersession reproducibility of mass spectrometry profiles and its effect on accuracy of multivariate classification models. *Bioinformatics* 23, 3065–3072.

3. Baggerly, K.A., Morris, J.S., Edmonson, S.R., and Coombes, K.R. (2005) Signal in noise: evaluating reported reproducibility of serum proteomic tests for ovarian cancer. *J. Natl. Cancer Inst.* 97, 307–309.

4. Tirumalai, R.S., Chan, K.C., Prieto, D.A., Issaq, H.J., Conrads, T.P., et al. (2003) Characterization of the low molecular weight human serum proteome. *Mol. Cell. Proteomics* 2, 1096–1103.

5. Washburn, M.P., Wolters, D., and Yates J.R. III. (2001) Large-scale analysis of the yeast proteome by multidimensional protein identification technology. *Nat. Biotechnol.* 19, 242–247.

6. McLerran, D., Grizzle, W.E., Feng, Z., Bigbee, W.L., Banez, L.L., et-al. (2008) Analytical validation of serum proteomic profiling for diagnosis of prostate cancer: sources of sample bias. *Clin. Chem.* 54, 44–52.

7. Traum, A.Z., Wells, M.P., Aivado, M., Libermann, T.A., Ramoni, M.F., et-al. (2006) SELDI-TOF MS of quadruplicate urine and serum samples to evaluate changes related to storage conditions. *Proteomics* 6, 1676–1680.

8. Villanueva, J., Philip, J., Chaparro, C.A., Li, Y., Toledo-Crow, R., et-al. (2005) Correcting common errors in identifying cancer-specific serum peptide signatures. *J. Proteome Res.* 4, 1060–1072.

9. Whistler, T., Rollin, D., and Vernon, S.D. (2007) A method for improving SELDI-TOF mass spectrometry data quality. *Proteome Sci.* 5, 4–14.

10. Seam, N., Gonzales, D.A., Kern, S.J., Hortin, G.L., Hoehn, G.T., Suffredini, A.F. (2007) Quality control of serum albumin depletion for proteomic analysis. *Clin. Chem.* 53, 1915–1920.

11. Sundsten, T., Eberhardson, M., Goransson, M., and Bergsten, P. (2006) The use of proteomics in identifying differentially expressed serum proteins in humans with type 2 diabetes. *Proteome Sci.* 4, 4–22.

12. Villanueva, J., Lawlor, K., Toledo-Crow, R., and Tempst, P. (2006) Automated serum peptide profiling. *Nat. Protoc.* 1, 880–891.

13. Aivado, M., Spentzos, D., Alterovitz, G., Out, H.H., Grall. F., et-al. (2005) Optimization and evaluation of surface-enhanced laser desorption/ionization time-of-flight mass spectrometry (SELDI-TOF MS) with reversed-phase protein arrays for protein profiling. *Clin. Chem. Lab. Med.* 43, 133–140.

14. McLerran, D., Grizzle, W.E., Feng, Z., Thompson, I.M., Bigbee, W.L., et-al. (2008) SELDI-TOF MS whole serum proteomic profiling with IMAC surface does not reliably detect prostate cancer. *Clin. Chem.* 54, 53–60.

15. Baggerly, K.A., Coombes, K.R., and Morris, J.S. (2005) Bias, randomization and ovarian proteomic data: A reply to "Producers and Consumers." *Canc. Informatics* 1, 9–14.

16. Semmes, O.J., Feng, Z., Adam, B.L., Banez, L.L., Bigbee, W.L., et-al. (2005) Evaluation of serum protein profiling by surface-enhanced laser desorption/ionization time-of-flight mass spectrometry for the detection of prostate cancer: I. Assessment of platform reproducibility. *Clin. Chem.* 51, 102–112.

17. Villanueva, J., Philip, J., DeNoyer, L., and Tempst, P. (2007) Data analysis of assorted serum peptidome profiles. *Nat. Protoc.* 2, 588–602.

18. Hendriks, M.M., Smit, S., Akkermans, W.L., Reijmers, T.H., Eilers, P.H., et-al. (2007) How to distinguish healthy from diseased? Classification strategy for mass spectrometry-based clinical proteomics. *Proteomics* 7, 3672–3680.

19. Wong, J.W., Cagney, G., and Cartwright, H.M. (2005) SpecAlign–processing and alignment of mass spectra datasets. *Bioinformatics* 21, 2088–2090.

20. Au, J.S.K., Cho, W.C.X., Yip, T.T., Yip, C., Zhu, H., et-al. (2007) Deep proteome profiling of sera from never-smoked lung cancer patients. *Biomed. Pharmacother.* 61, 570–577.

Chapter 9

Hormones as Biomarkers: Practical Guide to Utilizing Luminex Technologies for Biomarker Research

Faina Linkov, Zoya Yurkovetsky, and Anna Lokshin

Summary

Hormones are chemical messengers produced in one part of the body and released into the blood to trigger or regulate particular functions of the body in another part. Hormone actions vary widely, but can include stimulation or inhibition of growth, induction or suppression of apoptosis, activation or inhibition of the immune system, regulating metabolism, and preparation for a new activity or phase of life. There is a growing interest in the role that hormones may play in the development and progression of various cancers. Recent research suggests that hormone levels may explain differences in risk for some of the most commonly diagnosed cancers, including breast, ovarian, and others; however, additional studies utilizing novel hormone measurement technologies are needed to investigate the roles of common hormones in cancer. Increasing our understanding of the role of hormones and other biomarkers in the etiology and the course of different cancers has a great potential to facilitate the development of new treatment modalities. This chapter provides an overview on multiplexing xMAP technology by Luminex (Austin, TX) that can be used for simultaneous analysis of several biologic markers, e.g., hormones. The xMAP immunoassay technology combines the principle of a sandwich ELISA with the fluorescent-bead-based technology allowing individual and multiplex analysis of up to 100 different analytes in a single microtiter well. Serum assay described in the methods section is performed in 96-well microplate format according to the protocol provided by LINCO Research, Inc. (St. Louis, MO). Human Pituitary LIN-COplex Kit is utilized for simultaneous quantification of six pituitary hormones in serum, plasma, tissue lysate, and culture supernatant samples: Prolactin, FSH, LH, TSH, GH, and ACTH.

Key words: Hormones, Luminex, Biological markers, Cancer, ELISA.

1. Introduction

1.1. Hormones

Hormones are chemical messengers produced in one part of the body and released into the blood to trigger and regulate particular functions of the body in another part. Hormone actions

Michael A. Tainsky, *Methods in Molecular Biology, Tumor Biomarker Discovery, Vol. 520*
© Humana Press, a part of Springer Science+Business Media, LLC 2009
DOI: 10.1007/978-1-60327-811-9_9

vary widely, but can include stimulation or inhibition of growth, induction or suppression of apoptosis, activation or inhibition of the immune system, regulating metabolism, and preparation for a new activity or phase of life. There is a growing interest in the role that hormones may play in the development and progression of various cancers. Recent research suggests that hormone levels may explain differences in risk for some of the most commonly diagnosed female cancers and could be responsible for as many as 15% of cancers in the UK *(1)*. Hormones play a major role in the etiology of several of the commonest cancers worldwide, including cancers of the endometrium, breast and ovary in women, and cancer of the prostate in men. It is likely that the main mechanisms by which hormones affect cancer risk are by controlling the rate of cell division, the differentiation of cells, and the number of susceptible cells. Hormones have very marked effects on cell division in the endometrium; estrogens stimulate mitosis whereas progestins oppose this effect *(2)*. Multiple lines of evidence support a central role of hormones in the etiology of breast cancer. Accumulating data indicate a significant positive association of breast cancer development with prolactin levels, although additional confirmation is needed *(3)*.

In the last 10 years, scientists have increasingly identified changes in the levels, frequency, and types of endocrine hormones as important contributors to the major cancers faced by Western populations such as breast cancer (estrogen, progesterone, prolactin), prostate cancer (estrogen, testosterone), endometrial cancer (estrogen), and thyroid cancer (TSH, T3, T4) *(4)*.

Hormones secreted by pituitary gland including FSH, LH, TSH, prolactin, GH, and ACTH have been reported to associate with the development of malignancies. We have demonstrated differential expression of these hormones in serum of patients with different cancers, e.g., ovarian, pancreatic, breast, endometrial, as compared to matched cancer-free individuals (**Fig. 1**). Specifically, we found that LH was upregulated in all of these four cancers. TSH, prolactin, and GH were upregulated in ovarian, pancreatic, and endometrial cancers, while ACTH was upregulated in ovarian and endometrial cancers. *P* values < 0.05 were considered statistically significant. These findings are consistent with the "gonadotropin hypothesis," which postulates that gonadotropin overstimulation of epithelial cells results in their increased proliferation and subsequent malignant transformation.

Follicle-stimulating hormone (FSH) is a hormone synthesized and secreted by gonadotropes in the anterior pituitary gland. According to the "two cell, two gonadotropins" theory, both FSH and LH are necessary for ovarian follicular maturation and the syntheses of ovarian steroid hormones *(5)*. It has been previously demonstrated that human ovarian cancer cells express FSH receptor (FSHR). However, whether FSHR plays a role in

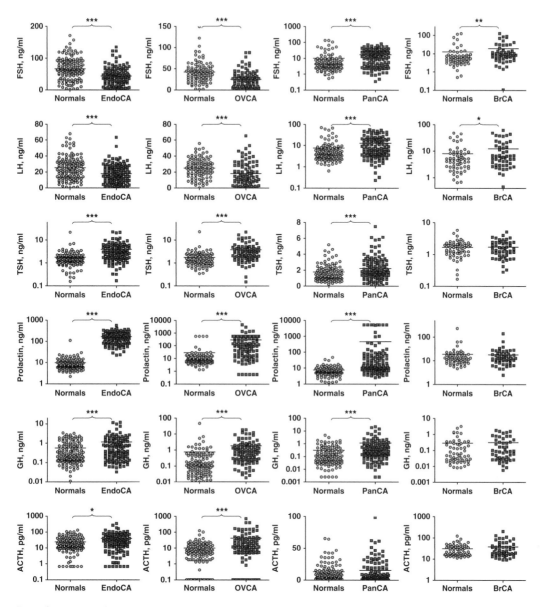

Fig. 1. Comparison of hormone levels in cancer patients vs. control groups: *$P < 0.05$; **$P < 0.01$; ***$P < 0.001$ (*See Color Plates*).

ovarian cancer development is still ambiguous *(6)*. Development, growth, and function of the ovary are controlled by endocrine and paracrine signals. These may also influence the development of ovarian cancer *(7)*. In addition to the importance of FSH in ovarian cancer development, previous research indicated that both luteinizing hormone (LH) and FSH may be implicated in endometrial cancer cell growth *(8)*.

Increasing evidence suggests that LH plays an important role in cancer development and progression. LH is a hormone synthesized and secreted by gonadotropes in the anterior lobe of the pituitary gland. In concert with the other pituitary gonadotropin FSH, it is necessary for proper reproductive function. Lower LH and higher E2 are reported in women with breast, endometrial, and ovarian cancer (before surgery) *(9)* Previous study also suggested that inhibition of the preovulatory LH surge might be a critical event in the tumor-induced cessation of reproductive cycling *(10)*.

Thyroid-stimulating hormone (also known as TSH or thyrotropin) is a hormone synthesized and secreted by thyrotrope cells in the anterior pituitary gland which regulates the endocrine function of the thyroid gland. The role of TSH has been investigated in great detail in the development of thyroid cancer *(4, 11–14)*. Experimental studies and clinical data have demonstrated that thyroid-cell proliferation is dependent on thyroid-stimulating hormone (TSH), thereby providing the rationale for TSH suppression as a treatment for differentiated thyroid cancer *(13)*. Although its role in the development of other cancers remains in question, it has been suggested that TSH and prolactin may play a role in breast cancer development *(15)*

Prolactin is classically considered to be a pituitary hormone mainly involved in milk protein production, and it has important functions for development of the mammary gland *(16)*. Prolactin is a peptide hormone synthesized and secreted by lactotrope cells in the anterior pituitary gland. Research suggests that receptors for sex steroids and prolactin are coexpressed and are crossregulated, providing a potential mechanism for the synergy among estrogen, progesterone, and prolactin in the control of tumor growth *(17)*. In addition, prolactin can be secreted by endometrium, myometrium, cervix, prostate cells, and T cells. Recently, prolactin was reported as a biomarker for ovarian cancer.

Growth hormone (GH) is a polypeptide hormone synthesized and secreted by the anterior pituitary gland which stimulates growth and cell reproduction in humans and other vertebrate animals. Insulin-like growth factors (IGF-1 and IGF-2) and the IGF-1 membrane receptor (IGF-1R) have been found to play a critical role in the carcinogenesis of several tumors, among them colorectal cancer *(18)* and prostate cancer *(19)*. The ability of GH, via its mediator peptide IGF-1, to influence regulation of cellular growth has been the focus of much interest in recent years *(20)*. IGF is highly associated with the risk of cancer because of its role in cell proliferation and tumor growth. In previous studies, high plasma levels of IGF-1, IGF-2, and IGFBP-3 were associated with good prognosis in patients with advanced nonsmall cell lung cancer *(21)*. There is a need for further validation of prognostic significance of IGF system in various types of cancers, as altered IGF levels may become a useful tool for the early detection of cancer.

Adrenocorticotropic hormone (ACTH or corticotropin) is a polypeptide hormone synthesized from POMC, (preopiomelano-cortin) and secreted from corticotropes in the anterior lobe of the pituitary gland in response to the hormone corticotropin-releasing hormone (CRH) released by the hypothalamus. Despite some evidence that ACHT may be important in the development of cancer *(22)*, both GH and ACTH were rarely investigated as potential biomarkers of endometrial, ovarian, pancreatic, or breast cancer. With growing importance of hormones in cancer detection and treatment, technologies that can measure levels of multiple hormones in one small samples are gaining popularity.

1.2. Background on Luminex

At the University of Pittsburgh, we utilized a novel multiana-lyte xMAP profiling technology (Luminex Corp., Austin, TX), that allows simultaneous measurement of multiple biomarkers in blood serum of cancer patients and matched healthy individuals *(23)*, to evaluate the utility of hormones and other biomarkers in the early diagnosis of cancer. Various studies at the University of Pittsburgh and nationally suggested that hormones could be potentially used as biomarkers of cancer progression and relapse.

Several years ago, Luminex Corporation introduced a novel protein array system (xMAP for Multianalyte Profiling), which allows for simultaneous quantitation of up to 100 soluble ana-lytes in one sample. xMAP technology uses polystyrene micro-spheres internally dyed with differing ratios of two spectrally distinct fluorophores to create a family of 100 differentially spec-trally addressed bead sets. Each of the 100 spectrally addressed bead sets can be conjugated with a capture antibody specific for a unique target protein. In a multiplexed assay, antibody-conjugated beads are allowed to react with sample (plasma, serum, or cell culture supernatant). After washing, secondary, or detection, antibodies are added to a microtiter plate well to form a cap-ture sandwich immunoassay. The assay solution is analyzed by the fluorometric array reader, which obtains two fluorescence read-ings for every single bead: one that identifies a bead as a mem-ber of one of the 100 possible sets, and another that measures the amount of fluorescent dye, phycoerythrin (PE) bound to the detection antibody in the assay. The amount of green fluores-cence is proportional to the amount of analyte captured in the immunoassay. Bio-Plex Manager software correlates each bead set to the assay reagent that has been coupled to it. Extrapolat-ing to a standard curve allows quantitation of each analyte in the sample. Using the xMAP assay, thousands of beads can be analyzed in seconds, allowing up to 100 analytes to be measured in a 96-well microplate in 1 h (**Fig. 2** provides a short outline of Luminex xMap technology principle).

In addition, since the fluorescence from each bead is meas-ured independently, enough statistics is accumulated to allow for

100 Unique Beads

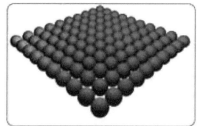

Two fluorescent dyes are combined in varying amounts to create 100 beads with unique fluorescent spectra. Each bead can be linked to a unique substrate or capture antibody.

Dual Laser Detection

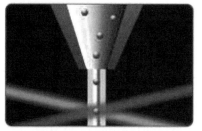

As each bead flows through a cuvette in single file, a red laser detects the identity of the bead. Simultaneously, a second green laser quantifies the fluorescence associated with analyte-bound reporter. The analyte being measured is unique to that bead set.

Luminex® 100 Instrument

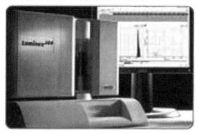

Fig. 2. Luminex technology overview. (From LUCERNACHEM http://www.lucerna-chem.ch/98.html).

assaying each sample in one well and not in duplicates. Recent published reports have provided experimental evidence that the xMAP technology offers an efficient method for antibody screening *(24–27)*. Several companies, such as Millipore/Linco Research/Upstate (St. Louis, MO), Invitrogen/Biosource International (Camarillo, CA), Qiagen (Valencia, CA), and others, are now manufacturing multiplex kits for simultaneous determinations of cytokines, growth factors, and hormones using the xMAP platform. Based on these features of the xMAP system, we consider it to be highly suitable for screening of protein arrays including multiplex screening of hormones.

2. Materials

2.1. Equipment: Luminex/Bio-Plex Workstation

The Luminex 100 IS System is a flexible analyzer based on the principles of flow cytometry that is designed to meet the needs of laboratory medicine and the care of patients, as well as being used in the research environment, including our Luminex Core Facility at the University of Pittsburgh Cancer Institute. The system enables multiplexing (simultaneous measurement) of up to 100 analytes in a single microplate well, using very small sample volumes, which is a very useful feature for conserving valuable specimens. The Luminex 100 IS System delivers fast and cost-effective bioassay results on many assay formats including nucleic acid assays, receptor-ligand assays, immunoassays, and enzymatic assays. The Luminex 100 IS System is the combination of two core xMAP technologies. The first is xMAP microspheres, a family of 100 fluorescently dyed 5.6 micron-sized polystyrene microspheres that act as both the identifier and the solid surface to build the assay. The second is a flow cytometry-based instrument, the Luminex 100, which integrates key xMAP detection components such as lasers, optics, advanced fluidics, and high-speed digital signal processors (http://www.luminexcorp.com/01_xMAPTechnology/). The Luminex Core at the University of Pittsburgh is equipped with the Luminex 100 reader with Bio-Plex (Bio-Rad Laboratories, Hercules, CA) software installed. It is designed for template-based data acquisition with robust data regression analysis, which is ideal for the clinical laboratory setting.

2.2. Software

Intuitive software is necessary to efficiently handle the large amount of data generated in multiplex assays. Bio-Rad has applied years of experience developing integrated system software and hardware to create Bio-Plex Manager, the first software package of its kind dedicated to the analysis of multiplexed assay data. This software yields maximum information from changes and correlations among analytes (http://www.luminexcorp.com/product_list.html?record_id = 6&product_type = SOFTWARE). Setting up Bio-Plex Manager Software is easy, as software comes with a guide that quickly leads the user through system setup and data analysis. This software is equipped with automated setup, run, and shutdown functions, and simple and flexible multiplex template formatting.

Additionally, Bio-Plex Manager Software features: automated system monitoring and error flags; data reduction programming to efficiently handle large amounts of data generated by multiplex assays; automated generation of standard curves; multiple curve-fitting analyses; automated calculation of concentration and coefficient of variation; sorting and screening tools for rapid analysis of only relevant samples; and standardized exportable Excel data files. The last feature makes it very easy to exchange data among collaborators, even with those who do not have Bio-Plex Manager Software.

2.3. Reagents

The following reagents are supplied with this kit (Cat. HPT-66K):

1. Antibody-Immobilized Beads (20×, 20 µL antibody beads/bottle; hFSH, hLH, hTSH, hProlactin, hGH, hACTH).
2. Human Pituitary Standard Cocktail.
3. Human Pituitary Quality Controls (Controls I and II).
4. Serum Matrix (Porcine Serum containing 0.08% Sodium Azide).
5. Bead Diluent (3.5 mL).
6. Human Pituitary Detection Antibodies (biotinylated, 5.5 mL).
7. Streptavidin-Phycoerythrin (5.5 mL).
8. LINCOplex Assay Buffer (50 mM PBS, 25 mM EDTA, 0.08% Sodium Azide, 0.05% Tween 20, 1% BSA, pH 7.4, 30 mL).
9. LINCOplex 10× Wash Buffer (1:10 dilution in deionized water to give 10 mM PBS, 0.05% Proclin, 0.05% Tween 20, pH 7.4, 30 mL).
10. Microtiter Filter Plate, Plate Sealers.
11. Mixing Bottle.

2.4. Collection and Storage of Blood Serum

Draw 10 µl of peripheral blood from tested subjects using standardized phlebotomy procedures. Collect blood samples without anticoagulant into red-top vacutainers (for sera) and allow blood to coagulate for 30 min at room temperature. Separate sera by centrifugation, immediately aliquot samples, and store in a dedicated –80°C freezer. Avoid multiple freeze-thaw cycles (> 2) for each sample.

3. Methods

3.1. Preparation of Reagents for the Assay

First, prepare antibody-immobilized beads. Sonicate each antibody-bead bottle for 30 s, vortex for 1 min, add 0.15 mL from each antibody-bead bottle to the Mixing Bottle, add 2.25 mL Bead Diluent, and vortex well. Next, prepare human pituitary standard cocktail. Reconstitute the human standard cocktail with

250 µL deionized water to give a final concentration of standards as follows: 100 mIU/mL FSH, 200 mIU/mL LH, 50 uIU/mL TSH, 100 ng/mL Prolactin, 50 ng/mL GH, and 12.5 ng/mL ACTH. Mix vial very well, vortex for 10 s, let it set for 5–10 min, and transfer to polypropylene microfuge tube. This is Standard 7. Then prepare working standards. **Figure 3** outlines preparation of serial dilutions of protein standards.

Label six polypropylene microfuge tubes as follows: Standard 1 (Std 1), Std 2, Std 3, Std 4, Std 5, and Std 6. Add 150 µL of Assay Buffer to each tube. Prepare serial dilutions by adding 50 µL of Std 7 to Std 6 tube, mix well and transfer 50 µL of Std 6 to Std 5 tube, mix well, add 50 µL of Std 5 to Std 4 tube, mix well, and so far (*see* **Fig. 1**). The background (Std 0) will be Assay Buffer. The serial dilutions result in the concentrations for each hormone presented in **Table 1**.

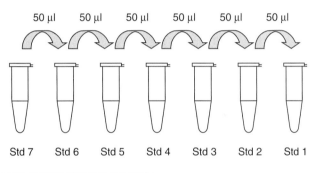

Fig. 3. Preparation of serial dilutions of protein standards.

Table 1
Human pituitary hormone concentrations

	FSH	LH	TSH	GH	Prolactin	ACTH
	mIU/mL	mIU/mL	µIU/mL	ng/mL	ng/mL	Ng/mL
Std 1	0.024	0.049	0.012	0.012	0.024	0.003
Std 2	0.098	0.195	0.049	0.049	0.098	0.012
Std 3	0.39	0.781	0.195	0.195	0.39	0.049
Std 4	1.563	3.125	0.781	0.781	1.563	0.195
Std 5	6.25	12.5	3.125	3.125	6.25	0.781
Std 6	25.0	50.0	12.5	12.5	25.0	3.125
Std 7	100.0	200.0	50.0	50.0	100.0	12.5

Next, prepare controls. Reconstitute Human Pituitary Control I and Human Pituitary Control II with 250-µL Deionized Water, mix well, vortex, let it set for 5–10 min, and transfer to appropriate polypropylene microfuge tubes. To prepare Wash Buffer, dilute 30 mL of 10× Wash buffer (mixed well at room temperature) with 270 mL deionized water. To prepare Serum Matrix, add 1.0 mL deionized water to the bottle containing lyophilized Serum Matrix, mix well, and let it reconstitute for 10 min.

3.2. Immunoassay Procedure

Block filter plate by pipetting 200 µL of Assay Buffer into each well of the plate. Mix the sealed plate well on a plate shaker at room temperature for 10 min. To remove Assay Buffer, first use vacuum, then, blot on paper towels. Next, add 25 µL of Assay buffer to the 0 Standard and to the Samples wells. Then, add 25 µL of each Standard or Control into the appropriate wells. Afterward, add 25 µL of Serum Matrix to the Background, Standards, and control wells. Consequently, add 25 µL of Sample into the appropriate wells. Finally, add 25 µL of the Mixed Beads to each well, seal plate, cover with aluminum foil, and incubate on a plate shaker for 2 h at room temperature.

Next, remove fluid by vacuum and wash twice with 200 µL/ well of Wash Buffer. To remove Assay Buffer, first used vacuum, then, gently blot on paper towels. Add 50 µL of Detection Antibody Cocktail into each well, seal, cover with aluminum foil, and incubate on a plate shaker for 1 h at room temperature.

After incubation, add 50 µL Streptavidin–Phycoerythin to each well containing the 50 µL of Detection Antibody Cocktail, seal, cover with aluminum foil, and incubate on a shaker for 30 min at room temperature.

Next, remove fluid by vacuum and wash twice with 200 µL/ well of Wash Buffer, by vacuum filtration between each wash. Excess fluid on the bottom of the plate can be wiped with a tissue. Then, add 100 µL of Sheath Fluid to all wells, cover with foil, and shake for 5 min. Finally, analyze sample on Luminex Instruments using five-parametric-curve-fitting method for calculating Pituitary Hormones concentrations in samples.

4. Notes

1. Luminex technology makes it possible to simultaneously detect the levels of multiple analytes. Bead-based approach permits this analysis to be performed in a single small sample (1–50 µL), thus allowing substantial conservation of valuable patient samples. Finally, due to liquid-phase incubation,

all reactions are completed within short periods of time compared with conventional ELISA. Thus, this technique is cost effective, saves time, and offers flexibility. However, the detection range could be not sensitive to circulating levels of some hormones. In these instances, high-sensitivity xMAP assays will have to be developed. As with ELISAs, the investigator must explore whether expected levels will fall within the standard range of the kit. Since some hormones may demonstrate optimal performance at serum dilutions that could be suboptimal for other hormones, more than one multiplexed assay will have to be performed.

2. Allow all reagents to warm to room temperature before use in the assay (20–25°C).Beads are light sensitive and must be covered with aluminum foil all the time.

3. Diagram placement of Background, Standards, Controls, and samples on Well Map Worksheet in a vertical configuration. The instrument will only read the 96-well plate vertically.

4. After hydration, all standards and controls must be transferred to polypropylene tubes.

5. The standards prepared by serial dilution must be used within 1 h of preparation.

6. In order to avoid settling, during addition of beads, shake bead mix occasionally.

7. Prior to performing any comparisons of blood proteins, a pattern of temporal changes in these proteins (reliability study) has to be determined in order to discriminate between meaningful changes and potential normal fluctuations.

8. Blood samples have to be collected in maximally uniform way to allow for comparisons among sera from different sources.

9. To enable the comparisons, subjects in experimental and control populations should be optimally matched. Matching should be performed based on at least gender and age. When hormones are studied in women, it is recommended to analyze postmenopausal and premenopausal populations separately. In some cases, matching is based on hormone replacement therapy (HRT) in women. Additionally, matching on smoking status, disease status, and other parameters has to be performed when possible.

10. Standard multiparametric curves developed by Bio-Rad Laboratories for Bio-Plex reader (http://www.bio-rad.com/LifeScience/pdf/Bulletin_2861.pdf)) are designed to provide optimal fit throughout the entire standard range. The type of logistic equation that will yield the best fit through a set of points is dependent on the shape of the standard curve.

If the curve is S-shaped and symmetrical (i.e., similar shapes on both ends of the "S"), a 4PL or 5PL regression will yield similar results. When the curve is not symmetrical, as in low- and high-response curves, a better fit will be achieved using a 5PL regression.

11. Therefore, the researcher has responsibility to provide adequate controls to be able to compare different analyses performed on different dates. When a large study is planned within 6–12 month period, it is best to preorder the appropriate number of kits so that the same lots of reagents are used throughout the study. However, even if all reagents utilized are of the same lot, the run-to-run (intra-assay) variability may occur due to the following reasons: a. Differences in reconstitution of lyophilized standards; b. Differences in day-to-day calibration of Bio-Plex reader, etc. To circumvent these problems, it is highly recommended to use a set of quality controls, i.e., serum samples representing the whole range of analyte concentrations that have to be analyzed with each run, preferably on each plate. There should be minimum 6 of such controls, 3 representing the low concentration range and 3 representing the high range. Including these quality controls will allow for scaling and normalization of run-to-run data to ensure low inter-run variability and allow run-to-run comparisons.

References

1. Doll, R., and R. Peto, Epidemiology of Cancer. Oxford Textbook of Medicine. ed. by Warrell, D., et al., 4th edition (2003). OUP: Oxford

2. Key, T.J., Hormones and cancer in humans. Mutat Res, (1995). 333(1–2): 59–67.

3. Hankinson, S.E., Endogenous hormones and risk of breast cancer in postmenopausal women. Breast Dis, (2005). 24: p. 3–15.

4. Portier, C.J., Endocrine dismodulation and cancer. Neuro Endocrinol Lett, (2002). 23 Suppl 2: p. 43–7.

5. Arslan, A.A., et al., Reliability of follicle-stimulating hormone measurements in serum. Reprod Biol Endocrinol, (2003). 1: p. 49.

6. Choi, J.H., et al., Overexpression of follicle-stimulating hormone receptor activates oncogenic pathways in preneoplastic ovarian surface epithelial cells. J Clin Endocrinol Metab, (2004). 89(11): p. 5508–16.

7. Chu, S., et al., FSH-regulated gene expression profiles in ovarian tumours and normal ovaries. Mol Hum Reprod, (2002). 8(5): p. 426–33.

8. Davies, S., et al., Regulation of endometrial cancer cell growth by luteinizing hormone (LH) and follicle stimulating hormone (FSH). Br J Cancer, (2000). 83(12): p. 1730–4.

9. Cramer, D.W., et al., Characteristics of women with a family history of ovarian cancer. II. Follicular phase hormone levels. Cancer, (1994). 74(4): p. 1318–22.

10. Krieg, R.J., Jr., J.P. Rogers, Jr., and H.R. Seibel, Influence of a prolactin- and ACTH-secreting tumour on oestrous cyclicity, the pro-oestrous surges of LH and prolactin and ovarian hypertrophy in the rat. J Endocrinol, (1987). 114(1): p. 41–8.

11. Hargadine, H.R., J.M. Lowenstein, and F.S. Greenspan, Elevated serum TSH in human thyroid cancer. Oncology, (1970). 24(3): p. 172–80.

13. Biondi, B., S. Filetti, and M. Schlumberger, Thyroid-hormone therapy and thyroid cancer: a reassessment. Nat Clin Pract Endocrinol Metab, (2005). 1(1): p. 32–40.

14. Chia, S.Y., et al., TSH receptor mRNA measurement in blood as a marker for circulating

thyroid cancer cells and its role in the preoperative diagnosis of thyroid cancer. J Clin Endocrinol Metab, (2007). 92(2): p. 468–75.

15. Tarquini, B., et al., Mammary cancer risk: circulating TSH and prolactin, fibrocystic breast disease in chronoepidemiologic perspective. Cancer Detect Prev, (1981). 4(1–4): p. 525–34.

16. Ormandy, C.J., et al., Null mutation of the prolactin receptor gene produces multiple reproductive defects in the mouse. Genes Dev, (1997). 11(2): p. 167–78.

17. Ormandy, C.J., et al., Coexpression and cross-regulation of the prolactin receptor and sex steroid hormone receptors in breast cancer. J Clin Endocrinol Metab, (1997). 82(11): p. 3692–9.

18. Peters, G., et al., IGF-1R, IGF-1 and IGF-2 expression as potential prognostic and predictive markers in colorectal-cancer. Virchows Arch, (2003). 443(2): p. 139–45.

19. Baffa, R., et al., Low serum insulin-like growth factor 1 (IGF-1): a significant association with prostate cancer. Tech Urol, (2000). 6(3): p. 236–9.

20. Jenkins, P.J., A. Mukherjee, and S.M. Shalet, Does growth hormone cause cancer? Clin Endocrinol (Oxf), (2006). 64(2): p. 115–21.

21. Han, J.Y., et al., The prognostic significance of pretreatment plasma levels of insulin-like growth factor (IGF)-1, IGF-2, and IGF binding protein-3 in patients with advanced non-small cell lung cancer. Lung Cancer, (2006). 54(2): p. 227–34.

22. Imura, H., Y. Nakai, and H. Takahashi, [Hormone production and abnormalities in gene expression in tumors]. Gan To Kagaku Ryoho, (1986). 13(3 Pt 2): p. 721–30.

23. Vignali, D.A., Multiplexed particle-based flow cytometric assays. J Immunol Methods, (2000). 243(1–2): p. 243–55.

24. Earley, M.C., et al., Report from a workshop on multianalyte microsphere assays. Cytometry, (2002). 50(5): p. 239–42.

25. Seideman, J. and D. Peritt, A novel monoclonal antibody screening method using the Luminex-100 microsphere system. J Immunol Methods, (2002). 267(2): p. 165–71.

26. Jones, L.P., et al., Multiplex assay for detection of strain-specific antibodies against the two variable regions of the G protein of respiratory syncytial virus. Clin Diagn Lab Immunol, (2002). 9(3): p. 633–8.

27. Pickering, J.W., et al., A multiplexed fluorescent microsphere immunoassay for antibodies to pneumococcal capsular polysaccharides. Am J Clin Pathol, (2002). 117(4): p. 589–96.

Chapter 10

High-Throughput Analysis of Serum Antigens Using Sandwich ELISAs on Microarrays

Shannon L. Servoss, Rachel Gonzalez, Susan Varnum, and Richard C. Zangar

Summary

Enzyme-linked immunosorbent assay (ELISA) microarrays promise to be a powerful tool for the detection and validation of disease biomarkers. ELISA microarrays are capable of simultaneous detection of many proteins using a small sample volume. Although there are many potential pitfalls to the use of ELISA microarrays, these can be avoided by careful planning of experiments. In this chapter we describe a high-throughput protocol for processing ELISA microarrays that will result in reliable and reproducible data.

Key words: ELISA microarray, Antibody microarray, High throughput.

1. Introduction

With the large amounts of data generated from the combined efforts of sequencing the genome and analyzing the genome via DNA microarrays, there is an increasing emphasis on relating these data to functional changes in key proteins *(1–6)*. Because mRNA expression levels and functional protein expression often do not correlate well *(7–9)*, these studies must be done at the protein level. Immunoassays, such as enzyme-linked immunosorbent assay (ELISA), are commonly used for single-protein detection, but require large sample volumes for detecting multiple proteins. In order to match the rapid progression of genomics, a high-throughput technique for analysis of the proteome is needed *(1–6)*.

Sandwich ELISA microarrays, a miniaturized version of the standard 96-well plate ELISA protocol, allow for the simultaneous

Michael A. Tainsky, *Methods in Molecular Biology, Tumor Biomarker Discovery, Vol. 520*
© Humana Press, a part of Springer Science+Business Media, LLC 2009
DOI: 10.1007/978-1-60327-811-9_10

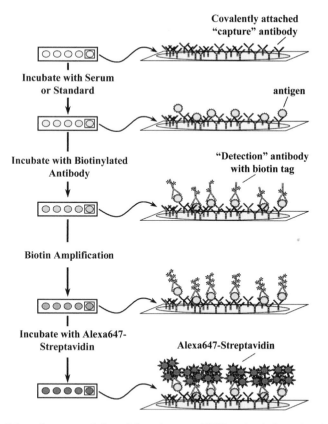

Fig. 1. Schematic representation of the microarray ELISA protocol. Reproduced with permission from *(13)*.

screening of many proteins (up to ~50) within a small sample volume (~15 μL after dilution). **Figure 1** shows a schematic overview of this protocol. For sandwich ELISAs, the target protein is captured via a surface-immobilized antibody. A second labeled antibody, specific for a different epitope on the same protein, is used for detection. The signal is amplified using an enzymatic reaction and is detected using fluorescence. ELISA microarrays have the potential to achieve pg/mL or better sensitivity with amplification *(6)*. ELISA microarrays promise to be an excellent method for the detection and validation of biomarkers.

2. Materials

2.1. Array Printing

1. Aminosilane-coated slides preprinted with hydrophobic patching – Erie Scientific (Portsmouth, NH).
2. Disuccinimidyl suberate or DSS – Pierce (Rockford, IL).

3. Dimethyl sulfoxide or DMSO – Sigma-Aldrich (St. Louis, MO).

4. HPLC-grade methanol – Fisher Scientific (Hampton, NH).

5. Slide rack: Tissue Tek H4465 24-slide holder – VWR (West Chester, PA).

6. Incubation chamber: Tissue Tek H4455 Staining dish – VWR.

7. GeSiM NanoPlotter 2.1 – Quantum Analytics (Foster City, CA).

8. Tip wash solution: 200 mM Sodium Hydroxide – Sigma-Aldrich.

9. Antibodies – multiple sources.

10. Orientation spot: IgG-conjugated Alexa633 – Invitrogen (Carlsbad, CA).

11. Block solution: 10 mg/mL casein in phosphate-buffered saline, or PBS – Bio-Rad (Hercules, CA).

12. PBS-T wash solution: 0.05% Tween 20 (Sigma Aldrich) in phosphate-buffered saline, pH ~ 7.2 (NERL Diagnostics; available through VWR).

2.2. Slide Processing

1. Antigens – multiple sources.

2. Biotinylated detection antibodies – multiple sources.

3. Tyramide Signal Amplification kit, containing streptavidin-conjugated horse radish peroxidase (StAv-HRP), biotinyltyramide, and amplification diluent – Perkin Elmer (Boston, MA).

4. Streptavidin-conjugated Alexa647 (StAv-A647) – Invitrogen.

5. ScanArray Express HT microarray scanner – Perkin Elmer.

2.3. Data Analysis

1. ScanArray Express software – Perkin Elmer.

2. ProMAT software – available for no charge at http://www.pnl.gov/statistics/ProMAT.

3. Methods

While the methods for sandwich ELISA microarray are well established, scale-up for high-throughput processing can be problematic. However, by following the steps outlined later it is possible to process 24 + slides (or 384 chips) in a single experiment and obtain reliable and reproducible data. All slide incubation and wash steps utilize the slide rack and incubation chamber unless otherwise noted.

3.1. Array Printing

1. In order to create a covalent binding site, the aminosilane slides can be activated with the homobifunctional crosslinker DSS (*see* **Note 1**). This activation results in the formation of amine reactive NHS-esters (*see* **Notes 2** and **3**).

2. Dissolve the desired amount (see next step) of DSS in 0.5–1.0 mL of DMSO (*see* **Note 4**).

3. Place the appropriate amount of HPLC-grade methanol in an incubation chamber, create a vortex using a magnetic stir bar, and add DSS-DMSO solution for a final concentration of 0.2 mg DSS/mL.

4. Place the slides in the slide rack and immerse in the DSS solution. Incubate the slides for 5 min at room temperature.

5. Rinse the slides twice in fresh HPLC-grade methanol (*see* **Note 5**) and centrifuge dry at $500 \times g$ for 30 s in a centrifuge that is designed to spin multiwelled microplates.

6. Suspend each antibody in PBS, or other amine-free buffer (*see* **Note 6**), to 0.5–1.0 mg/mL (*see* **Note 7**). Dispense 5–15 mL of antibody into a 384-well flat bottom plate in the order they are to be printed (*see* **Note 8**).

7. We recommend using a noncontact printer, such as the GeSiM NanoPlotter 2.1, for spotting antibodies. The humidity for this printer should be maintained at ~60% using an external humidifier and controller/sensor. In order to prevent reagent evaporation, the plate cooler should be set at 1–3°C above the dew point (*see* **Note 9**). Sixteen arrays can be printed on a single slide, with 9 mm spacing between arrays to allow for the use of a multichannel pipette for reagent addition. Set the pitch (spacing between spot centers) to 400–500 mm. Washing of the tips between spotting reagents is essential to preventing crosscontamination (*see* **Note 10**).

8. Leave the slides in the printer at ~60% humidity for 1 h after printing in order to allow for completion of the antibody immobilization reaction.

9. Using a ScanArray Express HT, scan with the Red Reflect setting to confirm successful spotting of reagents.

10. Quickly immerse slides in block solution (*see* **Note 11**). Incubate slides in block solution at room temperature for 1 h or at 4°C overnight.

11. Immerse slides in PBS-T. Transfer to fresh PBS-T and incubate for 2 min.

12. At this point the slides can either be used immediately, as described later, or stored for later use. For storage, quickly dip rinse slides twice in deionized water, spin dry at $500 \times g$ for 30 s on each side in a plate centrifuge, and place in vacuum-sealed bag with desiccant. Slides should be stored at −20°C

until ready to use. We have found that slides are stable for at least 3 months.

3.2. Slide Processing

All incubation steps are conducted at room temperature.

1. If slides were stored at –20°C, allow them to come to room temperature prior to opening sealed bag, removing the required slides, and resealing and freezing any unused slides.

2. Immerse slides in PBS-T and incubate for 2–5 min. Aspirate excess fluid from chips.

3. Prepare samples and standards, making all dilutions in 0.1× block solution. Standards should be diluted fourfold with at least seven dilutions plus an antigen-free blank. Serum samples should be run at multiple dilutions to cover the wide range of protein concentrations (e.g., 5×, 100×, and 2,000× dilutions). Add 15 μL of sample or standard to the chips, each in triplicate. Incubate with gentle mixing (on Belly Dancer), covered, in a humid chamber (*see* **Note 12**) overnight (12–16 h).

4. Aspirate sample from chips. Immerse slides in PBS-T. Transfer to fresh PBS-T and incubate for 2–5 min.

5. Immerse slides in detection antibody solution. For our studies, each biotinylated detection antibody is typically used at 25 ng/mL. Incubate the slides for 2 h.

6. Immerse slides in PBS-T. Transfer to fresh PBS-T and incubate for 2–5 min.

7. Immerse slides in StAv-HRP, diluted 1:99 in PBS-T. Incubate for 30 min.

8. Immerse slides in PBS-T. Transfer to fresh PBS-T and incubate for 2 min. Repeat wash twice. Aspirate excess fluid from chips.

9. To each chip, add 15 mL of biotinyltyramide, diluted 1:99 in amplification diluent (*see* **Note 13**). Incubate with rapid mixing on Belly Dancer, covered, in a humid chamber for 10 min (*see* **Note 14**).

10. Immerse slides in PBS-T. Transfer to fresh PBS-T and incubate for 2 min.

11. Immerse slides in StAv-A647, diluted to 1 mg/mL in PBS-T. Incubate for 30 min.

12. Immerse slides in PBS-T. Transfer to fresh PBS-T and incubate for 10 min. Rinse slides quickly twice in deionized water. Immediately centrifuge dry at $500 \times g$ for 30 s on each side. Dry for 30 min in a vacuum chamber (*see* **Note 15**).

13. Scan slides for A647 using Perkin Elmer ScanArray Express HT.

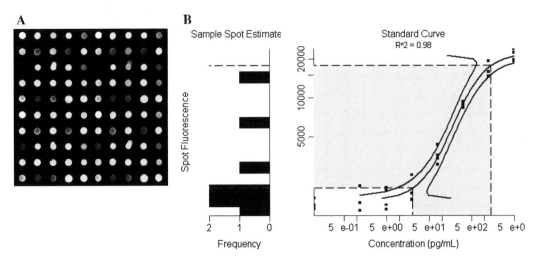

Fig. 2. (**A**) Representative image of an ELISA microarray chip and (**B**) ProMAT output image that can be used to quickly assess the data quality. The shaded area on the "Standard Curve" graph shows the optimal usable range of this curve. The "Sample Spot Estimate" histogram shows the distribution of the signal intensities for the samples and provides a rapid method for assessing how well these values fall within the usable range of the standard curve.

3.3. Data Analysis

1. Quantify images using ScanArray Express software (*see* **Note 16**). Save the resulting spreadsheet as a .csv file.

2. ProMAT version 2.0, a custom software we developed for the analysis of ELISA microarray data, is used to fit the standard curves and predict sample concentrations *(10, 11)*. Using ProMAT, the standard curves can be fit using various models, including 4-parameter logistic, power, linear, or spline. We find that the best fits are typically obtained by selecting 4-parameter logistic with spline back-up in the rare case that the data do not converge to the model. **Figure 2** shows an example of a typical standard curve and sample predictions as generated by ProMAT.

4. Notes

1. The water-soluble form of DSS, bis[sulfosuccinimidyl] suberate or BS3, can also be used. However, BS3 is significantly more expensive than DSS and is less practical for processing large numbers of slides.

2. NHS esters are liable to hydrolysis. Therefore, for optimal results, printing on activated slides should be completed within 12 h of activation.

3. Microarrays of comparable quality can also be obtained by using untreated aminosilane or poly-l-lysine slides (Seurynck-Servoss, Baird, Rodland, and Zangar; unpublished data). Therefore, the crosslinking step can be considered optional.

4. DSS is not readily soluble in methanol. Therefore, it is first dissolved in DMSO to allow for rapid dissolution.

5. The same methanol solutions can be used for multiple rinses. After repeated use, the second rinse should replace the first rinse and use fresh methanol for the second rinse. The use of HPLC-grade methanol is necessary to maintain residue-free surfaces, which in turn is essential for consistent printing results.

6. Amine-containing buffers, such as Tris–HCl, will compete for reactive sites and result in reduced antibody binding.

7. The inclusion of any agent that prevents spot drying or encourages spot spreading, such as glycerol or surfactant, to the antibody solution can result in poor spot morphology. Carrier proteins, such as albumin, should also be avoided as they will compete for binding sites on the slide surface and thereby reduce antibody binding.

8. For the GeSiM printer, it is best if capture antibodies are loaded left to right and top to bottom, leaving no gaps between wells. To ease the quantification process, always print an orientation spot in the upper left corner of each array.

9. A dew point calculator is available at http://www.decatur.de/javascript/dew/index.html.

10. We find that programming the GeSiM printer to wash the tips between spotting reagents with water for 30 s, followed by a 10-s incubation with 2 µL of 200 mM NaOH, and then a second wash with water for 30 s will prevent reagent carryover.

11. Immersing the slides in the block solution slowly can result in the formation of comets. For blocking, the slides should be immersed as rapidly as possible without causing major turbulence in the block solution.

12. A sealable plastic container with a damp paper towel in the bottom can be used as a humid chamber. Separate the slides from the paper towel using a thin sheet of plastic.

13. Biotinyltyramide should be diluted immediately prior to use to prevent side reactions.

14. Longer incubation times with biotinyltyramide may increase slide noise and/or background.

15. In order to obtain stable fluorescence, it is necessary to dry the slides completely.

16. During quantitation, only have one image opened at a time for data output to be compatible with ProMAT.

Acknowledgements

Supported by National Institutes of Health grants R01 EB006177 and U01 CA117378 and contract Y1-CN-5014.

References

1. Angenendt, P. (2005) Progress in protein and antibody microarray technology. Drug Discovery Today, 10, 503–511.

2. Barry, R. and Soloviev, M. (2004) Quantitative protein profiling using antibody arrays. Proteomics, 4, 3717–3726.

3. Kingsmore, S.F. (2006) Multiplexed protein measurement: Technologies and applications of protein and antibody arrays. Nature Reviews Drug Discovery, 5, 310–320.

4. Kreutzberger, J. (2006) Protein microarrays: A chance to study microorganisms? Applied Microbiology and Biotechnology, 70, 383–390.

5. Stoll, D., Templin, M.F., Schrenk, M., Traub, P.C., Vohringer, C.F. and Joos, T.O. (2002) Protein microarray technology. Frontiers in Bioscience, 7, C13–C32.

6. Zangar, R.C., Daly, D.S. and White, A.M. (2006) ELISA microarray technology as a high-throughput system for cancer biomarker validation. Expert Review of Proteomics, 3, 37–44.

7. Anderson, G.P., Jacoby, M.A., Ligler, F.S. and King, K.D. (1997) Effectiveness of protein A for antibody immobilization for a fiber optic biosensor. Biosensors and Bioelectronics, 12, 329–336.

8. Gygi, S.P., Rochon, Y., Franza, B.R. and Aebersold, R. (1999) Correlation between protein and mRNA abundance in yeast. Molecular and Cellular Biology, 19, 1720–1730.

9. Le Naour, F., Hohenkirk, L., Grolleau, A., Misek, D.E., Lescure, P., Geiger, J.D., Hanash, S. and Beretta, L. (2001) Profiling changes in gene expression during differentiation and maturation of monocyte-derived dendritic cells using both oligonucleotide microarrays and proteomics. Journal of Biological Chemistry, 276, 17920–17931.

10. Daly, D.S., White, A.M., Varnum, S.M., Anderson, K.K. and Zangar, R.C. (2005) Evaluating concentration estimation errors in ELISA microarray experiments. BMC Bioinformatics, 6, 17.

11. White, A.M., Daly, D.S., Varnum, S.M., Anderson, K.K., Bollinger, N. and Zangar, R.C. (2006) ProMAT: protein microarray analysis tool. Bioinformatics, 22, 1278–1279.

12. Woodbury, R.L, Varnum, S.M., Zangar, R.C. (2002) Elevated HGF levels in sera from breast cancer patients detected using a protein microarray ELISA. Journal of Proteome Research, 1, 233–237.

Chapter 11

Tissue Microarrays as a Tool in the Discovery and Validation of Tumor Markers

Stephen M. Hewitt

Summary

Tissue microarrays are a platform of condensed histopathology that has revolutionized the translation of basic science to clinical utility. Tissue microarrays have resulted in a paradigm shift from histopathology to immunopathology and moved analysis of small selected samples sets of tens of specimens to a high-throughput environment of hundreds of specimens. Tissue microarrays have influenced validation strategies, but have a role in discovery as well, allowing a pathways approach to analysis of tumors.

Key words: Tissue microarray, Immunohistochemistry, Pathology, Histology, Tumor, Formalin-fixed paraffin-embedded tissue.

1. Introduction

Identification of tumor markers is but one step of the process to improved patient outcomes in cancer. There are a plethora of tools and models for the identification of tumor markers. The discovery process for a tumor marker is a complex multistep process. An essential step in the process is generalization of any finding to a larger set of samples, ultimately within the context of the disease process (cancer).

With cancer, ultimately a tumor marker is related to the tumor – either the marker is derived from the tumor cells themselves or is in response to the tumor's presence. Cancer is a disease of proliferative cells, and hence the examination of tissue, via histopathology, is a key element of diagnosis, prognosis, and prediction of response to therapy. We have the inherent advantage

Michael A. Tainsky, *Methods in Molecular Biology, Tumor Biomarker Discovery, Vol. 520*
© Humana Press, a part of Springer Science + Business Media, LLC 2009
DOI: 10.1007/978-1-60327-811-9_11

of being able to visualize, with the aid of a microscope, the cancer cells, and distinguish how they are different for the normal tissue. Traditionally this has been purely based on histomorphology, the appearance of the cells at the light microscope level after the application of a simple stain, such as an H&E.

The tissue microarray (TMA) has revolutionized this process. The process remains cell based; however, the shift is now from histomorphology to presence of specific proteins as detected most commonly by immunohistochemistry. A TMA is a relatively simple construct of cores of tissue extracted from tissue blocks and reinserted into a recipient block *(1)*. This TMA block is then sectioned to yield a TMA slide which can then be subject to any analysis that is routinely applied to tissue. The key elements are that the selection of the tissue removed is directed and that its placement in the recipient is directed so that the array is an organized structure.

2. What Can Be Placed in a TMA?

Virtually any biologic specimen can be arrayed. Although rare, TMAs can be constructed of plant material and other biologic specimens. The majority of TMAs are constructed of archival human tissue obtained from departments of pathology *(2)*. This is the same tissue that is removed for therapeutic and diagnostic considerations in the process of medical care. Autopsy tissue is routinely encountered; however, the rate of autopsy in the US has declined significantly, not to mention issues of tissue quality with prolonged postmortem times (so-called warm ischemia times), making this tissue less useful and less plentiful than many researchers believe.

Use of human tissue requires appropriate ethical review and safeguards. The guidelines and rules for use of human diagnostic pathology material vary greatly at the local, state, and national levels. The subject is too complex to review here, but if you are constructing a TMA, it is imperative to obtain appropriate approvals and implement safeguards on patient identities. If you are obtaining a TMA, you must ensure you follow the rules and regulations of your institution, in addition to those of the source institution.

Just because a tumor has a described natural history, does not mean that samples of the tumor are available in the archives of your local pathology department. With the advances in diagnostic modalities, especially radiology, not to mention the advances of treatment for cancer beyond surgery (radio- and chemotherapy), many tumors, especially metastatic tumors are rarely resected, or even biopsied, and as a result are not available for inclusion in TMAs. For those interested in construction of progression-related TMA; multi-institutional studies, potentially with tissue procurement protocols, should be considered *(3)*.

Although human tumors are the most common source of tissue for TMAs, other tumor models systems are routinely encountered. Mouse tissue, is routinely utilized for the construction of TMAs, either consisting of tumors from transgenic lines, or other rodent tumor model systems. Dogs are routinely utilized as a model for some human cancers, including osteosarcoma and lymphoma. Typically these are companion animals, pets in the community, and their tissue is obtained in the same means as human tissue – from diagnostic and therapeutic interventions *(4)*.

Beyond tumor and normal tissue, the most commonly arrayed specimens are cell lines and xenografts. Cell line arrays (CMAs) are routinely constructed from panels of cell lines either as stand-alone platforms for research or inclusion as controls in other TMAs. The NCI60, a panel of 60 cell lines used by the NCI for screening of chemotherapeutic agents, has been arrayed *(2)*. As an extension of this, xenograft arrays (XMAs) can be constructed from tumors transplanted into mice *(2, 5)*.

3. What Is Appropriate Material for a TMA?

TMAs are routinely constructed of formalin-fixed, paraffin-embedded tissue *(1, 6)*. Frozen tissue can be utilized *(7)*; however, it is an extremely delicate resource, and the challenges of constructing a TMA of frozen tissue, let alone its storage, generally prevent the construction of frozen-tissue-based TMA. After reading this chapter, it should be apparent when a frozen tissue TMA is appropriate, and when not.

Alternative fixatives for paraffin-embedded tissues are routinely encountered both in research and clinical care environments. Ethanol as a fixative, typically employed as a 70% solution, in place of 10% neutral buffered formalin is an excellent choice for some studies *(8)*. Other fixatives have been utilized; however, they tend to result in hard tissues, which, especially in older archival material, tend to crumble and produce suboptimal arrays. Bouin's fixative is an acid-based fixative and should be avoided on this account *(6)*. Decalcification is a common issue. There are two common methods of decalcification: acid and EDTA. Neither are perfect and both are documented to damage some antigens; however; EDTA seems to be preferred in the construction of TMAs *(6)*.

Regardless of the choice of fixative, it is important, at a minimum to know which tissue samples are fixed in what fixative;

otherwise, appropriate staining conditions for immunohistochemistry are illusive. Differences in tissue handling and processing can impart enormous impacts on immunohistochemical assays, and these problems become magnified on TMAs *(9)*. Often there is little a researcher can do but be aware of these pitfalls. If possible, it is best to avoid mixing tissues with different types of fixation on a TMA. If this is not possible, grouping them by fixative may assist in debugging assays and interpretation.

4. What Assays Can Be Applied to a TMA?

If you can perform the assay on a piece of tissue on a microscope slide, you can probably apply it to a TMA. The vast majority of assays on TMAs are immunohistochemical stains. Routine histochemical stains, most commonly an H&E stain, are frequently applied.

In situ assays, either for RNA or DNA, visualized either by radioactivity, fluorescence, ECL, or chromagenic means, can be applied to a TMA *(10–12)*. In situ assays are less frequently employed as an application largely because the complexity of assay renders them rare in general, replaced by PCR, as well as the complexity of interpretation. Interpretation of in situ assays is frequently performed at high magnification, and the high density of TMAs makes data collection tedious in the absence of sophisticated imaging systems. Although DNA quality is rarely a problem, RNA quality in formalin-fixed tissue can be a limiting issue for low abundance transcripts; however, the literature does document detection and quantification of such transcripts by in situ hybridization *(10, 11)*.

Other assays, including Fourier transform infrared spectroscopy and Raman spectroscopy, have been applied to TMAs *(13)*. These are examples where the TMA platform has truly enabled the technology by providing the high-throughput platform required for analysis. Two assays that in general should not be interpreted on TMAs are mitotic counts and vessel density assays for angiogenesis *(14)*. Both of these assays depend on determining an average number of events per fields observed, and the core sizes are inadequate of an appropriate sampling.

5. Adequacy of Number and Size

One of the most common questions asked of those who work with TMAs routinely is how do you determine how many samples and what core size to construct the TMA. The simplest answer is "more is better." In general a larger number of samples is more important than larger cores. We typically do not construct TMAs of less than 25 samples and from a statistical point of view, for determining a difference between two groups, 50 total samples divided equally two groups is optimal. The TARP lab does not place more than 500 cores of 0.6-mm diameter on a single section for technical reasons in manufacture, assay performance, and interpretation. Rarely does an investigator have more than 500 samples, and as the number of samples dwindles, the core size should increase. With the advent of new arrayers and a larger community or researchers, guidelines are becoming more difficult to reach consensus on.

Arguments of adequate tissue sample size are common. The simple fact is that tissue always has some level of heterogeneity, and different cells are of different sizes, not to mention admixture with normal cells, blood vessels, and stroma. For any marker, the adequacy of sampling is independent and can only be determined by experimentation and comparison to whole sections, for which there is a reasonable outcome measure, most commonly survival. As a rule of thumb, a 0.6-mm core to tissue contains ~1,500 epithelial cancer cells. If 5% of the cells express the given marker, that is 75 positive cells. For reference, many CMAs are constructed to contain between 100 and 300 cells. There are two exceptions that require mention. TMAs of osteosarcoma are best constructed with 1.0-mm needles as the needle wall thickness is optimal for strength and the cores are not so large as to be excessively cracked. CMAs are frequently constructed with only 0.6-mm or 1.0-mm needles as the cores offer no histomorphology and are limited to cytomorphology, requiring a minimum of 200× total magnification.

6. Why Would I Need a TMA?

All roads lead to a TMA, or so it would seem in some instances. In fact, when working with tumor markers, all roads lead to testing in patient samples and most commonly today, before a tumor marker is tested in patient samples it is screened on a TMA *(2)*. The genesis of TMAs was to screen tumor markers against human samples *(1)*, and in general this remains the main use; however, how an investigator comes to interrogate a TMA has changed over time.

The schema of arriving at a TMA experiment can be described in two ways – mechanistically – what experiments lead you to a TMA, or theoretically, what is the utility of a TMA. The theoretic will be discussed first, followed by the common mechanistic examples.

Tumor markers are generally broken into three groups: diagnostic, prognostic, and predictive (15). Diagnostic markers are those that render a finding of the presence or type of disease. This was anticipated to be significant role for TMAs – identification of new tumor markers; however, there is limited need for new diagnostic markers. Cancer vs. benign is frequently easily distinguished, and few protein biomarkers have utility discriminating cancer vs. benign. There remain questions of tumor origin (lineage), and TMAs have demonstrated utility (16) in development of these markers but it is not a common use.

Prognostic markers are those that predict the natural behavior of a tumor. In clinical care, grade and stage of a malignancy are used to prognosticate the behavior of a tumor and guide the decision process of treatment. TMAs excel at the development of new tumor markers that are prognostic. There is a debate about the utility of prognostic markers, where they forecast the behavior of a tumor, but are not useful in making a medical decision. Nonetheless, TMAs are most commonly used in description of tumor behavior, either linked to outcome, or in some instances description of signaling pathways of growth and differentiation. The test of a marker for this utility is its capacity to add knowledge. Markers that provide information that is not greater than what can be determined by grade and stage are of little value (15).

Lastly are predictive markers: these are markers that can predict a response to a specific treatment, predict toxicity, or are used a decision point in clinical care. These biomarkers directly predict the individual's response to a set of conditions and are more commonly directed at drugable targets. Development of predictive markers is complex and multistep, and is central to the approach of personalized medicine.

Mechanistically, how investigators find themselves needing a TMA is even more complex. Routinely TMAs are used more as a validation tool than a discovery tool; however, they can be applied for raw discovery. The process of discovery with a TMA is to collect a series of markers and apply them to a TMA in an effort to discern some function. Typically this is accomplished by applying antibodies of markers that have been described in the literature as having a theoretic or predicted interaction, or the antibody reagent is new. Currently a wide-scale screening approach is underway with the human protein atlas, where antibodies to all predicted peptides are being generated and screened on TMAs of normal tissue and tumors (www.proteinatlas.org).

More commonly the approach for an investigator is to carry out some discovery method (described in the other chapters of this text) then seeking to confirm and generalize the finding. Although that appears to be a common path, different discovery approaches alter the nature of validation.

Most commonly expression microarrays have been the discovery platform that generate interest in the application of a TMA. The general advantage is that if immunohistochemistry is employed, the validation moves from transcriptional to proteomic *(17, 18)*. The downside to this is twofold, (a) you have to have an antibody to the encoded protein and (b) the correspondence of transcriptional upregulation to upregulation at the protein level is limited. Simply put, for every target shown upregulated at the transcriptional level, flip a coin to predict its status at the protein. There are multiple levels of biologic control between transcription and the presence of protein in a cell, compounded with the nature of detection of the protein with immunohistochemistry. One advantage of the TMA approach is that it significantly extends the number of specimens examined. Expression array experiments are typically performed on limited numbers of samples (tens), while validation on a TMA will routinely involve hundreds of samples which can easily cover the spectrum of tumor grade and stage. In the event an antibody is not available, or cannot be logically developed, RNA in situ hybridization can be utilized to validate the expression array. As assays for mRNA have had limited clinical adoption, the approach of porting a discovery from the transcriptome to proteome has been more popular.

Increasingly proteomic methodologies are being applied to discovery of tumor biomarkers, and TMAs again are called on to validate results. For those methods that are not based on the use of antibodies, the approach and utility is similar to expression arrays: identification of an antibody against the target and validation against a larger cohort of tissue. In the instance where the original discovery methodology included the use of an affinity reagent, the tumor marker is already at the proteomic level. Here the success of validation seems improved, as the issues of transcriptome and proteome concordance are not at play *(19)*. Most commonly antibody array and reverse-phase array discovery methods are supplying targets for the TMA analysis.

Lastly, there is the issue of where discovery begins and validation ends. Demonstration of a tumor marker having utility in a single cohort is not sufficient to see its introduction into clinical care *(2)*. Most candidate tumor markers are first screened on TMAs without clinical information that allows simple determination of expression pattern and prevalence in a statistically relevant number of specimens. If they warrant further investigation, they are typically tested on a specific tumor panel for which clinical information (outcome) is available to determine utility. If the tumor marker is a predictive marker, additional cohorts from clinical trials of patients who did and did not respond to the therapy are generally pursued. Lastly, and unfortunately not commonly enough, a tumor marker should be screened on population-based tumor TMAs that allow calculation of real prevalence rates for the marker and identification of populations with specific profiles *(20)*.

7. Building, Buying, or Collaborating on a TMA?

Investigators have typically one of two reactions to planning to use a TMA: "I will build my own," or "I will buy one," but fail to consider collaboration. There are pros and cons of each, outlined as follows. Ultimately the answer should be at least two of the three options, as revalidation on a second independent cohort is an essential element of generalizing a novel finding.

Although construction of a TMA is not particularly challenging, obtaining the tissue is not simple, and optimally a histopathologist should review slides of the donor blocks before construction of the TMA. The instrumentation for array construction is becoming more common and more affordable; however, purchase of an arrayer is a poor investment if only one array or a few targets are to be explored. From an economic point of view, TMAs are best produced in high-volume environments where the appropriate team of researchers, pathologists, and technical staff can be assembled. This is not to dissuade construction of a TMA, but rather to temper the enthusiasm with the challenges.

Purchase of a TMA is simple: get on the web and go. Numerous vendors offer TMAs of a wide variety of tumors and normal tissues. You get what you paid for. TMAs with large numbers of specimens and extensive clinical information are very expensive. Vendors are only able to obtain a limited number of high-quality (> 90% of cores present) sections and have cost associated with obtaining the material, annotation of outcome, and construction of the TMA. Other TMAs of good quality are generally available, but may lack clinical information. For some purposes, this is fine, and in other instances, will not address the question. Unfortunately there are too many cut-rate TMAs constructed of tissue obtain from undocumented sources. The phrase "junk in, junk out" best describes these TMAs. Tissue is fundamentally a reagent and must be of appropriate quality to yield valid results. In general commercial TMAs are a useful resource and provide a stepping stone in the process of confirming a finding, but fail to produce a strong test in a clinically relevant cohort of patients.

The best analogy of TMA slides is that they are like baseball trading cards. You do not need ten identical Mickey Mantles, and would happily trade a Mantle for a Hank Aaron, if you do not have one in your collection. Very few projects require all the TMA sections that are produced, and collaboration via sharing TMAs is an effective means of leveraging the expense and effort that goes into construction of a high-quality TMA. Currently there are no TMA "clearing houses," but in general it is not difficult to identify a group that might have an appropriate TMA from the literature. Alternatively, if tissue is available, a researcher should investigate developing a collaboration with a TMA core lab to produce a new TMA. Often the TMA core lab will retain a block for their own use, or to develop other collaborations, and produce one or more for the collaborator who initiates the project and provides the tissue.

Mentioned previously was the issue of ethical approval to use human tissue in research, but equally important, and too frequently ignored are the contractual obligations of sharing research tissue that are an element of academic collaborations. Typically referred to as Material Transfer Agreements (MTAs) these are the contractual agreements that stipulate ownership, intellectual property rights, allowed uses, and agreements on publication of material obtained from collaboration. Many investigators tend to ignore them, at their own peril. Large multi-institutional collaborative TMAs are frequently delayed because of issues in obtaining the MTAs. In some instances one MTA is required for construction of the array, and a separate MTA will be utilized for distribution of the TMA slides.

8. Have TMA, What Next?

Once a researcher has the TMA and has chosen the assay to perform, the real work begins. TMAs have taught researchers more about assays and specimen quality than anticipated *(18)*. It is very easy and common to discover a failure in the reagents and assays that was previously unanticipated. All assays on TMAs should be repeated in some fashion. Pilot arrays on sections of lower quality (fewer cores) are highly recommended as a means of fine tuning an assay and not wasting valuable resources.

Regardless of the assay, the real challenge is interpretation of the results and analysis of the data. TMAs are tissues and contain cytomorphologic and histomorphologic information. Although not all stains require analysis by a pathologist, consultation is highly recommended. It is not possible to a priori determine the means of categorizing the results of a TMA before the staining has been done. For well-described tumor markers the literature is certainly a starting point. This certainly creates complexity in marrying results from some discovery platforms with TMA results *(18)*.

Evaluation of immunohistochemistry relies on appreciation of location and intensity of staining within a specific cell population.

In clinical use, this is most commonly simplified to interpretation as positive or negative, which has the advantages of simplified analysis and high reproducibility. However that is not the nature of science, where quantification is desired. Frequently two parameters – the percentage of cells expressing a marker and the intensity of the marker – are reported. When performed manually, the data are qualitative and often reported on scales of 0– 3 or 4. When quantified with software, more quantitative (continuous scale) results are possible.

Ultimately it is not the raw data that is key, but the analysis *(18)*. Analysis of TMA results frequently confuses researchers, and well it should. Clinically immunohistochemistry is most robust as a positive/negative assay, and if a real clinical utility is envisioned, this must be kept in mind. Kaplan–Meier survival curves are typically generated on binary data (positive/negative) or a limited number of categories. At the other end of the spectrum, pathway analysis based on correlation, heat maps, and hazard proportion models are best carried out on quantitative data with dynamic range not adequately obtained with qualitative analysis. In the end, the analysis stands depends on the greatest amount of information that can be obtained from the combination of clinical parameters and characterization of the expression pattern.

9. Conclusions

The tissue microarray has become an indispensable tool in biomedical research. As the embodiment of high-throughput pathology and the means of translating tumor markers from discoveries to tools of clinical relevance they have advanced biomedical research significantly over the last decade. The TMA platform remains challenging because working with tissue remains challenging – at the level of collection, annotation, assay performance, and most importantly interpretation.

References

1. Kononen J, Bubendorf L, Kallioniemi A, Bärlund M, Schraml P, Leighton S, Torhorst J, Mihatsch MJ, Sauter G, Kallioniemi OP. Tissue microarrays for high-throughput molecular profiling of tumor specimens. *Nat Med.* 1998 Jul;4(7):844–7.
2. Braunschweig T, Chung JY, Hewitt SM. Tissue microarrays: bridging the gap between research and the clinic. *Expert Rev Proteomics.* 2005 Jun;2(3):325–36.
3. Becker D, Mihm MC, Hewitt SM, Sondak VK, Fountain JW, Thurin M. Markers and tissue resources for melanoma: meeting report. *Cancer Res.* 2006 Nov 15;66(22):10652–7.
4. Khanna C, Wan X, Bose S, Cassaday R, Olomu O, Mendoza A, Yeung C, Gorlick R, Hewitt SM, Helman LJ. The membrane-cytoskeleton linker ezrin is necessary for osteosarcoma metastasis. *Nat Med.* 2004 Feb;10(2):182–6.

5. Whiteford CC, Bilke S, Greer BT, Chen Q, Braunschweig TA, Cenacchi N, Wei JS, Smith MA, Houghton P, Morton C, Reynolds CP, Lock R, Gorlick R, Khanna C, Thiele CJ, Takikita M, Catchpoole D, Hewitt SM, Khan J. Credentialing preclinical pediatric xenograft models using gene expression and tissue microarray analysis. *Cancer Res.* 2007 Jan 1;67(1):32–40.

6. Hewitt SM. Design, construction, and use of tissue microarrays. *Methods Mol Biol.* 2004;264:61–72.

7. Schoenberg Fejzo M, Slamon DJ. Frozen tumor tissue microarray technology for analysis of tumor RNA, DNA, and proteins. *Am J Pathol.* 2001 Nov;159(5):1645–50.

8. Gillespie JW, Best CJ, Bichsel VE, Cole KA, Greenhut SF, Hewitt SM, Ahram M, Gathright YB, Merino MJ, Strausberg RL, Epstein JI, Hamilton SR, Gannot G, Baibakova GV, Calvert VS, Flaig MJ, Chuaqui RF, Herring JC, Pfeifer J, Petricoin EF, Linehan WM, Duray PH, Bova GS, Emmert-Buck MR. Evaluation of non-formalin tissue fixation for molecular profiling studies. *Am J Pathol.* 2002 Feb;160(2):449–57.

9. Goldstein NS, Hewitt SM, Taylor CR, Yaziji H, Hicks DG; Members of Ad-Hoc Committee On Immunohistochemistry Standardization. Recommendations for improved standardization of immunohistochemistry. *Appl Immunohistochem Mol Morphol.* 2007 Jun;15(2):124–33.

10. Wang Y, Hewitt SM, Liu S, Zhou X, Zhu H, Zhou C, Zhang G, Quan L, Bai J, Xu N. Tissue microarray analysis of human FRAT1 expression and its correlation with the subcellular localisation of beta-catenin in ovarian tumours. *Br J Cancer.* 2006 Mar 13;94(5):686–91.

11. Geiszt M, Lekstrom K, Brenner S, Hewitt SM, Dana R, Malech HL, Leto TL. NAD(P)H oxidase 1, a product of differentiated colon epithelial cells, can partially replace glycoprotein 91phox in the regulated production of superoxide by phagocytes. *J Immunol.* 2003 Jul 1;171(1):299–306.

12. Huang HE, Chin SF, Ginestier C, Bardou VJ, Adélaïde J, Iyer NG, Garcia MJ, Pole JC, Callagy GM, Hewitt SM, Gullick WJ, Jacquemier J, Caldas C, Chaffanet M, Birnbaum D, Edwards PA. A recurrent chromosome breakpoint in breast cancer at the NRG1/neuregulin 1/heregulin gene. *Cancer Res.* 2004 Oct 1;64(19):6840–4.

13. Fernandez DC, Bhargava R, Hewitt SM, Levin IW. Infrared spectroscopic imaging for histopathologic recognition. *Nat Biotechnol.* 2005 Apr;23(4):469–74.

14. Takikita M, Chung JY, Hewitt SM. Tissue microarrays enabling high-throughput molecular pathology. *Curr Opin Biotechnol.* 2007 Aug;18(4):318–25.

15. Hewitt SM, Takikita M, Braunschweig T, and Chung J-Y. (2007) Predictive tissue biomarkers: The promise & the challenge. *Biomarkers Med.* 1(2): 313–318.

16. Nishizuka S, Chen ST, Gwadry FG, Alexander J, Major SM, Scherf U, Reinhold WC, Waltham M, Charboneau L, Young L, Bussey KJ, Kim S, Lababidi S, Lee JK, Pittaluga S, Scudiero DA, Sausville EA, Munson PJ, Petricoin EF 3rd, Liotta LA, Hewitt SM, Raffeld M, Weinstein JN. Diagnostic markers that distinguish colon and ovarian adenocarcinomas: identification by genomic, proteomic, and tissue array profiling. *Cancer Res.* 2003 Sep 1;63(17):5243–50.

17. Chuaqui RF, Bonner RF, Best CJ, Gillespie JW, Flaig MJ, Hewitt SM, Phillips JL, Krizman DB, Tangrea MA, Ahram M, Linehan WM, Knezevic V, Emmert-Buck MR. Post-analysis follow-up and validation of microarray experiments. *Nat Genet.* 2002 Dec;32 Suppl:509–14.

18. Hewitt SM. The application of tissue microarrays in the validation of microarray results. *Methods Enzymol.* 2006;410:400–15.

19. Braunschweig T, Kaserer K, Chung J-Y, Bilke S, Krizman D, Knezevic V, Hewitt SM. (2007) Proteomic expression profiling of thyroid neoplasms with antibody arrays. *Proteomics Clin Appl.* 1:264–271.

20. Goodman MT, Hernandez BY, Hewitt S, Lynch CF, Coté TR, Frierson HF Jr, Moskaluk CA, Killeen JL, Cozen W, Key CR, Clegg L, Reichman M, Hankey BF, Edwards B. Tissues from population-based cancer registries: a novel approach to increasing research potential. *Hum Pathol.* 2005 Jul; 36(7):812–20.

Chapter 12

Quantitative, Fluorescence-Based *In Situ* Assessment of Protein Expression

Christopher B. Moeder, Jennifer M. Giltnane, Sharon Pozner Moulis, and David L. Rimm

Summary

As companion diagnostics grow in prevalence and importance, the need for accurate assessment of *in situ* protein concentrations has increased. Traditional immunohistochemistry (IHC), while valuable for assessment of context of expression, is less valuable for quantification. The lack of rigorous quantitative potential of traditional IHC led to our development of an immunofluorescence-based method now commercialized as the AQUA® technology. Immunostaining of tissue samples, image acquisition, and use of AQUA software allow investigators to quickly, efficiently, and accurately measure levels of expression within user-defined subcellular or architectural compartments. IHC analyzed by AQUA shows high reproducibility and demonstrates protein measurement accuracy similar to ELISA assays. The process is largely automated, eliminating potential error, and the resultant scores are exported on a continuous scale. There are now numerous published examples where observations made with this technology are not seen by traditional methods.

Key words: Immunohistochemistry, Quantitative analysis, Biomarkers, AQUA, Tissue microarrays,

1. Introduction

Quantitative assessment of protein and RNA has been increasing in accuracy and multiplicity for years, but nearly all quantitative techniques require dissolution of the substrate and hence loss of spatial information. Immunohistochemistry can be both quantitative and maintain the spatial information. The decreased size of clinical pathology specimens and the increased need for accuracy have Progressively pushed the tissue biomarker field into quantitative immunohistochemistry. Currently, semiquantitative pathological

Michael A. Tainsky, *Methods in Molecular Biology, Tumor Biomarker Discovery, Vol. 520*
© Humana Press, a part of Springer Science + Business Media, LLC 2009
DOI: 10.1007/978-1-60327-811-9_12

scoring of markers is important in disease management decisions. Scores include one of four discrete, ordinal categories (0, 1+, 2+, and 3+) for HER-2 staining or estimated percent positivity for estrogen and progesterone receptor. Some groups use a combination of intensity and area staining as in the Hscore *(1)* or the Allred system *(2)*. However, all of these systems suffer from the problems of subjectivity, noncontinuity, and variable reproducibility. These problems and related issues have led to the first effort at standardization published recently as the ASCO/CAP guidelines for assessment of HER2 expression *(3)*. Since the results of this assay in the clinical setting determine whether or not a patient will receive a course of therapy (often costing over $100,000) *(4)*, it seems likely that this will be the first of a number of such efforts toward standardization of critical companion diagnostic assays.

Historically, quantitative assessment has been done using both chromagens and fluorescent methods. While chromagens have the advantage of providing context, through the addition of hematoxylin counterstains, they also have disadvantages. Fluorescence-based detection systems can be multiplexed and can generally provide a broader dynamic range than chromagens. Here we focus on a system developed by our lab, but now commercially available, that allows quantitative assessment of protein expression with accuracy comparable to an ELISA assay but without loss of spatial information.

AQUA® (originally an abbreviation for Automated QUantitative Analysis but now trademarked) technology uses multiple fluorescent labels on conventional formalin-fixed, paraffin-embedded histology material. Images are then captured at all appropriate wavelengths to measure expression based on the colocalization and intensity of the immunostain *(5)*. AQUA analysis of IHC staining has shown comparable accuracy to protein detection by ELISA assay *(6)* and is currently being used to quantify expression on both tissue microarrays (TMAs) *(7)* and whole sections *(8)*. TMAs have facilitated the development of AQUA since they have facilitated standardization by arraying of cell lines and multiple samples on the same slides for assessment of reproducibility. This protocol describes the use of AQUA in assessment of a TMA, but it can be similarly used for whole sections.

2. Materials

2.1. Immunohisto-chemical Staining of Formalin-Fixed, Paraffin-Embedded Tissue for Fluorescence Microscopy

1. Xylenes, use in hood.
2. *Citrate Buffer*. 3.84 g sodium citrate dehydrate in 2 L double deionized water, pH to 6.
3. *Pressure cooker*: 6-quart aluminum pressure cooker (Presto).
4. *Peroxidase Blocking Buffer*. 10 mL 30% H_2O_2 in 390 mL Methanol.

5. *Tris-buffered saline (10× TBS)*. For 5 L stock, 438 g NaCl, 121.8 g Trizma Base (Sigma), 4,500 mL deionized H_2O, pH to 8 with concentrated HCL, bring up to 5 L with H_2O).

6. *TBS wash buffer (1×TBS)*. From 10×TBS stock.

7. *TBS with Tween 20 wash/diluent buffer (TBS-T)*. TBS (1×) with 0.05% (v/v) Tween 20 (Sigma).

8. *Primary antibody dilution buffer*. 0.3% (w/v) Albumin Bovine Serum, Fraction V, $\geq$ 96% (Sigma) in TBS/T, (BSA/TBS-T).

9. *Primary target antibody*. For example, mouse antihuman $ER\alpha$ clone 1D5; (DAKO, Carpinteria, CA).

10. *Primary mask antibody*. Rabbit antibovine cytokeratin (wide-spectrum screening, WSS; Z0622, DakoCytomation, for use with mouse target primaries) or Mouse AntiHuman Cytokeratin (Clone AE1/AE3 DakoCytomation, for use with rabbit target primaries are used here for detecting breast cancer, appropriate masks should be determined for different tissue types (see discussion of masking later).

11. *Secondary target antibody*. DAKO EnVision™ + System, HRP, goat antimouse for mouse target primaries or antirabbit for rabbit against target primaries.

12. *Secondary mask antibody*. Goat antirabbit (secondary to rabbit cytokeratin) or goat antimouse (secondary to mouse cytokeratin); Alexa-546 (Invitrogen; Eugene, OR) applied in low-light conditions.

13. *Target flourophor*. Cy5-Tyramide Reagent Pack with amplification diluent (PerkinElmer; Boston MA) applied in low-light conditions.

14. *Mounting medium with nuclear stain*. Prolong Gold antifade reagent with DAPI "4′6-diamidino-2-phenylindole" (Invitrogen).

15. Dark slide chamber with moistened filter paper and supports to hold slides for humid incubation.

2.2. AQUA ® Image Acquisition and Analysis System

Image acquisition is now performed on the HistoRx PM-2000 platform (HistoRx, New Haven, CT). This platform is the professional optimization of the original platform developed in our lab around an Olympus BX51 microscope, a Cooke Sensicam High Performance camera, and a Prior Proscan automated stage control. The PM-2000 captures images from either TMAs or whole sections and provides a stack of high-resolution monochromatic images for analysis by the AQUA software. The images are viewable, but examination of the images by "eye" is not part of the scoring system.

The images are then analyzed by the AQUA program, which generates a table of AQUA scores and associated sample coordinates. The software operational details are available from HistoRx.

3. Methods

3.1. Immunohisto-chemical Staining

Staining procedures listed have been optimized for use with the AQUA automated image acquisition system and analysis software. Other than changes to target antibody dilution, manipulations are rarely made. As an example, Images and data shown in this chapter are for ER-α on breast carcinomas. Adjustments for antibody dilution, incubation time and selection of antibodies for tumor mask, and compartment selection should be made according to the question of interest and tissue under study.

1. *Day 1.* Melt paraffin off slides in 60°C incubator for 20 min or until slides are translucent. Remove residual paraffin by incubating in two changes of Xylenes for 20 min each. Wash slides two times in 100% ethanol for 1 min each time, followed by one wash in 70% ethanol also for 1 min. Transfer slides to tap water with a slow gradient under running water, and transfer to 100% water for at least 5 min for rehydration. Pressure cook slides in citrate buffer for 10 min from the time lock pin slides up, indicating the unit has pressurized. Cool under running tap water for 10 min. Incubate slides in peroxidase block for 30 min. Wash with two changes of tap water for 30 s each and transfer to (1×) TBS wash buffer. Dry slides carefully around the array edge with a fresh Kimwipe, adding enough BSA/TBS-T to fully cover array area. Incubate in humidity chamber with BSA/TBS-T for 30 min at room temperature. Decant off BSA/TBS-T by tipping slide along its long edge against a paper towel, and again dry the edges with a fresh Kimwipe. Store in (1×) TBS while preparing cytokeratin antibody (1:100) in BSA/TBS-T. Add enough to each slide to cover array area and incubate overnight at 4°C. (Note: typically, primary target antibodies are applied with cytokeratin antibody and incubated overnight. For some antibodies, such as ERα/ 1D5, however, this is too long and nonspecific staining increases).

2. *Day 2.* Make primary ERα antibody solution (1:50) in BSA/TBS-T and cover all tissue on slide, incubating in humidity chamber for 1 h at room temperature. Decant off antibodies and rinse briefly with TBS-T. Wash all slides twice in (1×) TBS-T for 10 min each and once in (1×) TBS for another 10 min. Dry slides around edge with fresh Kimwipe and apply goat antirabbit Alexa-546 solution (1:100) in goat antimouse

Envision (neat) to all slides. Incubate in humidity chamber for 1 h at room temperature. Decant off secondary antibodies and repeat washing procedure as described above. Dry slides around edge with fresh Kimwipe, and apply Cy5-tyramide solution (1:50) in reagent pack amplification diluent to each slide. Wash all slides twice in TBS-T, first for 10 min, then for 5. Wash a final time in (1×) TBS for 5 min. Dry slides around edge with fresh Kimwipe, and apply Prolong Gold with DAPI (50–75 µL). Gently place cover slip over array and let dry overnight in the complete absence of light.

3. Clean surface of coverslip with ethanol if necessary, and seal around edges of the cover slip with clear nail polish to further preserve stain and prevent fading. Note: We have successfully removed coverslips applied in this manner using acetone to remove sealing polish and incubating slides in warmed phosphate-buffered solution.

3.2. Image Acquisition

Capturing images of the spots on a TMA or fields from a whole slide uses a software package that comes with the PM2000 platform for image collection. Specific instructions are included and training and support is available from the vendor (HistoRx, New Haven CT). Although the process is somewhat automated with some human intervention, the key steps are enumerated as follows.

Initially, the software acquires a series of low-resolution (4×) images, producing a scan of the entire slide using a fluorescence cube set selected by the user (often the channel marking tissue nuclei). For TMAs, signal from the low-resolution image is optimized to produce image acquisition coordinates reflecting areas of interest across the array, represented by spots, which are validated by the user. Aligning the resulting spots into corresponding rows and columns, as well as assigning the order with which image files will be created, creates a text file with saved spot coordinates. At each individual spot, the script takes an in-focus image and an additional out-of-focus image 8 µm below the original focal plane for all fluorophores selected by the user. For example, an in and out-of-focus image is taken with the blue filter (DAPI/ nuclear compartment) filter before rotating to repeat with emission filters for the mask (Orange, Alexa-546) and the target protein (Red, Cy5). According to the coordinates assigned in **step 3**, the microscope continues this procedure for all spots on the array, saving all images to a chosen computer directory**.

3.3. AQUA and Expression Quantification

The underlying basic assumptions of AQUA are that any entity must be defined by a molecular interaction, rather than a contrast-generated edge (as is seen in feature extraction software). For example, nuclei are defined by colocalization with DAPI pixels, rather than by sphericity or roundness. A second basic premise is that every concentration is composed of a numerator and a denominator. Thus to generate an *in situ* concentration, we measure the amount of signal (the sum or the intensities in the target pixels) as the numerator and divide by the area of the pixels of interest (or the user-defined compartment). We define the following terms for use of AQUA (**Fig. 1**):

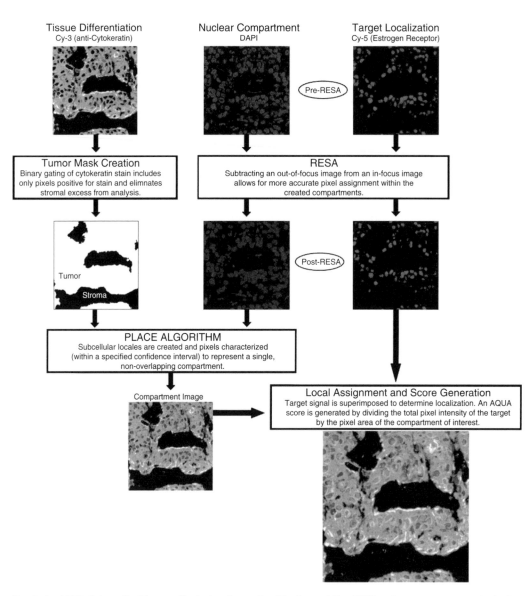

Fig. 1. An AQUA Schematic Diagram illustrates the main objectives of the AQUA software components including identifying tumor, creating subcellular compartments, and localizing/measuring target protein expression within these compartments (*See Color Plates*).

1. *Mask.* The user-defined region of interest as selected by a molecular interaction. For example for epithelial tumors, cytokeratin is used as a mask. For neural tumors, we use GFAP, etc. The goal is that the mask excludes stromal tissue or blank space.

2. *Compartment.* The compartment is also defined by a molecular interaction, but ultimately results in a set of pixels that represent the desired entity (for example a pan-cadherin antibody might be used to define a membrane compartment). To quantify tumor protein expression, the compartment pixels must be within the Mask. The definition of which pixels are within a compartment is subject to either manual or automated threshold determination, and can be assisted by the RESA process defined later. Compartments may be traditional subcellular membrane-bound structures (like nuclei or golgi) or virtual structures (like a kinase) as long as there is a molecular interaction to uniquely define a set of pixels. Compartments can also be cellular or architectural features like T-cells, vessels, or lymphatics.

3. *Target.* The target is the protein being measured. The intensity is measured and summed over all of the pixels within the defined compartment. Usually long-wavelength fluorophores (emission peaks greater than 650 nm) are used for targets to minimize interference due to autofluorescence.

With the acquired in-and out-of-focus images, AQUA software is used to generate scores (equivalent to *in situ* concentrations) for each of the user-defined targets in each of the user-defined compartments. Initially, the tumor mask is designated by the binary gating of pixels in which staining exceeds the threshold. Setting an intensity threshold assigns positively stained pixels as "on" and discards the rest as "off," followed by slight dilation and hole-filling algorithms to produce a mask which is an accurate representation of tumor area within the histospots or fields (**Fig. 1**). For ERα, the DAPI stains of the nuclei are used in generating nuclear compartments. Subtracting the generated nuclear compartment from the tumor mask creates a non-nuclear compartment, which includes both the cytoplasm and the membrane, which is sufficient for addressing many issues that require resolution only in the 1 μm range.

Since we do not use confocal or convolution/deconvolution imaging to remove out-of-focus light, the accurate assignment of compartments requires an extra step. We take a second out-of-focus image for each filter for application of the rapid exponential subtraction algorithm (RESA). The RESA algorithm works by utilizing the out-of-focus image for each histospot or field to subtract the light in a manner inversely proportional to the intensity in the out-of-focus image. Details of the exact methods are in US patent #7,219,016. New extensions of RESA are in development to reduce nonspecific background in all channels. The PLACE algorithm uses the remaining signal and ensures the most accurate compartmental assignment possible. Applied to the target, it assigns pixels to nonoverlapping user-created compartments within a 95% confidence interval. AQUA scores are then generated as the sum of the total pixel intensity of the target within the compartment of interest (the numerator) divided by the pixel area of that same compartment within the tumor mask (the denominator) *(5)* (**Fig. 2**).

After all spots or fields in an array have been run through the script, intensity thresholds set, and compartments created, the final step in the quantification process includes validation of each individual spot. This includes adjusting thresholds, cropping out adjacent histospots, and refining percent of remaining values of the RESA algorithm. Data quality is improved by having trained investigators review each image to either be included in, or discarded from overall, final analysis. There is also automated validating software available from HistoRx that can review images for inclusion or exclusion. The extent and aggressiveness of the validation process varies with the specific biological question being addressed. To completely remove any subjectivity, this step is performed by the HistoRx software.

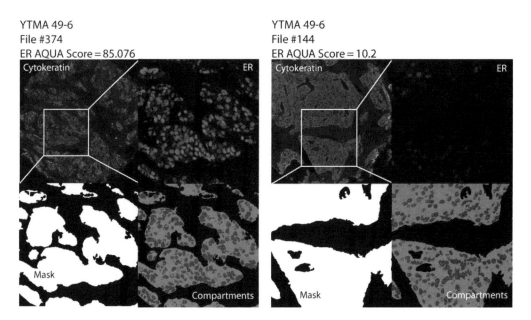

Fig. 2. Two examples of estrogen receptor expression based on AQUA analysis are shown using a set of images that illustrates the monochromatic cytokeratin image, the mask, the compartments, and the target at two magnifications so the reader can evaluate all of the features that generate the AQUA score. File #374 on the left with a nuclear compartment AQUA score of 85 is an example of a high expression level. File #144 on the right, with an AQUA score of 10.2, is an example of low expression of ER (*See Color Plates*).

3.4. Standardization and Assessment

After completion of AQUA-based analysis the results need to be assessed for reproducibility and standardization. These are key features that can show the rigor of results obtained using this method, but are very difficult to assess on conventionally stained material. Reproducibility is best assessed by reading multiple spots (or fields) from the same tumor in independent experiments. The collection of two- or three-fold information generates increased confidence in both the experimental result and the method. Many studies have been done to address the issue of the number of spots required to be representative of a whole section *(9–11)*, and most suggest between 2 and 4 depending on tumor type. Collection of at least 2 spots allows linear regression and/or evaluation of Spearman's ρ to assess the reproducibility of the assay. **Figure 3** shows an example of the reproducibility we have seen in a cohort of breast cancer cases assessed for estrogen receptor. Generally ρ values between 0.6 and 0.9 are seen in high quality, reproducible assays, where values nearer 0.6 suggest high degrees of marker heterogeneity within the tumor. Serial sections from the same TMA block typically give ρ values in the 0.95–0.98 range. When the ρ value drops below 0.5, there is usually a systematic error to be discovered and we have seen this between different lots of antibody from the same vendor *(12)*. This assessment is generally applied to TMAs, but can also be applied to fields within whole sections *(8)*.

Standardization is also important for rigorous assessment of *in situ* protein expression. To achieve standardization, we have used cell lines, prepared as tissue. By creating a series of TMA

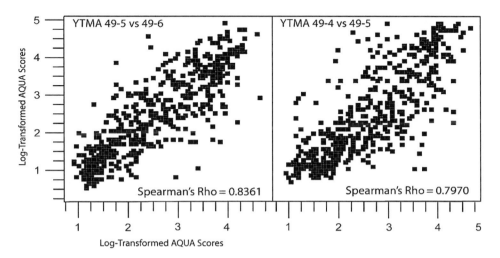

Fig. 3. Assessment of reproducibility using linear regression shows high levels of correlation with Spearman's ρ values around 0.8. These arrays contain regions of tumor cored at different times and locations for each patient, showing the level of marker heterogeneity and assay reproducibility. ρ values range from 0.6 to 0.9 depending on tumor heterogeneity. Values below 0.5 often are a sign of systematic error or low-quality antibody.

spots from cell lines, absolute values can be obtained in pg/ mg total protein *(6)*. This can be done by standardizing against ELISA assays or other methods of measurement of protein within cell lines. This method can also be used to find the "biological" cutpoint for the threshold of expression. **Figure 4** shows a number of cell lines that are ER negative or ER positive, thus allowing selection of the AQUA score that is the threshold for positive for any given performance of the assay.

The method for preparation of formalin-fixed paraffin-embedded cell lines for standardization controls is as follows:

Cell preparation varies with cell lines used; however for all cell lines, immediate fixation is critical. Thus cells are grown in flasks to desired density, fixed by removing medium and then directly adding formalin to the culture flask. Cells should not be trypsinized or pretreated prior to fixation as that may generate artifacts of hypoxia or other cellular stress. Adherent cell lines can be disassociated from the flask using a cell scraper after fixation.

1. Start with a generous amount of cells (often 6–8 T150 flasks) suspended in 10% neutral buffered formalin in a 50-mL conical.

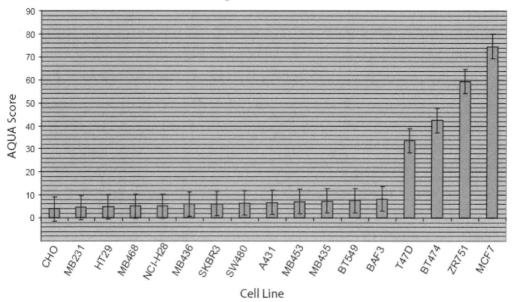

Fig. 4. This histogram shows expression levels of a number of cell lines ranked by expression level of ER. This allows visualization of a plateau of negative cases, suggesting the threshold of AQUA scores associated with system noise. When the curve breaks, levels of expression rise above background. Based on the AQUA scores of cell lines on the array, a cutpoint can be determined based on ELISA assays or other in vitro assays of the same cell lines. Even without knowing the exact concentration, graphing in this manner allows determination of a biological cutpoint for the threshold of ER expression (in this case at an AQUA score of 10).

2. Prepare 10 mL of 1% Low Melt agarose in 1× phosphate-buffered saline (PBS). Incubate for at least 1 h at 55°C to get solution to a consistent temperature.

3. Prepare 0.6-mL Eppendorf tubes, each with approximately 50 μL of paraffin (Surgipath, Blue Ribbon Tissue Embedding Infiltration Medium), liquefying paraffin in bottom of tube by incubating for 5 min at 60°C. Remove from incubator and refrigerate to harden. (This makes a flat surface at the bottom of the tube and a pellet that is easier to work with in **step 5**.)

4. Centrifuge 50-mL conicals with fixed cells at 1,200 rpm for 5 min.

5. Gently aspirate supernatant and wash with approximately 30 mL of 1× PBS. Repeat twice, resuspending in 1× PBS and centrifuging each time.

6. Remove 1× PBS from final wash and resuspend in approximately 0.4 mL of 80% ethanol. Transfer to 0.6-mL Eppendorf tube from **step 2** (or 1.5-mL tubes for large volumes of cells).

7. Pack cells by centrifugation at 12,000 rpm for 5 min.

8. Gently remove ethanol, leaving pellet of cells in the bottom. Repeat by adding 0.4 mL of 80% ethanol and centrifuging again for 5 min. (This removes the last traces of PBS and helps the cells remain stuck together).

9. Again, gently aspirate off ethanol. Using a Heyman probe or a similar small tool, transfer cell pellet to a labeled Eppendorf cap (removed from its tube with a razor blade). Mold pellet into cap with the Heyman probe.

10. If pellet does not fill the cap, use approximately 75 μL of 1% agarose (from **step 1**) to fill voids around the edges of the cap. Work quickly and put caps immediately into a freezer. Let sit overnight.

11. Pop the pellets of cap-molded cells into labeled tissue cassettes (Therm-Fisher). Store overnight submerged in 80%ethanol before taking to histology department for embedding.

12. Embed pellets in vertical position in the center of a paraffin block without eosin as eosin increases autofluorescence.

4. General Notes

1. To see a broad range of expression it is important to titer antibodies to optimal dilutions prior to image acquisition.

This issue and its implications for accurate measurement of protein expression are addressed in McCabe et al. *(6)*.

2. The most frequently altered steps of the staining protocol involve incubation time adjustments for BSA/TBS-T block and primary target antibodies. If primary target antibodies do not stain optimally at 4°C overnight, they are usually incubated at room temperature for 1–2 h.

3. Because compartmentalization is so dependent on successful stains for each of the deposited fluorophores, when a spot does not show a DAPI or Mask protein stain, it must be discarded. The strict application of validation can result in elimination of as many as 20% of the spots on an array.

4. For some tissues, it is difficult to find appropriate masking proteins. For example, melanoma is masked with anti-S100 antibody, which stains some other cells as well, that should not be considered in analysis.

5. Catenin and cadherin family proteins can be used to construct more accurate membrane compartments, as cytokeratin can only be localized with AQUA to the cortical cytoplasm. We have had the most success with alpha-catenin since it seems to be preserved in most tumors, where cadherins and beta-catenin is often reduced or lost.

6. During AQUA validation, spots with extremely small compartmental/tumor mask areas may show inaccurately high AQUA scores due to such a small denominator. Consequently, tumor mask areas less than 5% of the total histospot's area are generally excluded from analysis.

References

1. McCarty, K. S., Jr., Szabo, E., Flowers, J. L., Cox, E. B., Leight, G. S., Miller, L., Konrath, J., Soper, J. T., Budwit, D. A., Creasman, W. T., et al. (1986) Use of a monoclonal anti-estrogen receptor antibody in the immunohistochemical evaluation of human tumors. Cancer Res 46, 4244s–48s.

2. Allred, D. C., Harvey, J. M., Berardo, M., and Clark, G. M. (1998) Prognostic and predictive factors in breast cancer by immunohistochemical analysis. Mod Pathol 11, 155–68.

3. Wolff, A. C., Hammond, M. E., Schwartz, J. N., Hagerty, K. L., Allred, D. C., Cote, R. J., Dowsett, M., Fitzgibbons, P. L., Hanna, W. M., Langer, A., McShane, L. M., Paik, S., Pegram, M. D., Perez, E. A., Press, M. F., Rhodes, A., Sturgeon, C., Taube, S. E., Tubbs, R., Vance, G. H., van de Vijver, M., Wheeler, T. M., and Hayes, D. F. (2007) American Society of Clinical Oncology/College of American Pathologists guideline recommendations for human epidermal growth factor receptor 2 testing in breast cancer. J Clin Oncol 25, 118–45.

4. Elkin, E. B., Weinstein, M. C., Winer, E. P., Kuntz, K. M., Schnitt, S. J., and Weeks, J. C. (2004) HER-2 testing and trastuzumab therapy for metastatic breast cancer: a cost-effectiveness analysis. J Clin Oncol 22, 854–63.

5. Camp, R. L., Chung, G. G., and Rimm, D. L. (2002) Automated subcellular localization and quantification of protein expression in tissue microarrays. Nat Med 8, 1323–7.

6. McCabe, A., Dolled-Filhart, M., Camp, R. L., and Rimm, D. L. (2005) Automated quantitative analysis (AQUA) of *in situ* protein expression, antibody concentration, and prognosis. J Natl Cancer Inst 97, 1808–15.

7. Cregger, M., Berger, A. J., and Rimm, D. L. (2006) Immunohistochemistry and quantitative analysis of protein expression. Arch Pathol Lab Med 130, 1026–30.

8. Chung, G. G., Zerkowski, M. P., Ghosh, S., Camp, R. L., and Rimm, D. L. (2007) Quantitative analysis of estrogen receptor heterogeneity in breast cancer. Lab Invest 87, 662–9.

9. Nielsen, T. O., Hsu, F. D., O'Connell, J. X., Gilks, C. B., Sorensen, P. H., Linn, S., West, R. B., Liu, C. L., Botstein, D., Brown, P. O., and van de Rijn, M. (2003) Tissue microarray validation of epidermal growth factor receptor and SALL2 in synovial sarcoma with comparison to tumors of similar histology. Am J Pathol 163, 1449–56.

10. Torhorst, J., Bucher, C., Kononen, J., Haas, P., Zuber, M., Kochli, O. R., Mross, F., Dieterich, H., Moch, H., Mihatsch, M., Kallioniemi, O. P., and Sauter, G. (2001) Tissue microarrays for rapid linking of molecular changes to clinical endpoints. Am J Pathol 159, 2249–56.

11. Camp, R. L., Charette, L. A., and Rimm, D. L. (2000) Validation of tissue microarray technology in breast carcinoma. Lab Invest 80, 1943–9.

12. Pozner-Moulis, S., Cregger, M., Camp, R. L., and Rimm, D. L. (2007) Antibody validation by quantitative analysis of protein expression using expression of Met in breast cancer as a model. Lab Invest 87, 251–60.

Chapter 13

Tumor Marker Discovery by Expression Profiling RNA from Formalin-Fixed Paraffin-Embedded Tissues

Maureen T. Cronin, Debjani Dutta, Mylan Pho, Anhthu Nguyen, Jennie Jeong, and Mei-Ian Liu

Summary

Clear identification among early-stage cancer patients of those at highest risk of having metastatic disease would be of great benefit in treatment planning and management. Considerable additional benefit would accrue to high-risk patients if their responses to specific therapeutic alternatives could be predicted. Molecular biomarkers in the form of gene expression profiles are proving to be more effective tools for both prognostic and predictive patient stratification than more traditional methods such as patient demographics and histopathology indicators. Such biomarkers must be clinically validated before they can be effectively used to manage patients in clinical studies or clinical practice. This can be most efficiently accomplished by analyzing archived clinical samples with well-characterized clinical outcomes. Doing studies of this type requires reoptimization of traditional molecular expression profiling techniques to analyze RNA from fixed paraffin-embedded tissues. We have modified molecular methods for RNA extraction, RNA quantification, reverse transcription, and quantitative PCR to work optimally in archived clinical samples in order to develop a clinically validated assay for breast cancer prognosis and prediction of patient response to hormonal and chemotherapy.

Key words: Breast cancer, Formalin-fixed paraffin-embedded tissue, Quantitative RT-PCR, Expression profiling, Molecular biomarkers, Prognosis, Prediction.

1. Introduction

Over the last decade, more than a dozen different laboratories have demonstrated that mRNA levels can be measured in fixed, paraffin-embedded (FPE) tumor specimens, despite the fact that RNA extracted from FPE tissue is often present in fragments less than ~300 bases in length *(1–8)*. This methodology is now being

Michael A. Tainsky, *Methods in Molecular Biology, Tumor Biomarker Discovery, Vol. 520*
© Humana Press, a part of Springer Science + Business Media, LLC 2009
DOI: 10.1007/978-1-60327-811-9_13

actively applied to the discovery and development of tumor markers as diagnostic assays. This focus on developing biomarkers from FPE specimens has been for two main reasons: first, the prognostic/predictive potential of gene expression profiles has been clearly demonstrated *(9–19)*; and second, FPE tissue represents by far the most abundant supply of solid tissue specimens associated with clinical records that can be used for this type of development work *(20)*. The standard process for handling biopsy and surgical specimens is to treat tissues in a fixing agent such as formalin and then embed them in paraffin so they can be easily handled for sectioning and staining. RT-PCR (reverse transcription, polymerase chain reaction) assay of FPE RNA can result in rapid, large-scale analysis of specimens from completed clinical trials to identify and validate biomarkers as routine clinical diagnostic assays.

Creating a standard, controlled set of methods, including all process steps from tissue extraction through reverse transcription and PCR, allows sensitive, precise, panels of RT-PCR assays to be optimized to FPE specimen analysis and then applied to clinical research to generate diagnostic tests *(21)*. Variables such as pathology fixation and the extent of RNA fragmentation in FPE tissue due to archive storage time can be compensated for by assay design and data normalization strategies. Probe and primer sets for RT-PCR assays should be designed to be short and homogeneous in length for effective reference gene-based data normalization *(2)*.

RNA extracted from archival breast cancer specimens using a proteinase K tissue digestion allows maximum recovery of short RNA species. Normalizing the amount of RNA used in multiplexed gene-specific reverse transcription further supports specimen-to-specimen comparisons. Distributing the cDNA products of reverse transcription into parallel quantitative PCR reactions allows maximum sensitivity and straightforward analysis of gene expression.

2. Materials

2.1. Sample Preparation

1. Microtome.
2. Polypropylene 1.5-mL microcentrifuge tubes, nuclease-free grade.

2.2. RNA Extraction

1. MasterPure RNA Purification Kit (Epicentre Biotechnologies, Madison, WI) containing 1× Tissue and Cell Lysis Solution, Proteinase K (50 µg/µL), MPC Protein Precipitation Reagent, RNase-free DNase I enzyme (1 unit/µL), 1× DNase I buffer, 2× Tissue and Cell Lysis Solution (*see* **Note 1**).
2. 75% Ethyl alcohol, molecular biology grade.
3. Ethyl alcohol, 200 proof, molecular biology grade.
4. Isopropanol (Omnisolv, EM Science, Gibbstown, NJ).

5. Nuclease-free water.

6. Xylene.

2.3. RNA quantitation

1. NanoDrop ND-1000 Spectrophotometer (NanoDrop Technologies, Willmington, DE).

2. Nuclease-free water.

2.4. Reverse Transcription

1. Hard-Shell Thin-Wall 96-well Microplate or 96-well Twin-tec PCR, Skirt-C.

2. Nuclease-Free Water.

3. PCR Strip Tubes with Cap.

4. Polarseal Foil.

5. Universal Human Reference RNA (Stratagene, San Diego, CA).

6. Gene-specific oligonucleotide primers.

7. Omniscript RT Kit containing RNase-Free Water, 5 mM dNTP Mix, 10× RT Buffer, 4 U/µL Omniscript RT (Qiagen, Valencia, CA).

8. RNase Inhibitor (20 unit/µL) (Applied Biosystems, Foster City, CA).

2.5. CR

1. 384-Well Clear Optical Reaction Plate or 384-well Clear Twin-tec Plate.

2. ABI PRISM 7900HT Sequence Detection System (Applied Biosystems, Foster City, CA).

3. Hard-Shell Thin-Wall 96-Well Microplate or 96-well Twin-tec PCR, Skirt-C.

4. Nuclease-Free Water.

5. Optical Adhesive Covers.

6. Polarseal Foil.

7. Sealing Tape for 96-Well Plates.

8. Oligonucleotide primers and dual-labeled TaqMan probe for each gene assay.

9. 2× TaqMan® Universal PCR Master Mix, no AmpErase UNG (Applied Biosystems).

3. Methods

Expression profiling RNA from archival samples is challenging due to the generally fragmented state of the RNA. However, fixed paraffin-embedded samples are easily and safely handled at room temperature since the fixation process stabilizes the biomolecules in these samples and destroys pathogens. Most protocols for isolating RNA and preparing it for molecular analysis have been developed and optimized for RNA isolated from fresh tissue or cultured cells. RNA from these sources is typically of kilobase length with intact polyadenylated tails suitable for oligo-dT primed cDNA synthesis. However, these methods are typically unsuccessful when applied to extracting RNA from fixed tissues and preparing cDNA from it for molecular analysis.

Successful extraction from fixed tissues requires that protocols be reoptimized to recover a smaller class of RNA than typically obtained from fresh tissue and cell lines. Priming for cDNA synthesis must be based on random primers and gene-specific oligonucleotide primers rather than oligo dT priming. In addition, amplicon lengths for RT-PCR targets must be constrained to be of a similar size as the lower average length of RNA recovered from the sample population under study. Often for fixed, paraffin-embedded tissues, this is less than 100 nucleotides.

An RNA extraction method based on proteinase K tissue digestion, such as the MasterPure Kit available from Epicentre Biotechnologies (Madison, WI), followed by nucleic acid precipitation is recommended. This method is effective since it tends to efficiently recover small-sized RNA molecules. The nucleic acid extract is then DNase treated to remove residual genomic DNA which could interfere with accurate RT-PCR expression analysis.

The RNA is quantified so that a standard amount of RNA can be added to the cDNA synthesis and consequently the PCR reactions. Optical density reading using the ND1000 microspectrophotometer (NanoDrop Technologies, Wilmington, DE) is an accurate and effective way to measure RNA concentration for small numbers of samples. However, the RiboGreen fluorescent dye assay based on a standard curve made using ribosomal RNA (RiboGreen Assay, Molecular Probes, Invitrogen, Carlsbad, CA) can be assembled in 96-well plates and read on a plate reader in fluorescence mode (SpectraMax, Molecular Devices, Sunnyvale, CA) when large numbers of samples must be processed. The direct spectrophotometer method of RNA quantitation will be described here.

The RT-PCR method given in this protocol is the TaqMan method run on the ABI PRISM 7900HT real-time detection system (Applied Biosystems, Foster City, CA). This platform permits flexibility in scaling to handle different sets of samples since the 7900HT instrument can be used in either 96-well or 384-well formats. In addition, the assay plates can be assembled by hand using multichannel pipettes or on a larger scale with robotic liquid handing systems such as the Beckman Bio-Mek or the Tecan Aquarius. The protocol versions described here are the manual methods that can be done in any laboratory without relying on robotic systems.

Color Plates

a

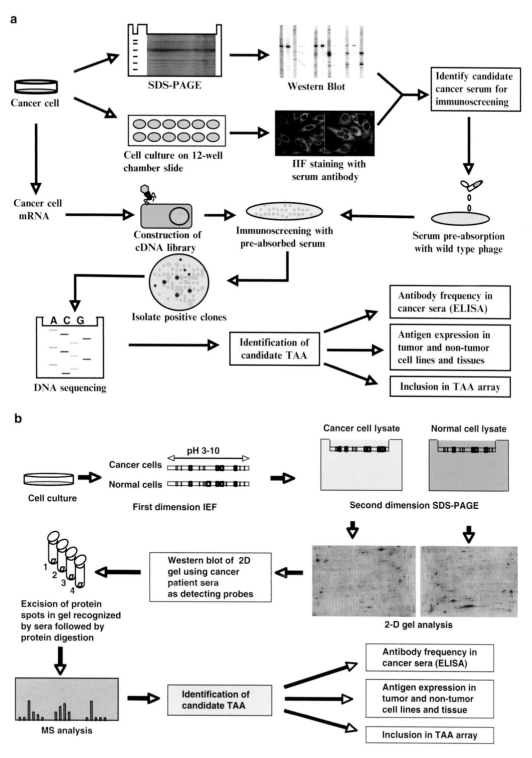

SDS-PAGE Western Blot Identify candidate cancer serum for immunoscreening

Cancer cell

Cell culture on 12-well chamber slide IIF staining with serum antibody

Cancer cell mRNA Construction of cDNA library Immunoscreening with pre-absorbed serum Serum pre-absorption with wild type phage

Isolate positive clones

ACG

DNA sequencing Identification of candidate TAA

Antibody frequency in cancer sera (ELISA)

Antigen expression in tumor and non-tumor cell lines and tissues

Inclusion in TAA array

b

Cancer cell lysate Normal cell lysate

pH 3-10

Cancer cells
Normal cells

Cell culture

First dimension IEF Second dimension SDS-PAGE

1 2 3 4

Western blot of 2D gel using cancer patient sera as detecting probes

Excision of protein spots in gel recognized by sera followed by protein digestion

2-D gel analysis

MS analysis Identification of candidate TAA

Antibody frequency in cancer sera (ELISA)

Antigen expression in tumor and non-tumor cell lines and tissue

Inclusion in TAA array

Chapter 1, Fig. 1. Schematic representation of TAA identification. (*For complete caption refer page 4 and 5*)

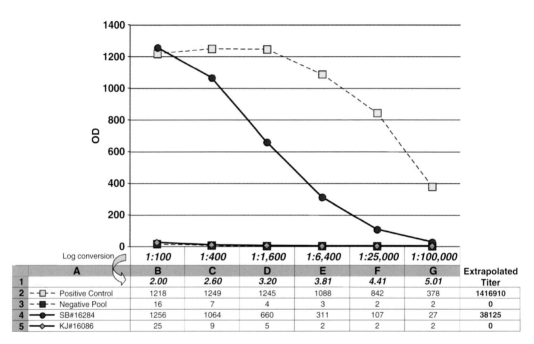

	A	B	C	D	E	F	G	Extrapolated
	Log conversion	*1:100*	*1:400*	*1:1,600*	*1:6,400*	*1:25,000*	*1:100,000*	
1		*2.00*	*2.60*	*3.20*	*3.81*	*4.41*	*5.01*	**Titer**
2	– ☐ – Positive Control	1218	1249	1245	1088	842	378	**1416910**
3	– ■ – Negative Pool	16	7	4	3	2	2	**0**
4	—●— SB#16284	1256	1064	660	311	107	27	**38125**
5	—◇— KJ#16086	25	9	5	2	2	2	**0**

Chapter 2, Fig. 1. Representative example of ELISA results with four serum samples tested in serial dilutions, shown in OD values, against full-length protein antigen NY-ESO-1. All samples were obtained with informed consent under IRB approved protocols: positive control serum is from melanoma patient NW-29 (from Dr. E. Jäger, Frankfurt, Germany), negative control is from a pool of 6 healthy donor sera from the blood bank, and serum samples SB#16284 and KJ#16086 are from ovarian cancer patients (from Dr. K. Odunsi, Buffalo, NY).

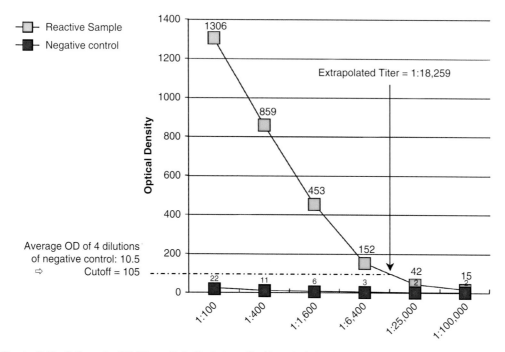

Chapter 2, Fig. 2. Example of ELISA results to illustrate method for calculating titers.

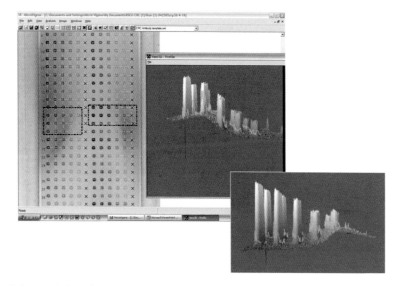

Chater 7, Fig. 3. Data analysis performed by MicroVigene (VigeneTech, MA) software program. Spot finding, regional and local background subtraction, and linear dynamic range finding are performed by the software program. Combined with the calibrator, this method provides for a reproducible and quantifiable value for every sample.

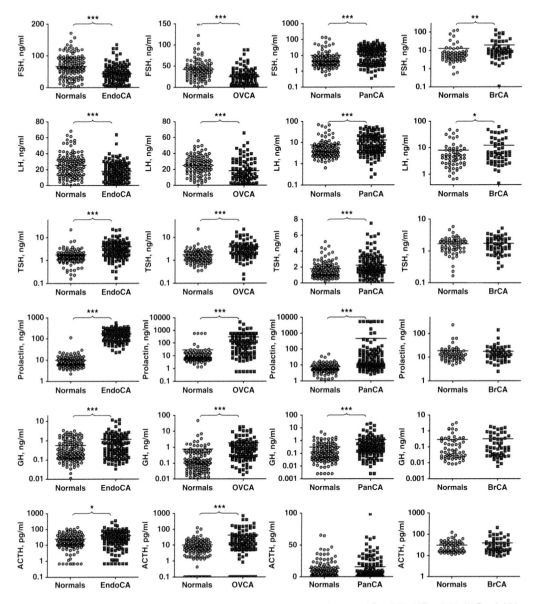

Chapter 9, Fig. 1. Comparison of hormone levels in cancer patients vs. control groups: *P < 0.05; **P < 0.01; ***P < 0.001.

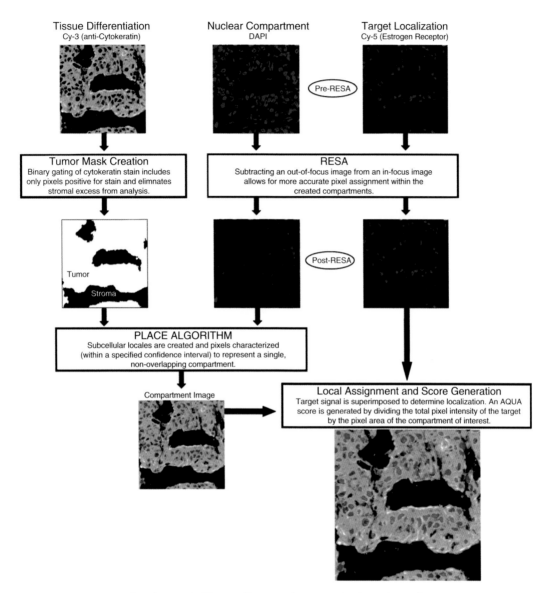

Chapter 12, Fig. 1. An AQUA Schematic Diagram illustrates the main objectives of the AQUA software components including identifying tumor, creating subcellular compartments, and localizing/measuring target protein expression within these compartments.

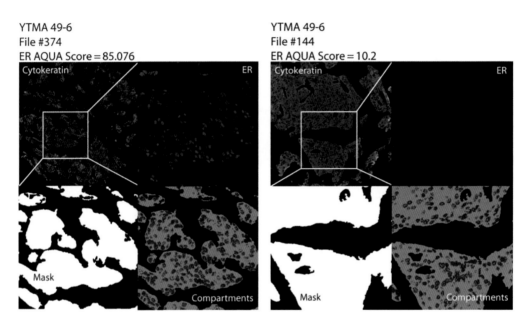

YTMA 49-6
File #374
ER AQUA Score = 85.076

YTMA 49-6
File #144
ER AQUA Score = 10.2

Chapter 12, Fig. 2. Two examples of estrogen receptor expression based on AQUA analysis are shown using a set of images that illustrates the monochromatic cytokeratin image, the mask, the compartments, and the target at two magnifications so the reader can evaluate all of the features that generate the AQUA score. File #374 on the left with a nuclear compartment AQUA score of 85 is an example of a high expression level. File #144 on the right, with an AQUA score of 10.2, is an example of low expression of ER.

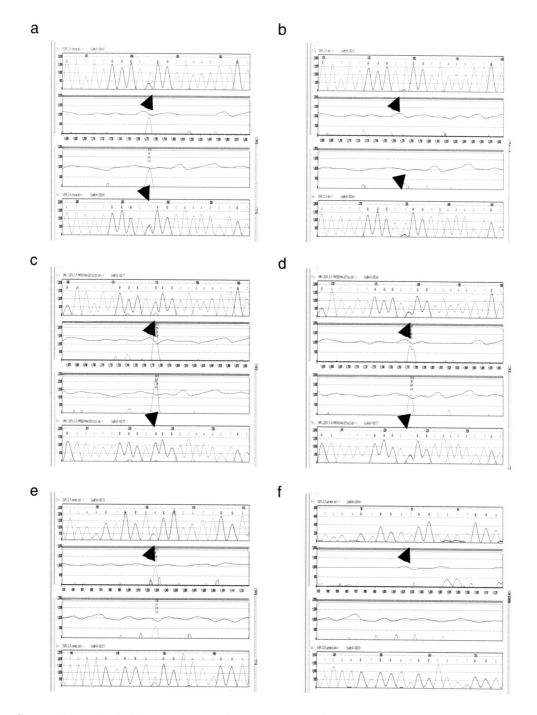

Chapter 15, Fig. 2. Sample DNA sequence chromatograms, as viewed using Mutation Surveyor. The upper chromatogram in each image represents the forward strand and the lower chromatogram represents the reverse strand (**a**, **b**) Comparison of a typical missense mutation observed in a lung tumor tissue sample (**a**, *arrows*) with that of one with weak missense mutation signal detectable (**b**, *arrows*). The mutation observed in both samples, 2573T > G (L858R) in EGFR is observed in approximately 4% of all lung adenocarcinomas. The mutation and level of intensity observed in B was reproducible. (**c**, **d**) Allele amplification bias can result in loss of signal beyond detection. Chromatograms (**c**) and (**d**) represent independent PCR reactions from the same DNA sample. In chromatogram (**c**), the 2573G allele was preferentially amplified (*arrows*) as compared with chromatogram (**d**), where both the 2573G and 2573T alleles were comparatively amplified (*arrows*). (**e**, **f**) Comparison of a chromatogram derived from tumor tissue (**e**) with that of a blood sample (**f**) from the same individual. The missense mutation detected in tumor (**e**, *arrow*) is not detected in the blood sample (**f**, *arrow*); therefore, it is unique to tumor tissue.

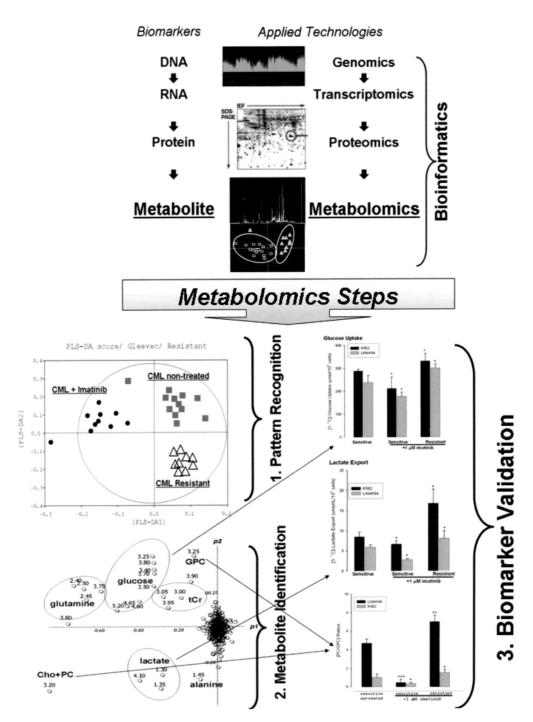

Chapter 20, Fig. 1. (**a**) Potential applications of genomics, proteomics, and metabolomics technologies in cancer research; (**b**) Three steps of NMR-based metabolomics analysis (as an example for imatinib treatment in chronic myeloid leukemia cells) using principal component analysis: pattern recognition ('black box" using PCA scores) → metabolite identification ('biomarker" using PCA plot) → metabolite quantification ('validation').

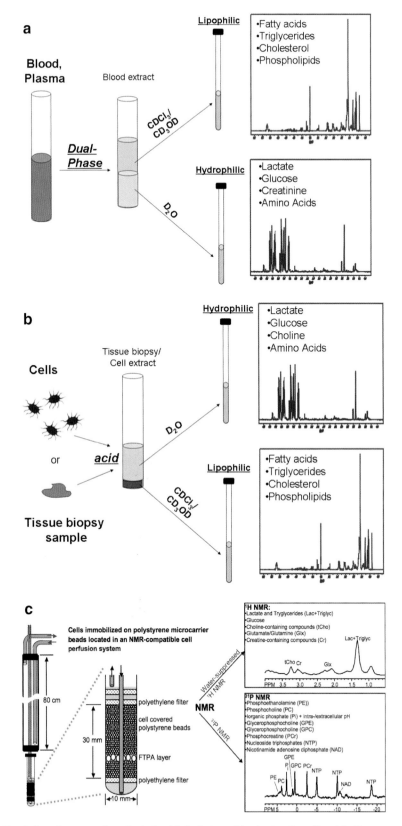

Chapter 20, Fig. 2. Sample preparation charts for (**a**) dual-phase blood extraction; (**b**) acidic tissue or cell extraction; (**c**) perfused cells.

Chapter 21, Fig. 3. (**a**) is a *T*2-weighted turbo spin-echo image showing the VOI from which 1H MRS images were acquired with a 2D PRESS pulse sequence. The three spectra (**b**, **c**, and **d**) labeled in **a** were extracted from the corresponding voxels in the normal brain tissue (**b**), and two Gd-enhanced area (**c**) and (**d**). The spectra were acquired with an echo time (TE) of 135 ms and an elliptical 16 ×16 phase encoding scheme. The acquisition time for the 2D data set was 4:45 min.

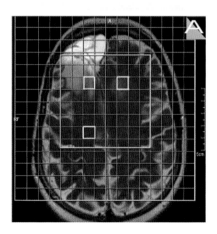

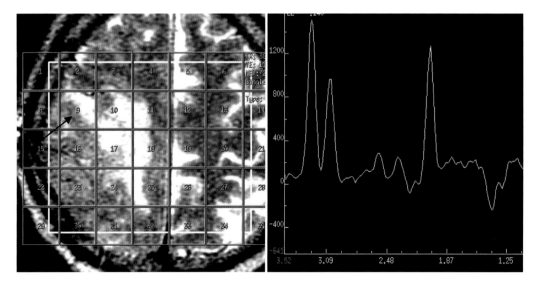

Chapter 21, Fig. 10. MRS image of the GBM in the right frontal lobe. It is not the case shown in **Fig. 6**. The MRS spectrum for pixel #9 in the tumor area is shown on the right. The GBM has a characteristic spectrographic signature for a malignant tumor, demonstrating an increase in the choline (CHO) peak (3.2 ppm), a decrease in the *n*-acetylaspartate (NAA) peak (2.02 ppm), an increased CHO/creatine (3.0 ppm) ratio, and double inversed lactate peaks (1.35 ppm) in the left end of the spectrum.

Chater 21, Fig. 11. rCBV image generated from perfusion-weighted DSE for the GBM in the right frontal lobe shown in **Fig. 10**. Usually a GBM will show a high rCBV, displayed as "hot" *red* color in the tumor core. In this case, due to prior surgical removal of the tumor, the high rCBV signal in the area was lost for the susceptibility artifact by using the *T2**-weighted GE pulse sequence.

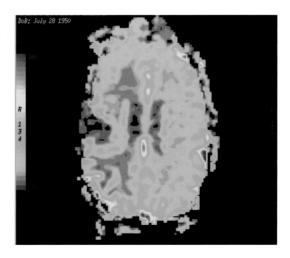

Chapter 21, Fig. 14. Ktrans map (~permeability map) generated from PWI DCE for a GBM in the left frontal lobe. The tumor core shows "hot" *yellow* color in the middle of the WM (the "cold" *pink*) area. The vessels serving the GBM exhibit poor integrity due to angiogenesis and there is marked leakage, seen as a hyperintense signal on the map.

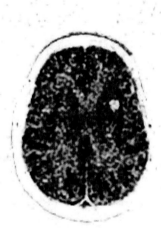

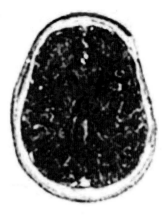

Chapter 21, Fig. 15. fBV map generated from PWI DCE for the GBM in the left frontal lobe shown in **Fig. 14**. The portion of the GBM seen as hyperintense on the fBV map has a higher vascular density, resulting from angiogenesis. The center of the tumor is hypointense and may correspond to necrosis, which is always present in GBM.

Chapter 22, Fig. 1. Animal positioning, T_2-weighted brain MRI and localized ^{1}H-MRS of the brain. *Cho* Total cholines, *Glx* Glutamate + glutamine + GABA, *mI* myo-inositol, *NAA* N-acetyl aspartate, *PCr* Phosphocreatine + creatine.

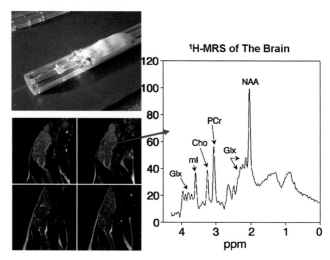

3.1. Gene Selection and Assay Design

For each gene candidate to be used in the study, identify the appropriate mRNA reference sequence using LocusLink and the correct LocusID for the gene of interest. Access the consensus sequence through the NCBI Entrez nucleotide database and download. When selecting candidate genes, both biomarker and reference normalization genes should be considered.

Design RT-PCR primers and probes using Primer Express® software (Applied Biosystems, Foster City, CA) or the publicly available Primer3 program (http://frodo.wi.mit.edu/cgi-bin/primer3/primer3_www.cgi) *(22)* (*see* **Note 2**).

Order the oligonucleotide primers and fluorogenic TaqMan probes dual labeled with 5′-FAM as a reporter and a 3' quencher molecule (*see* **Note 3**) from a commercial supplier.

3.2. Sample Preparation

1. Preparing formalin-fixed paraffin-embedded samples for RNA extraction requires using a microtome to cut sections from paraffin blocks in which the fixed tissues have been embedded (*see* **Note 4**). Although the dimensions of embedded tissues vary widely, three 10-μm FPE sections cut from one paraffin block from each patient case are a good rule of thumb for obtaining microgram amounts of RNA. Cut the three sections sequentially, allowing them to curl as the microtome blade moves over the block surface.

2. Using a fine brush and/or tissue forceps, place all three 10-μm sections into one 1.5-mL polypropylene microcentrifuge tube for extraction.

3. Add 1 mL of xylene to each tube containing a tissue sample. Invert the tube until the tissue sample is dislodged from the bottom of the tube. Mix the samples for 5 min. Centrifuge the samples in a microcentrifuge set between +18°C and +25°C for 5 min at approximately 14,000 rpm. Carefully aspirate and discard the supernatant without disturbing the tissue on the bottom of the tube.

4. Repeat the steps for a total of two xylene extractions. Visually inspect the sample for evidence of paraffin. If residual paraffin exists, repeat the xylene extraction process until the paraffin is completely removed.

5. Add 1 mL of 100% ethanol to each sample tube. Invert and shake each tube until the tissue sample is dislodged from the bottom of the tube. Loosening the tissue increases the surface area exposed to the ethanol. Invert the sample tubes 10–15 times to ensure adequate mixing. Centrifuge the sample tubes in a microcentrifuge set between +18°C and +25°C for 5 min at approximately 14,000 rpm. Repeat for a total of two clean-up washes.

3.3. RNA Extraction Using the Masterpure RNA Purification Kit

1. Calculate and prepare the amount of T&C Lysis Solution (1×) needed including a 10% overage when samples will be processed as a batch: (Number of samples × 1.1) × 298 μL.

Table 1
Preparation of Proteinase K Solution

Reagent	1 reaction (µL/reaction)
1× T&C Lysis Solution	298 µL
Proteinase K	2 µL

2. Calculate and prepare the amount of Proteinase K (50 µg/µL) needed including a 10% overage when samples will be processed as a batch: (Number of samples × 1.1) × 2 µL (*see* **Table 1**)

3.4. Preparation of Proteinase K/T&C Lysis Solution

1. Dispense the required volume of Tissue and Cell Lysis Solution (1×) into a centrifuge tube.

2. Add the required volume of Proteinase K to the centrifuge tube containing the 1× Tissue and Cell Lysis Solution. Important: Do not store the Proteinase K/T&C Lysis solution on ice.

3. Add 300 µL of Proteinase K/T&C Lysis solution to each sample extraction tube. Tightly cap each tube. Vortex each tube for approximately 5–10 s.

4. Incubate the samples at +65°C for 2 h. Shake down or centrifuge the tubes in a microcentrifuge set at +20°C for 5–30 s at no more than 14,000 rpm. Transfer the samples to an ice bucket. Allow the samples to incubate on ice for 3–5 min.

5. Add 150 µL of MPC Protein Precipitation Reagent to each sample. Vortex the samples for approximately 10 s. Centrifuge the samples in a microcentrifuge set at +20°C for 10 min at approximately 14,000 rpm.

6. Obtain a new 1.5-mL microcentrifuge tube for each sample. Dispense 500 µL of isopropanol (at +4°C) into each tube. Aspirate the supernatant from the sample tube and transfer it to the matching 1.5-mL microcentrifuge tube containing the isopropanol.

7. Mix the sample for approximately 3 min. Centrifuge the samples in a microcentrifuge set at +4°C for 10 min at approximately 14,000 rpm. Discard the supernatant without disturbing the precipitated nucleic acid pellet (DNA and RNA).

8. Calculate the amount of 1× DNase I buffer needed as follows: (Number of samples × 1.1) × 180 µL.

9. Calculate the amount of RNase-free DNase I enzyme (1 U/µL) needed as follows: (Number of samples × 1.1) × 20 µL (*see* **Table 2**).

Table 2
Preparation of DNase 1 Solution

Reagent	1 reaction (μL/reaction)
1× DNase I buffer	180 μL
RNase-free DNase I enzyme	20 μL

3.5. Preparation of DNase I Solution

1. Dispense the required volume of 1× DNase I buffer into a centrifuge tube.

2. Add the required volume of RNase-free DNase I enzyme to the test tube containing the 1× DNase I buffer. Important: Prepare the DNase I Solution immediately before dispensing it into the samples.

3. Add 200 μL of the DNase I Solution to each sample. Flick the sample tubes until the pellet is dislodged from the tube. Centrifuge the samples in a microcentrifuge set between +18°C and +25°C for approximately 30–60 s at approximately 3,000 rpm.

4. Incubate the samples with shaking at +37°C for 1 h.

5. Add 200 μL of 2× Tissue and Cell Lysis Solution to each sample. Vortex the samples for approximately 5 s to mix. Centrifuge the tubes in a microcentrifuge set at +20°C for 5–30 s at no more than 14,000 rpm.

6. Add 200 μL of MPC Protein Precipitation Reagent to each sample. Vortex the samples for approximately 10 s to mix. Incubate the samples on ice for 3–5 min. Centrifuge the samples in a microcentrifuge set at +20°C for 10 min at approximately 14,000 rpm to pellet the protein precipitate.

7. Label a new 1.5-mL microcentrifuge tube for each sample. Dispense 500 μL of isopropanol (at +4°C) into each tube. Aspirate the supernatant from the sample tube and transfer it to the matching 1.5-mL microcentrifuge tube containing the isopropanol. Invert the tube for approximately 1–2 s to ensure the supernatant and the isopropanol are mixed. Continue mixing for approximately 3 min.

8. Centrifuge the samples in a microcentrifuge set at +4°C for 10 min at approximately 14,000 rpm. The precipitated RNA will form a pellet at the bottom of the tube. Discard the supernatant.

9. Add 1 mL of 75% ethanol (at +4°C) to each sample tube. Invert the sample tubes for 1–2 s to mix. Centrifuge the samples in a microcentrifuge set at +4°C for 2 min at approximately 14,000 rpm. Discard the ethanol without disturbing the pellet on the bottom of the tube.

10. Repeat the steps for a total of two washes. Incubate the samples at +37°C for 1–2 min until the pellet is dry.

11. Resuspend the RNA in 30 µL of nuclease-free water.

12. Store the RNA at –20°C for periods of less than 1 day, or at –80°C for periods greater than a day.

3.6. RNA Quantification

1. Quantify each sample using the ND-1000 spectrophotometer. The instrument should first be initialized using water and then the background blank reading taken with the sample diluent, in this case also water. Add 1–1.5 µL of the RNA solution to the sample pedestal and take the optical density 260 nm reading.

2. Calculate the sample concentration as follows:

3. For nucleic acids, the solution's absorbance at 260 nm is used to calculate the concentration as follows

4. $C = (A \times e) / b$

   where C is the nucleic acid concentration (in ng/µL), A is the absorbance (in absorbance units, or AU), e is the wavelength-dependent extinction coefficient (in ng-cm/µL; 40 for RNA, 50 for dsDNA, 33 for ssDNA), and b is the cm path length The default NanoDrop path length = 1 mm; adjustable to 2 mm for highly concentrated samples.

3.7. Reverse Transcription

Reverse transcription is done in a 96-well plate as a batch process scalable from one sample up to 94 samples along with one positive control sample and one negative control sample. Any RNA source known to express the candidate genes to be used in the study can act as a positive control. Commercially available standard RNA mixtures made from cell line extracts such as the Universal Human Reference RNA (Stratagene, San Diego, CA) can serve the purpose of a positive control. The negative control uses water in place of the RNA template and tests for laboratory contamination of reagents with target sequences.

Create the gene-specific primer (GSP) pool for specifically priming the genes of interest during the reverse transcription reaction or, alternatively, use random primers. Random hexamers up to random nonamers have been shown to be successful in random primed reverse transcription.

1. To prepare a GSP pool, remove the appropriate reverse PCR primer stock tubes from –20°C storage. Allow the tubes to remain at room temperature until fully thawed, then vortex the reagent tubes for approximately 5 s until thoroughly mixed. Centrifuge in a microcentrifuge set at +4°C for 5–30 s at no more than 14,000 rpm. Store the thawed tubes on ice while in use.

2. Using the concentration on the reverse primer vendor certificate of analysis, calculate the volume of reverse primer to be added using the following equation: (*see* **Note 5**)

$$(C_1)(V_1) = (C_2)(V_2)$$

where C_1 is the starting concentration of each reverse primer stock solution, V_1 is volume of each reverse primer stock solution to be added, C_2 is final concentration of each reverse primer (1 μM), V_2 is the total volume of the GSP pool.

Example: To create 1 mL of the GSP pool with reverse primer each having a starting concentration of 200 μM:

$$(200\,\mu M)(V_1) = (1\,\mu M) \times (1{,}000\,\mu L),$$

$$V_1 = [(1\,\mu M) \times (1{,}000\,\mu L)] / [200\,\mu M],$$

$$V_1 = 5\,\mu L.$$

3. Calculate the volume of nuclease-free water to be added using the following equation:

Vol. of Nuclease – free water = Total vol. of GSP pool – (No. of reverse primers × vol. of each reverse (*see* **Table 3**).

3.8. GSP Priming Pool Preparation

1. Dispense the required volume of nuclease-free water into a microcentrifuge tube. Pipette the required volume of each reverse primer into the tube containing the water. Vortex the tube for approximately 5 s until thoroughly mixed. Centrifuge for approximately 5 s to remove any reagent from the tube lid.

2. Obtain the following reagents from –20°C storage: Omniscript RT Kit, including: dNTP Mix, 5 mM, 10× RT Buffer, RNase-Free Water.

3. Allow the reagents listed to thaw at room temperature until no crystals are visible. Vortex all the tubes containing 10× buffer, dNTP mix, RNase-free water, and GSP pool for approximately 5 s at a medium-high speed until thoroughly mixed. Shake down or spin down each tube to remove condensation from the tube lid, if necessary. Store the reagents on ice if the reagents will not be used immediately after it is thawed.

4. Calculate number of RT reactions to be run as follows:

5. Number of RT reactions = (Number of samples + 1 positive control + 1 negative control) + 5 sample reactions as overage.

Table 3
Calculation of nuclease free water to be added to reverse transcription priming pool.

Number of genes	Total pool volume	Vol per reverse primer	Nuclease-free water
192	1,000 μL	5 μL	40 μL

Table 4
Calculation of reagent volumes for preparing reverse transcription reaction

Reagents	1 reaction (μL/reaction)	94 samples (99 reactions includes five sample overage)
10× Buffer RT	4	396
dNTP mix, 5 mM each dNTP	4	396
Nuclease-free water	4	396
GSP pool,1 μM	2	198
ABI RNase inhibitor, 20 U/μL	1	99
Omniscript RT, 4 U/μL	1	99
Total volume	16	1,584

6. Based on the number of RT reactions, use **Table 4** to calculate the volume of each reagent required to make the Master Mix.

3.9. Master Mix Preparation for RT Reaction

1. Pipette the reagents listed into a labeled tube. Return the component reagents to the –20°C storage after use. Vortex the Master Mix tube at medium-high speed for approximately 2–5 s until thoroughly mixed. Shake down or centrifuge the tubes in the mini centrifuge for approximately 5 s to remove any reagent from the tube lids. Place the Master Mix tube on ice.

2. Obtain the sample RNA and positive RT control (e.g., Universal Human Reference RNA) from –20°C storage. Thaw the sample RNA and positive control RNA completely. Flick the tubes for 2–5 s to mix the RNA. Centrifuge the tubes in a microcentrifuge set at +4°C for 5–30 s at no more than 14,000 rpm.

3. Calculate the amount of RNA to use in each reaction using **Table 5**. The standard qPCR reaction will be 10 μL with the equivalent of 2 ng of cDNA per reaction well. RNA required = [Number of genes + overage wells] × 2 ng/well. The RNA must be at a concentration that the required amount is contained in, 24 μL since the standard reaction volume is 40 μL and 16 μL of reagent mix will be added.

3.10. Sample RNA Requirements

1. Assemble the reverse transcription reactions in a hard-shell thin-wall 96-well microplate or strip tubes (*see* **Note 6**).

2. To assemble the Positive Control dispense 21.9 μL of nuclease-free water into the positive control well or tube. Dispense 2.1 μL of the positive control RNA (at 200 ng/μL) into the positive control well.

Table 5
Calculation of RNA required for reverse transcription reaction.

No. of genes	No. of replicates	Overage wells	RNA required	Volume
192	1	18	420 ng/sample	24 μL

3. To assemble the Negative Control (no-template control) dispense 24 μL of nuclease-free water into the negative control well.

4. To assemble sample reverse transcription reactions dispense 221.9 μL of nuclease-free water into the positive control well or tube. Dispense 2.1 μL of each normalized RNA sample into a reaction well. Repeat the steps for the remaining RNA samples (*see* **Note** 7)

5. Add 16 μL of RT Master Mix to each well. Total reaction volume for each reaction is 40 μL. Mix the contents of the plate or strip tubes. When using plates, pipette the solution up and down 2–3 times to mix. When using strip tubes, flick the tubes for 2–5 s to mix. Seal plates with polarseal film or cap strip tubes with the attached caps. Centrifuge the plate in a plate centrifuge set at +10°C for approximately 2 min at approximately 2,000 rpm or pulse-spin the strip tubes in a minicentrifuge for approximately 5 s (*see* **Note 8**).

6. Thermocycle the RT reactions at +37°C for 60 min followed by +93°C for 5 min, followed by +10°C until the instrument is stopped. Reaction volume is 40 μL.

7. If the samples will be processed through quantitative PCR the same day, store them on ice. If the samples will be processed at a later time, store the samples in –20°C storage.

8. Preparation of the PCR Reactions.

9. PCR assay reagent preparation includes combining the Master Mix Reagent-cDNA mixture with the primer and probe mixtures. The protocol given here assumes 10 μL reactions for 192 genes with an equivalent of 2 ng of RNA (cDNA) per reaction run in a 384-well plate. Nevertheless, this protocol is very scalable and can be adapted to different numbers of candidate genes, modified for reactions run at different volumes, or reactions run with different amounts of RNA in each reaction. Similarly, the process can be adapted for using 96-well reaction plates rather than 384-well reaction plates. One qPCR Master Mix is prepared for each of the following: each test sample, the negative (no template) control for each test sample, the reverse transcription positive control sample, and the reverse transcription negative control sample. In this

process, 2× TaqMan® Universal PCR Master Mix solution is combined with a cDNA sample or nuclease-free water. All steps described here can be done using multichannel pipettors or with automated liquid handling robots such as the Tecan Aquarius robot or Beckman Biomek workstation.

10. Obtain a bottle of 2× TaqMan Universal PCR Master Mix reagent from +4°C storage. Store the 2× TaqMan Universal PCR Master Mix on ice, protected from light, when in use (*see* **Note 9**).

11. Obtain the samples from +4°C storage or –20°C storage. If stored in the –20°C, store the samples on ice until thawed. If the samples are in plates, spin down using the plate centrifuge set at +10°C for approximately 2 min at approximately 2,000 rpm. Centrifuge strip tubes in the mini centrifuge for approximately 5 s to remove any reagent from the tube lid. Store the thawed sample on ice while in use.

12. Obtain an appropriate tube for preparing the sample Master Mix for one sample to be tested for 192 genes (210 wells to allow for an overage) of 10 µL reactions. Pipette the reagents listed in **Table 6**, Quantitative PCR Master Mix Preparation for one sample.

3.11. Quantitative PCR Master Mix Preparation for One Sample

1. Cap the Master Mix tube and invert for 2–5 s until fully mixed. Centrifuge the tube for approximately 5 s to remove any reagent from the lid if necessary. Place the Master Mix tube on ice.

   To prepare the negative (no-template control) for each sample obtain an appropriate tube for use in preparing the Master Mix. Prepare enough reagent for 192 gene negative controls plus a pipetting overage as shown in **Table 7**, Quantitative PCR Master Mix Preparation for one Negative Control into the labeled microcentrifuge tube.

3.12. Quantitative PCR Master Mix Preparation for One Negative Control

1. Cap the Master Mix tube and invert for 2–5 s until fully mixed. Centrifuge the tube in a mini centrifuge for approximately 5 s to remove any reagent from the lid if necessary. Place the Master Mix tube on ice.

Table 6
Preparation of PCR Master Mix for each test sample

2× Universal PCR master mix	1,050 mL
RT reaction mix (sample)	40 µL
Nuclease-free water	590 µL
Total volume	1,680 µL

Table 7
Preparation of PCR reaction negative control sample.

2× Universal PCR master mix	1,050 µL
Nuclease-free water	630 µL
Total volume	1,680 µL

2. To prepare the Master Mix containing the reverse transcription positive and negative control samples, label an appropriate tube for each and prepare each exactly as a test sample.

3. To prepare the primer and probe (P3) pools, thaw the primer and probe stock reagent tubes completely. Vortex the primer and probe tubes for approximately 30 s until thoroughly mixed. Centrifuge at +4°C for 5–30 s at no more than 14,000 rpm. While in use, store the thawed primer and probe tubes on ice.

4. Obtain an amber microcentrifuge tube, centrifuge tube, or other equivalent container and label it with the primer and probe set name.

5. Using the concentration provided on the certificate of analysis for the primers, calculate the volume of each primer to be added as follows (*see* **Note 10**).

6. Volume of forward or reverse primer = [(Final concentration of primer) × (Total volume of P3 pool)]/[(Initial Concentration of primer)].

7. *Example.* To create 600 µL of the P3 pool with each forward and reverse primers having a starting concentration of 200 µM:

8. Volume of forward or reverse primers = [(4.5 µM) × (Total volume of P3 pool)]/[(200 µM)]

9. Using the concentration provided on the certificate of analysis for the probes, calculate the volume of probe to be added as follows (*see* **Note 11**).

10. Volume of Probe = [(Final concentration of Probe) × (Total volume of P3 pool)]/[(Initial Concentration of Probe)]

11. *Example.* To create 600 µL of the P3 pool with each probe having a starting concentration of 100 µM:

12. Volume of Probe = [(1 µM) × (Total volume of P3 pool)]/[(100 µM)]

13. Determine the volume of nuclease-free water as follows.

14. Volume of Nuclease-Free Water = (Total Vol. of P3 mix) [(Vol. of Forward Primer) + (Vol. of Reverse Primer) + (Vol. of Probe)]

Vol. of forward primer (μL)	13.5
Vol. of reverse primer (μL)	13.5
Vol. of probe (μL)	6
Vol. of nuclease-free water (μL)	567
Total volume (μL)	600

Sample Calculation for Preparing 600 μL of P3 Pool

15. Pipette the calculated volumes of the required reagents into a microcentrifuge tube. Vortex the P3 pool for approximately 30 s until thoroughly mixed. Centrifuge in a microcentrifuge set at +4°C for 5–30 s at no more than 14,000 rpm. Store the P3 pool tube on ice while in use.

16. Distribute the P3 mixtures into a 96-well plate using 2 μL/well for 10 μL reactions. A plate layout should be predetermined where each primer and probe mix is deposited into two reaction wells: one for the test sample, one for the negative control. Once the P3 mixtures have been deposited, the master mix-cDNA and master mix-negative control should be distributed into the plate, each into one of the 192-well pairs.

17. Spin down the plate in a plate centrifuge set at +10°C for approximately 2 min at approximately 2,000 rpm. Ensure no air bubbles are trapped at the bottom of the plate. If air bubbles are seen, spin down the plate in the plate centrifuge set at +10°C for approximately 2 min at 2,000 rpm. Repeat until no air bubbles are trapped at the bottom of the plate. Hand seal the plate with polar seal film.

18. Run the Plate on the PRISM 7900 HT Sequence Detection System using the following selections: Assay: Absolute Quantitation; Container: 384-Well Clear Plate; Template: TaqMan 10 μL; Cycling Conditions: +95°C, 10 min; (+95°C, 20 s, +60°C, 45 s) for 40 cycles; Assay Volume: 10 μL.

3.13. Data Analysis   At the conclusion of the run, use the ABI PRISM 7900HT Sequence Detection System User Guide to export and process the data following the instructions for Real-Time Analysis for absolute quantification.

4. Notes

1. It is important to store and handle the components of the Epicentre MasterPure Kit appropriately. It contains: 1× Tissue and Cell Lysis Solution, Proteinase K (50 μg/μL),

MPC Protein Precipitation Reagent, RNase-free DNase I enzyme (1 U/μL), 1× DNase I buffer, 2× Tissue and Cell Lysis Solution. Proteinase K and DNase I enzymes must be kept at –20°C. Store the remaining components at +18°C to +25°C. Before using any buffers in the kit, ensure they have completely thawed (i.e., no particles or crystals are visible in the solutions) and are well mixed.

2. Amplicon sizes should be constrained to less than 100 bases total in length, including primer sequences. This design parameter should be adjusted in the Primer Express or Primer3 settings since the default usually permits amplicons as long as 300 bases to be designed. It is generally easier to get a design that meets all necessary criteria by not demanding the amplicon span an exon junction. DNase treatment of the RNA extracts and inclusion of the no-template controls eliminates the necessity to design RNA-specific assays.

3. The ABI PRISM 7900HT system is capable of detecting a number of different fluorescent reporter dyes, but the fluorescein-based dye FAM is the most robust and widely available. There are also multiple different quencher molecules that can be paired with the FAM dye on the dual-labeled probes. Although TAMARA dye was often used in the original form of the TaqMan assay, the newer "dark" (nonfluorescent) quenchers give much better assay results due to better quenching and lower assay backgrounds. Commercial oligonucleotide vendors offer a variety of TaqMan probe configurations.

4. Pathology fixation procedures are widely variable depending on tissue type and each laboratory's optimized practices. RNA can be successfully extracted from nearly all types and ages of fixed tissues; however, yield will vary with sample quality and age. The quality of the extracted RNA (degree of fragmentation) will also vary with sample age and fixation method. If tissue is available, a test extraction can be very helpful for estimating how much RNA to expect from a sample.

5. The concentration of each reverse primer stock solution is typically 100 μM or 200 μM. The reverse primers will be mixed with nuclease-free water to bring the final concentration of each reverse primer in the GSP pool to 1 μM.

6. Keep all reverse transcription reaction components cold throughout the qPCR reaction assembly process, including the plate or strip tubes by keeping them on ice, in a cooler, or equivalent.

7. Assembling the reverse transcription reactions can be done more easily if at the time each RNA sample is quantified, it is also normalized to a standard concentration of 200 ng/μL

using nuclease-free water. Alternatively, each reverse transcription reaction can be individually calculated and the final volumes normalized with nuclease-free water to compensate for any differences in added RNA volume.

8. When carrying out temperature-sensitive reactions in microtiter plates, it is very important to ensure no air bubbles are trapped at the bottom of the plate so that enzymatic mixtures are exposed uniformly to correct temperature conditions. If air bubbles are seen, tap the plate to dislodge the bubbles. Spin down the plate in the plate centrifuge set at +10°C for approximately 2 min at approximately 2,000 rpm. Repeat the previous step until no air bubbles are trapped at the bottom of the plate.

9. This section describes the steps used to prepare Master Mix for one sample. One Master Mix is prepared for each cDNA test sample, the RT-positive control sample and the RT-negative control sample. Similarly, one negative control Master Mix is prepared as a no-template control for each sample where nuclease-free water is substituted for the cDNA products of the reverse transcription reaction. It is recommended that the positive and negative reverse transcription samples be assembled and processed through PCR prior to assembling the test sample PCR plates to ensure the reverse transcription reaction was successful and no contaminations occurred.

10. The concentration of each forward and reverse primer stock solution is typically 100 μM or 200 μM. The primers will be mixed with probe and nuclease-free water to bring the final concentration of the primer in the P3 pool to 4.5 μM. Final primer concentrations in the PCR reaction are 900 nM.

11. The concentration of each probe stock solution is typically 100 μM. The probes will be mixed with primer and nuclease-free water to bring the final concentration of the probe in the P3 pool to 1 μM. The final PCR reaction probe concentration is 200 nM.

References

1. Abrahamsen, H.N., Steiniche, T., Nexo, E., Hamilton-Dutoit, S.J. and Sorensen, B.S. (2003) Towards quantitative mRNA analysis in paraffin-embedded tissues using real-time reverse transcriptase-polymerase chain reaction: a methodological study on lymph nodes from melanoma patients. J Mol Diagn, 5, 34–41.
2. Cronin, M., Pho, M., Dutta, D., Stephans, J.C., Shak, S., Kiefer, M.C., Esteban, J.M. and Baker, J.B. (2004) Measurement of gene expression in archival paraffin-embedded tissues: development and performance of a 92-gene reverse transcriptase-polymerase chain reaction assay. Am J Pathol, 164, 35–42.
3. Finke, J., Fritzen, R., Ternes, P., Lange, W. and Dolken, G. (1993) An improved strategy and a useful housekeeping gene for RNA analysis from formalin-fixed, paraffin-embedded tissues by PCR. Biotechniques, 14, 448–453.

4. Godfrey, T.E., Kim, S.H., Chavira, M., Ruff, D.W., Warren, R.S., Gray, J.W. and Jensen, R.H. (2000) Quantitative mRNA expression analysis from formalin-fixed, paraffin-embedded tissues using 5' nuclease quantitative reverse transcription-polymerase chain reaction. J Mol Diagn, 2, 84–91.

5. Rupp, G.M. and Locker, J. (1988) Purification and analysis of RNA from paraffin-embedded tissues. Biotechniques, 6, 56–60.

6. Sheils, O.M. and Sweeney, E.C. (1999) TSH receptor status of thyroid neoplasms–TaqMan RT-PCR analysis of archival material. J Pathol, 188, 87–92.

7. Specht, K., Richter, T., Muller, U., Walch, A., Werner, M. and Hofler, H. (2001) Quantitative gene expression analysis in micro-dissected archival formalin-fixed and paraffin-embedded tumor tissue. Am J Pathol, 158, 419–429.

8. Stanta, G. and Bonin, S. (1998) RNA quantitative analysis from fixed and paraffin-embedded tissues: membrane hybridization and capillary electrophoresis. Biotechniques, 24, 271–276.

9. Chang, J., Powles, T.J., Allred, D.C., Ashley, S.E., Clark, G.M., Makris, A., Assersohn, L., Gregory, R.K., Osborne, C.K. and Dowsett, M. (1999) Biologic markers as predictors of clinical outcome from systemic therapy for primary operable breast cancer. J Clin Oncol, 17, 3058–3063.

10. Davis, R.E. and Staudt, L.M. (2002) Molecular diagnosis of lymphoid malignancies by gene expression profiling. Curr Opin Hematol, 9, 333–338.

11. Gianni, L., Zambetti, M., Clark, K., Baker, J., Cronin, M., Wu, J., Mariani, G., Rodriguez, J., Carcangio, M., Watson, D., et-al. (2005) Gene expression profiles in paraffin-embedded core biopsy tissue predict response to chemotherapy in women with locally advanced breast cancer. J Clin Oncol, 23, 7265–7277.

12. Golub, T.R., Slonim, D.K., Tamayo, P., Huard, C., Gaasenbeek, M., Mesirov, J.P., Coller, H., Loh, M.L., Downing, J.R., Caligiuri, M.A., et-al. (1999) Molecular classification of cancer: class discovery and class prediction by gene expression monitoring. Science, 286, 531–537.

13. Habel, L.A., Shak, S., Jacobs, M.K., Capra, A., Alexander, C., Pho, M., Baker, J., Walker, M., Watson, D., Hackett, J., et-al. (2006) A population-based study of tumor gene expression and risk of breast cancer death among lymph node-negative patients. Breast Cancer Res, 8, R25.

14. Paik, S., Shak, S., Tang, G., Kim, C., Baker, J., Cronin, M., Baehner, F.L., Walker, M.G., Watson, D., Park, T., et-al. (2004) A multigene assay to predict recurrence of tamoxifen-treated, node-negative breast cancer. N Engl J Med, 351, 2817–2826.

15. Paik, S., Tang, G., Shak, S., Kim, C., Baker, J., Kim, W., Cronin, M., Baehner, F.L., Watson, D., Bryant, J., et-al. (2006) Gene expression and benefit of chemotherapy in women with node-negative, estrogen receptor-positive breast cancer. J Clin Oncol, 24, 3726–3734.

16. Ramaswamy, S., Ross, K.N., Lander, E.S. and Golub, T.R. (2003) A molecular signature of metastasis in primary solid tumors. Nat Genet, 33, 49–54.

17. Rosenwald, A., Wright, G., Wiestner, A., Chan, W.C., Connors, J.M., Campo, E., Gascoyne, R.D., Grogan, T.M., Muller-Hermelink, H.K., Smeland, E.B., et al. (2003) The proliferation gene expression signature is a quantitative integrator of oncogenic events that predicts survival in mantle cell lymphoma. Cancer Cell, 3, 185–197.

18. Sorlie, T., Perou, C.M., Tibshirani, R., Aas, T., Geisler, S., Johnsen, H., Hastie, T., Eisen, M.B., van de, R.M., Jeffrey, S.S., et-al. (2001) Gene expression patterns of breast carcinomas distinguish tumor subclasses with clinical implications. Proc Natl Acad Sci U.S.A, 98, 10869–10874.

19. van de Vijver, M.J., He, Y.D., van't Veer, L.J., Dai, H., Hart, A.A., Voskuil, D.W., Schreiber, G.J., Peterse, J.L., Roberts, C., Marton, M.J., et-al. (2002) A gene-expression signature as a predictor of survival in breast cancer. N Engl J Med, 347, 1999–2009.

20. Lewis, F., Maughan, N.J., Smith, V., Hillan, K. and Quirke, P. (2001) Unlocking the archive–gene expression in paraffin-embedded tissue. J Pathol, 195, 66–71.

21. Cronin, M., Sangli, C., Liu, M.L., Pho, M., Dutta, D., Nguyen, A., Jeong, J., Wu, J., Langone, K.C. and Watson, D. (2007) Analytical validation of the Oncotype DX genomic diagnostic test for recurrence prognosis and therapeutic response prediction in node-negative, estrogen receptor-positive breast cancer. Clin Chem, 53, 1084–1091.

22. Rozen, S. and Skaletsky, H. (2000) Primer3 on the WWW for general users and for biologist programmers. Methods Mol Biol, 132, 365–386.

Chapter 14

High-Throughput Mutation Screening Using a Single Amplification Condition

Lijia Shi and John E. Landers

Summary

Numerous innovative and high-throughput techniques have been established to identify human disease genes. However, DNA sequencing of candidate genes still remains as a major limitation in the identification of causative mutations. Much of this limitation is due to the time and labor needed for the polymerase chain reaction (PCR) optimization and reaction setup. Toward this end, we have established a simplified protocol that utilizes a single PCR amplification condition. PCR purification is accomplished via enzymatic digestion and all products can be sequenced using universal primers. This combination of a single amplification condition, single-step purification, and sequencing setup using universal primers all contribute to a simple and high-throughput mutation screen.

Key words: DNA sequencing, Mutation screening, PCR, Polymorphism detection.

1. Introduction

The search for human disease genes typically involves narrowing the list of candidate genes to a manageable number that can be intensely analyzed on an individual level. For example, linkage analysis studies can often restrict the location of a disease gene to a region of several megabases *(1–4)*. Allelic imbalance studies, using high-density SNP arrays or genome-wide microsatellite scans, can also identify localized regions displaying loss of heterozygosity that may harbor potential tumor suppressor genes *(5–8)*. More recently, the use of whole genome association studies have been used to identify candidate human disease genes *(9–12)*. Typically, in each of these cases, the candidate genes are then screened for mutations by DNA sequencing.

Michael A. Tainsky, *Methods in Molecular Biology, Tumor Biomarker Discovery, Vol. 520*
© Humana Press, a part of Springer Science + Business Media, LLC 2009
DOI: 10.1007/978-1-60327-811-9_14

DNA sequencing can be an expensive, time-consuming, and labor-intensive process. The abundance of sequencing companies and core facilities has reduced the price and effort such that outsourcing DNA sequencing is usually more economical than maintaining the procedure within the laboratory. However, there is still considerable effort involved in the amplification optimization for each locus to be sequenced. Additional efforts are also involved in polymerase chain reaction (PCR) purification and sequencing reaction setup. Toward this end, we have outlined a sequencing approach that allows a majority of loci (>85%) to be amplified with a single amplification condition *(13)*. Furthermore, the protocol outlines a simple process for DNA purification and sequencing reaction setup that can be performed quickly and efficiently. Additionally, due to the reduction of optimization and setup steps, the labor, cost, and time to achieve the project goals are significantly reduced.

2. Materials

2.1. Preparations and Storage of PCR and Sequencing Primers

1. Sequencing primer SeqForward (5′ TAG TAA AAC GAC GGC CAG T 3′) and SeqReverse (5′ TAG GAA ACA GCT ATG ACC ATG 3′) (Integrated DNA Technologies (IDT), Skokie, IL).

2. 96-well PCR primer plate (IDT) in which the forward and reverse primers are premixed to a final concentration of 25 μM (each primer) (*see* **Notes 2** and **3**). Each forward primer should be tagged at the 5′ end with the sequence of SeqForward, and each reverse primer should be tagged at the 5′ end with the sequence of SeqReverse. Lastly, wells H11 and H12 should contain the identical sequence as wells H9 and H10, respectively. These wells will be used as negative controls for the PCR reaction (*see* **Note 4**).

3. TE Buffer: 10 mM Tris, 1 mM EDTA, pH 8.0 (Fisher Scientific). Store at room temperature.

2.2. Polymerase Chain Reaction

1. 2× AmpliTaq Gold PCR Master Mix (Applied Biosystems, Foster City, CA) stored in 800 μL aliquots at 4°C.

2. Reduced TE buffer: 10 mM Tris, 0.1 mM EDTA, pH 8.0 (Fisher Scientific). Store at room temperature.

3. Molecular-Biology-Grade Water (Fisher Scientific). Store at room temperature.

4. High-quality genomic DNA diluted in reduced TE Buffer at 5 ng/μL. Store aliquots of 800 μL at –20°C.

5. Multipurpose centrifuge capable of handling 96-well plates.

6. 96-well GeneAmp PCR System 9700 (Applied Biosystems) or comparable thermocycler.

7. Aluminum Sealing Tape (Fisher Scientific).

8. Adhesive PCR Film (Fisher Scientific).

9. Hard-Shell 96-well Plate (BioRad, Hercules, CA).

10. Thermo-Fast 96 Detection Plate (Fisher Scientific).

11. 8-channel pipettor, 2–125 µL (Matrix Technologies, Hudson, NH).

2.3. Agarose Gel Electrophoresis

1. E-Gel Low Range Quantitative DNA Ladder (Invitrogen, Carlsbad, CA).

2. 2% E-Gel 96 Agarose (Invitrogen).

3. E-Holder Platform (Invitrogen).

4. Research multichannel pipette, 0.5—10 µL, 12-channel (Eppendorf, Westbury, NY).

5. Thermo-Fast 96 Low Profile Plate (Fisher Scientific).

6. UV Transilluminator (USA Scientific).

7. Photograph apparatus (Fisher Scientific).

2.4. Post-PCR Purification and Sequencing Reaction Setup

1. Exo-SAP IT (USB Corp., Cleveland, OH).

3. Methods

The methodology described here is toward the simultaneous amplification 94 distinct loci from a single DNA sample in a 96-well format. The ability to amplify each locus under a single condition is based on two PCR techniques. Touchdown PCR (TD-PCR) is an approach in which the annealing thermocycling temperature in the initial cycles is well above the T_m of the PCR primers *(14)*. However, in subsequent cycles, the annealing temperature is incrementally decreased. Eventually, the maximal annealing temperature will be reached in which amplification can occur. Mispriming is minimized due to the high temperature of the initial amplification. As the temperature decreases further and additional product is created, mispriming is minimized due to the abundance of the correct amplicon over the original genomic DNA template. This approach is very successful as a single-step PCR optimization procedure. In combination, we have added a 5′ tag-primer approach *(15)*. All forward and reverse PCR primers are tagged at their 5′ ends with a unique sequence. By doing so, we have observed a further increase in the success rate of TD-PCR to typically >90%. Furthermore, all PCR products can be sequenced with the same set of sequencing primers directed toward the 5′ tags, thus simplifying the sequencing reaction setup. Purification of the PCR products using Exo-SAP digestion *(16, 17)* also provides a simple one-step method that yields much more consistent results as compared to column purification methods.

3.1. Preparations and Storage of PCR and Sequencing Primers

1. The PCR primer stock plate from IDT should contain the tagged-forward and reverse primers premixed to a concentration of 25 μM. The last two wells (H11 and H12) represent negative controls.

2. Spin down primer stock plate at ~1000g for 2 min before opening the cover.

3. Dilute PCR primer stock plate into a Hard-Shell 96-well plate by adding 4 μL of 25 μM of stock primer mix to 96 μL of PCR-Grade water to make 100 μL of 1 μM primer working solution.

4. Mix the diluted primers well with an 8-channel pipettor.

5. Cover the 1 μM PCR primers plate with Aluminum seal and spin the plate at 2,500 rpm for 2 min.

6. Place the 1 μM diluted primer plate at 4°C for short-term storage or –20°C for long-term storage.

7. Sequencing primer stocks are received in tubes as dried powder. Before opening the cap for stock tubes, briefly spin tubes in a centrifuge to bring down all primers to the bottom of tube.

8. Resuspend each stock primer in TE buffer at concentration of 500 ng/μL based on the information sheet provided by the vendor.

9. Dilute the Sequencing Primers in PCR-Grade water to 8 ng/μL.

10. Dispense the diluted Sequencing Primers into 1.25 mL aliquots and store at –20°C.

3.2. Polymerase Chain Reaction Setup

1. Each PCR reaction volume is to be setup as seen in **Table 1**

2. Transfer 7.5 μL of 1 μM diluted PCR primer mix into each well of the PCR plate using an 8-channel pipettor.

3. Transfer 15 μL of 2× Amplitaq Gold Master Mix on PCR Plate with 8-channel pipettor (*see* **Note 5**).

4. Add 7.5 μL of PCR water to the negative control wells H11 and H12. Temporarily cover PCR plate, move to PCR staging area to add the DNA template.

Table 1
PCR Reaction Setup

Reagents and template	1× reaction (30 µL)	100× reactions (µL)
2× AmpliTaq master mix	15	1,500
1 µM PCR primer mix	7.5	–
10 ng/µL Genomic DNA	7.5	750
Total	30	–

5. Add 7.5 µL of 10 ng/µL genomic DNA to each well of the PCR plate (except H11 and H12). Be sure to change tips for each DNA transfer and avoid adding any DNA to wells H11 and H12.

6. Mix all wells by pipetting up and down several times.

7. Seal the PCR plate with PCR film and spin down plate at 2,500 rpm for 2 min.

8. Place the PCR plate into the thermocycler (*see* **Note 6**) and perform the following cycling method (*see* **Note 7**):

9. Following thermocycling, the PCR plate can be stored at 4°C.

95°C for 1 min	
95°C for 30 s	40 cycles
65°C – 0.5°C per cycle for 30 s	
72°C for 1 min	
95°C for 30 s	10 cycles
50°C for 30 s	
72°C for 1 min	
72°C for 10 min	
4°C Hold	

3.3. Agarose Gel Electrophoresis

1. After completion of PCR, the products are run on an E-Gel for quality checking (*see* **Note 8**).

2. Add 20 µL of water into each well of a 96-well low profile plate with an 8-Channel pipettor.

3. Spin down the PCR plate at 2,500 rpm for 2 min before opening the cover.

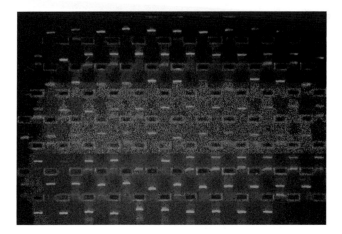

Fig. 1. Agarose Gel Electrophoresis of 94 Distinct PCR Reactions. Forward and reverse primers were selected from 94 distinct loci and 5′ tagged with the sequence SeqForward and SeqReverse, respectively, as indicated in **Subheading 2**. Amplification reactions were setup in a 96-well plate using a single DNA template and thermocycled using Touchdown-PCR conditions. The resultant products were subjected to electrophoresis using the E-Gel system (Invitrogen). As shown, >90% of the loci yield a single distinct amplicon. The last two wells of the bottom row represent negative control PCR reactions (wells H11 and H12).

4. Transfer 2 μL of the PCR products to the water and mix well with an 8-Channel pipettor.

5. Briefly spin down the low profile plate at 2,500 rpm.

6. Load 20 μL of each sample row from above on E-Gel with 12-channel pipettor.

7. Load 15 μL of Low Range DNA ladder into the last well of each row.

8. Electrophoresis the samples for 6 min.

9. Take a picture to record PCR result. An example of typical results is shown in **Fig. 1** (*see* **Notes 9** and **10**).

3.4. Post-PCR Purification and Sequence Reaction Setup

1. Prepare a thermocycling program for Exo-SAP digestion using the following conditions: 37°C for 15 min, 80°C for 15 min, 4°C Hold.

2. Dispense 4 μL of Exo-SAP into each well of new PCR plate.

3. Transfer 11 μL of each PCR to the Exo-SAP containing plate using a 12-channel pipettor.

4. Cover the plate with an Aluminum Seal and spin down briefly at 2,500 rpm.

5. Put the plate into the thermocycler and start the program for Exo-SAP digestion.

6. Dispense 12.5 μL of SeqPrimer Forward into each well of a new PCR plate.

7. Spin down Exo-SAP digestion plate at 2,500 rpm for 2 min before opening the cover.

8. Transfer 7.5 μL of Exo-SAP cleaned PCR products to the SeqPrimer Forward plate.

9. Dispense 12.5 μL of SeqPrimer Reverse into each well of the Exo-SAP digestion plate.

10. Label each plate with the sequencing primer name, the DNA sample amplified, and the PCR primer plate used for amplification.

11. Spin the plates briefly at 2,500 rpm and store at –20°C until submitting for sequencing (*see* **Note 11**).

4. Notes

1. As with all PCR procedures, it is recommended that the lab be divided into three different areas. Reagents should be prepared in a pre-PCR clean area to avoid contaminations. This area should be free of DNA template and PCR amplicons, and all PCR primers and master mix are stored in this room. The PCR staging area should be used to setup the PCR reaction and handle genomic DNA. Lastly, PCR thermocycling, post-PCR Cleanup, agarose gel electrophoresis, and sequencing setup can be done in the main lab area. Gloves and clean lab coats should be worn for all procedures.

2. Successful μL amplification is dependent on primer selection. It is highly recommended to select primers using the application Primer3 *(18)* (http://frodo.wi.mit.edu/primer3/input.htm). Primers should be selected using the default settings for primer length (min. 18/ opt. 20/ max 27), T_m (min. 57°C/ opt. 60°C/ max. 63°C), and %GC content (min. 20%/ max. 80%). Smaller-length PCR products are preferred. Larger-length PCR products should be subdivided with a minimal overlap of 50 base pairs. It is also recommended that the primers be verified by using UCSC Genome Browser In-Silico PCR *(19)* (http://genome.ucsc.edu/cgi-bin/hgPcr?org=Human&db=hg18&hgsid=93066 109) to insure only a single product will be amplified.

3. For exon screening sequencing, the application ExonPrimer (http://ihg.gsf.de/ihg/ExonPrimer.html) provides a very simple interface to select primers. Users of the UCSC Genome Browser can easily link to the ExonPrimer interface through the Gene Description pages.

4. Although other companies provide premixed primers resuspended at a normalized concentration, we have found that IDT provides the highest-quality oligonucleotides.

5. We have found that 2× AmpliTaq Gold PCR Master Mix yields the most consistent results as compared to other PCR master mixes. However, if another master mix is used, it is essential that a hot-start method be employed. Spurious PCR often occur when using Touchdown-PCR protocols without a hot-start procedure.

6. We have also tested thermocyclers from MJ Research and have observed similar results.

7. The procedure described here is based on PCR products less than 1,000 base pairs. Alterations of the protocol may be necessary for larger products, including cycling conditions, DNA/primer concentrations, and enzymes used for amplification.

8. Other 96-well agarose gel electrophoresis units are available and can be used for this step. However, the well layout of the E-gel 96 and the bufferless system is highly advantageous to high-throughput situations. Furthermore, the E-gel system can be easily incorporated into a liquid handling system to allow for automated analysis.

9. A single intense amplicon is representative of a successful amplification. Multiple bands are often due to related genes or attempting to use primers homologous to a repetitive sequence. We have observed typical success rates for PCR are ~85–95% which are influenced by GC-rich or highly repetitive regions. Poor experimental technique, such as incomplete mixing of reactions, poor-quality DNA/primers, substandard enzymes, can also result in low success rates.

10. Negative control wells (H11 and H12) should be compared to their corresponding experiment wells (H9 and H10, respectively) to insure no PCR product was generated. Appropriately sized bands in the negative controls wells are typically due to contaminating genomic DNA. Replacement of all reagents is recommended to eliminate contamination.

11. Nearly all PCR reactions that generated a single amplicon should yield excellent sequencing results. High percentages of failed sequencing reaction can be due to post-PCR cross-contamination. Alternatively, failed Exo-SAP purification can result in a high percentage of failed reactions. If this is suspected, replace the Exo-SAP enzyme mix and repeat the procedure.

12. The protocol as described utilizes the sequencing primers at a final concentration of 5 ng/μL in a 20 μL volume. This is

based on the submission recommendations of our sequencing core. However, it is necessary to consult your sequencing companies' submission requirements and alter this protocol appropriately.

13. Nearly all of the steps described here can be automated on the simplest of liquid handlers. We have automated this protocol on a Multiprobe II Automated Liquid Handling System (Perkin Elmer, Waltham, MA). Automating the procedures yields a higher level of throughput and reproducibility, and decreases the amount of labor needed to perform the desired tasks. If a liquid handler is not available, it is highly recommended to obtain single and multichannel electronic pipettors. Many of the steps described in this procedure require repeated pipetting and thus can benefit greatly from such instruments.

14. If the number of plates to be sequenced is high, it is recommended that barcoded plates be utilized. Barcode readers are inexpensive and can be directly attached to a lab computer. By using a simple program, like Microsoft Excel or Access, detailed information can be recorded for each plate (e.g., plate name, sequencing primer used, DNA used, date, operator). Sample tracking also becomes very simplified and human error is greatly reduced.

15. For the comparison of multiple DNA samples, the procedure just needs to be repeated for each new sample. Additionally, sequence alignment can be simplified by aligning corresponding wells on each plate to each other. For example, well A1 of all sequencing plates should be aligned to each other.

16. If the sequencing results are to be used for mutation detection, we recommended utilizing the PolyPhred software application *(20)* (http://droog.mbt.washington.edu/PolyPhred.html). Our group has found that PolyPhred has performed superior as compared to other commercially available software packages for mutation detection.

References

1. Sawcer, S., Ban, M., Maranian, M., Yeo, T.W., Compston, A., Kirby, A., Daly, M.J., De Jager, P.L., Walsh, E., Lander, E.S., et al. (2005) A high-density screen for linkage in multiple sclerosis. Am J Hum Genet 77:454–467

2. Janecke, A.R., Thompson, D.A., Utermann, G., Becker, C., Hubner, C.A., Schmid, E., McHenry, C.L., Nair, A.R., Ruschendorf, F., Heckenlively, J., Wissinger, B., Nurnberg, P., Gal, A. (2004) Mutations in RDH12 encoding a photoreceptor cell retinol dehydrogenase cause childhood-onset severe retinal dystrophy. Nat Genet 36:850–854

3. Puffenberger, E.G., Hu-Lince, D., Parod, J.M., Craig, D.W., Dobrin, S.E., Conway, A.R., Donarum, E.A., Strauss, K.A., Dunckley, T., Cardenas, J.F., Melmed, K.R., Wright, C.A., Liang, W., Stafford, P., Flynn, C.R., Morton, D.H., Stephan, D.A. (2004) Mapping of sudden infant death with dysgenesis of the testes syndrome (SIDDT) by a SNP

genome scan and identification of TSPYL loss of function. Proc Natl Acad Sci U S A 101:11689–11694

4. Sellick, G.S., Garrett, C., Houlston, R.S. (2003) A novel gene for neonatal diabetes maps to chromosome 10p12.1-p13. Diabetes 52:2636–2638

5. Cvetkovic, D., Pisarcik, D., Lee, C., Hamilton, T.C., Abdollahi, A. (2004) Altered expression and loss of heterozygosity of the LOT1 gene in ovarian cancer. Gynecol Oncol 95:449–455

6. Koppert, L.B., van der Velden, A.W., van de Wetering, M., Abbou, M., van den Ouweland, A.M., Tilanus, H.W., Wijnhoven, B.P., Dinjens, W.N. (2004) Frequent loss of the AXIN1 locus but absence of AXIN1 gene mutations in adenocarcinomas of the gastro-oesophageal junction with nuclear beta-catenin expression. Br J Cancer 90:892–899

7. Maris, T., Androulidakis, E.J., Tzagournissakis, M., Papavassiliou, S., Moser, H., Plaitakis, A. (1995) X-linked adrenoleukodystrophy presenting as neurologically pure familial spastic paraparesis [see comments]. Neurology 45:1101–1104

8. Stephens, L.A., Powell, N.G., Grubb, J., Jeremiah, S.J., Bethel, J.A., Demidchik, E.P., Bogdanova, T.I., Tronko, M.D., Thomas, G.A. (2005) Investigation of loss of heterozygosity and SNP frequencies in the RET gene in papillary thyroid carcinoma. Thyroid 15:100–104

9. Steinthorsdottir, V., Thorleifsson, G., Reynisdottir, I., Benediktsson, R., Jonsdottir, T., Walters, G.B., Styrkarsdottir, U., Gretarsdottir, S., Emilsson, V., Ghosh, S., et al. (2007) A variant in CDKAL1 influences insulin response and risk of type 2 diabetes. Nat Genet 39:770–775

10. Klein, R.J., Zeiss, C., Chew, E.Y., Tsai, J.Y., Sackler, R.S., Haynes, C., Henning, A.K., SanGiovanni, J.P., Mane, S.M., Mayne, S.T., Bracken, M.B., Ferris, F.L., Ott, J., Barnstable, C., Hoh, J. (2005) Complement factor H polymorphism in age-related macular degeneration. Science 308:385–389

11. Sladek, R., Rocheleau, G., Rung, J., Dina, C., Shen, L., Serre, D., Boutin, P., Vincent, D., Belisle, A., Hadjadj, S., Balkau, B., Heude, B., Charpentier, G., Hudson, T.J.,

Montpetit, A., Pshezhetsky, A.V., Prentki, M., Posner, B.I., Balding, D.J., Meyre, D., Polychronakos, C., Froguel, P. (2007) A genome-wide association study identifies novel risk loci for type 2 diabetes. Nature 445:881–885

12. Saxena, R., Voight, B.F., Lyssenko, V., Burtt, N.P., de Bakker, P.I., Chen, H., Roix, J.J., Kathiresan, S., Hirschhorn, J.N., Daly, M.J., et al. (2007) Genome-wide association analysis identifies loci for type 2 diabetes and triglyceride levels. Science 316:1331–1336

13. Jordan, B., Charest, A., Dowd, J.F., Blumenstiel, J.P., Yeh, R.F., Osman, A., Housman, D.E., Landers, J.E. (2002) Genome complexity reduction for SNP genotyping analysis. Proc Natl Acad Sci U S A 99:2942–2947

14. Don, R.H., Cox, P.T., Wainwright, B.J., Baker, K., Mattick, J.S. (1991) 'Touchdown' PCR to circumvent spurious priming during gene amplification. Nucleic Acids Res 19:4008

15. Tsang, S., Sun, Z., Stewart, C., Lum, N., Frankenberger, C., Subleski, M., Rasmussen, L., Munroe, D.J. (2004) Development of multiplex DNA electronic microarrays using a universal adaptor system for detection of single nucleotide polymorphisms. Biotechniques 36:682–688

16. Werle, E., Schneider, C., Renner, M., Volker, M., Fiehn, W. (1994) Convenient single-step, one tube purification of PCR products for direct sequencing. Nucleic Acids Res 22:4354–4355

17. Hanke, M., Wink, M. (1994) Direct DNA sequencing of PCR-amplified vector inserts following enzymatic degradation of primer and dNTPs. Biotechniques 17:858–860

18. Rozen, S., Skaletsky, H. (2000) Primer3 on the WWW for general users and for biologist programmers. Methods Mol Biol 132:365–386

19. Kent, W.J., Sugnet, C.W., Furey, T.S., Roskin, K.M., Pringle, T.H., Zahler, A.M., Haussler, D. (2002) The human genome browser at UCSC. Genome Res 12:996–1006

20. Nickerson, D.A., Tobe, V.O., Taylor, S.L. (1997) PolyPhred: automating the detection and genotyping of single nucleotide substitutions using fluorescence-based resequencing. Nucleic Acids Res 25:2745–2751

Chapter 15

DNA Sequencing of Cancer-Related Genes for Biomarker Discovery

Lisa M. Farwell and Victoria A. Joshi

Summary

Dideoxy DNA sequencing is routinely used in research and, increasingly, in clinical care for the detection of DNA sequence variants, single nucleotide changes, or small insertions or deletions, when the spectrum of DNA variation is unknown. DNA sequence variation can be present in tumor tissue that is not present in the normal tissue from the same individual. This somatic DNA sequence variation is often the cause of abnormal cell growth and/or regulation and, ultimately, tumorigenesis. Identification of these oncogenic DNA sequence variants has successfully led to the development of cancer therapies, since the abnormal protein products created from genomic DNA containing mutations can serve as targets for pharmacologic inhibition. Somatic DNA sequence analysis will continue to be a valuable technique for biomarker discovery until the complete spectrum of DNA variation observed in tumor tissue is understood.

Key words: Tumor, Sequencing, Cancer, Biomarker discovery, Sanger.

1. Introduction

Somatic alteration of DNA is a major mechanism of tumorigenesis. Two means by which this can be accomplished are by the inactivation of tumor suppressor genes and the activation of oncogenes. DNA sequencing efforts can be successful in identifying molecular defects that both drive and are the products of tumorigenesis. One successful example is that of BRAF. Activating BRAF mutations were identified in 70% of malignant melanomas, 10% of colon cancer, and a fraction of other cancers by investigators at the Wellcome Trust Sanger Institute who, as part of the

Michael A. Tainsky, *Methods in Molecular Biology, Tumor Biomarker Discovery, Vol. 520*
© Humana Press, a part of Springer Science+Business Media, LLC 2009
DOI: 10.1007/978-1-60327-811-9_15

Cancer Genome project, made the discovery within the first 20 tumor candidate genes sequenced (1). Inhibition of the activated version of BRAF could effectively treat these cancers, and BRAF inhibitors are currently in various stages of clinical development. The recently announced Cancer Genome Anatomy Project (National Cancer Institute and National Human Genome Research Institute) aims to create a complete atlas of the molecular alterations present in different tumors of different cancer types. Until this project is completed, sequencing of candidate genes in tumor tissue will remain a robust method of biomarker discovery.

Dideoxy sequencing is the most commonly used DNA sequencing methodology today. DNA polymerase adds deoxynucleotides to the free 3'OH end of a primer with sequence specific to the region of interest. When a fluorescent-labeled dideoxy nucleotide is incorporated, chain extension is terminated. These labeled fragments are separated by capillary electrophoresis, and the fluorescent signal of the terminating nucleotide can be detected by a software program that will determine the DNA sequence (2). Many of the procedures involved in DNA sequencing are routine and commercial kits are available for many steps of the process. We will highlight the procedures unique to the handling of tumor tissue for DNA sequencing which include DNA extraction from fixed or frozen tissue, primer design, PCR amplification and product clean-up, cycle sequencing and product clean-up, and data analysis and interpretation.

2. Materials

2.1. Equipment

1. Pipettors or liquid handling robotics.
2. Pipette tips – 10 μL, 20 μL, 200 μL, 1,000 μL (filtered, unfiltered).
3. 1.5-mL microcentrifuge tube.
4. 15-mL conical tubes.
5. Reagent reservoirs.
6. PCR tubes or 96- or 384-well plates (we use ABgene Thermofast 384-well Diamond Plate for PCR and cycle sequencing).
7. Velocity11 Plate Sealer (optional).
8. Applied Biosystems 3730 DNA Analyzer (or equivalent).
9. SPRIPlate 96-well or 384-well Magnet Plate (Agencourt product #000219 or 000222; if using MagBead clean-up).

2.2. DNA Extraction (All Reagents Stable for 1 Year Unless Otherwise Noted)

1. Qiagen QIAamp DNA Micro Kit (Qiagen #51104), stored at room temperature, columns stored at 4°C.

2. Xylene, Histological Grade.

3. Ethanol.

4. Molecular-biology-grade water.

5. Disposable Pellet Pestle with 1.5-mL microcentrifuge tubes (RNase-, DNase-, pyrogen-free, for frozen tissue).

2.3. PCR Amplification (All Reagents Stable for 1 Year Unless Otherwise Noted)

1. Positive amplification control (high-quality DNA) mL snap-cap tubes, 96-well or 384-well skirted plates.

2. Adhesive Seals (if using plates).

3. Taq DNA Polymerase and Buffers (we use AmpliTaq Gold, Applied Biosystems Catalog #4311858 – stored at –20°C).

4. 100 μM dNTP (Invitrogen Catalog #10297018) – stored at –20°C.

5. AMPure Magnetic Beads (Agencourt #000134) or equivalent stored at 4°C.

6. DMSO stored at room temperature.

7. Primers – Synthesized oligonucleotides (100 μM).

8. Agarose.

9. Agarose gel buffer (TE or TBE).

10. LowRange Molecular ladder – stored at room temperature.

11. 6× Loading Buffer - stored at room temperature.

12. 10 mg/mL Ethidium Bromide stored at room temperature.

2.4. DNA Sequencing

1. 1.5 mL, 96-well, or 384-well plates for PCR and cycle-sequence reaction and sequencing.

2. 20 μL Nonbarrier Tips.

3. Big Dye Terminator v3.1 stored at –20°C.

4. 5× Dilution Buffer (80 mM Tris-HCl, 2 mM $MgCl_2$) (ABI #4390253) stored at –20°C.

5. DMSO stored at room temperature.

6. M13 Universal Primer (100 μM) stored at –20°C.

7. Big Dye Terminator v3.1 Standard Kit stored at –20°C.

8. CleanSEQ® magnetic beads (Agencourt®, #000136) stored at 4°C.
   DNA sequence analysis software

3. Methods

3.1. DNA Extraction

3.1.1. Formalin-Fixed, Paraffin-Embedded Tissue

For discussion on selection of tissue source, *see* **Note 1**.

1. Add 1,200 µL of xylene to a labeled 1.5-mL microcentrifuge tube (one per sample).

2. Using a scalpel coated (but not dripping) with xylene, scrape the appropriate area of several sections of tissue to the 1.5-mL Eppendorf tube containing xylene.

3. Invert tube 15–20 times or until paraffin has completely dissolved.

4. Centrifuge the sample at $7,000 \times g$ (10,000 rpm) for 5 min. Carefully pipette off 600 µL of xylene at a time, avoiding the delicate tissue pellet.

5. Add 1,200 µL of 100% ethanol to each tube containing a tissue pellet. Invert tubes 5–10 times or until the tissue pellet is disrupted.

6. Centrifuge for 5 min at full speed (14,000 rpm). Carefully pipette off 600 µL of ethanol at a time, avoiding the delicate tissue pellet.

7. Again add 1,200 µL of 100% ethanol to the tissue pellet and invert to disrupt pellet. The tissue pellet will be tight at this stage and may be difficult to disrupt. Complete disruption is not necessary.

8. Centrifuge for 5 min at full speed. Carefully pipette off 600 µL of ethanol at a time, avoiding the delicate tissue pellet. Remove as much 100% ethanol as is possible.

9. Allow the tissue pellets to dry at room temperature under a PCR hood until ethanol has evaporated.

10. The tissue pellet should be resuspended in a buffer (Buffer ATL, if using Qiagen QIAamp DNA Micro Kit) and Proteinase K treated at 62°C (by adding 5 µL of Proteinase K) overnight to disrupt the cells. It may be necessary to add additional Proteinase K the following morning and continue incubation for an additional period depending upon the size of the tissue.

11. Proceed to the DNA extraction method of choice (for example, Qiagen QIAamp DNA Micro Kit).

12. DNA quantity and quality should be assessed by measuring the A260 and A260/280. In addition, the quality can be assessed visually by running a small aliquot of the DNA on an agarose gel. Intact DNA will not migrate into the gel and will appear as a single large fragment. DNA that is sheared will appear as a smear on the gel. It may be difficult to PCR-amplify sheared DNA.

13. DNA can be stored temporarily at 4°C, but long-term storage should be at –20° or –80°.

3.1.2. Frozen Tissue

1. Add 180 μL of buffer (ATL if using Qiagen QIAamp DNA Micro Kit) to a 1.5-mL microcentrifuge tube for homogenization.

2. Transfer frozen tissue to tube containing buffer as quickly as possible so that the tissue does not thaw.

3. Grind tissue in microcentrifuge tubes using a pestle.

4. If the sample is not adequately covered by the buffer, add an additional 180 μL to the sample. Transfer approximately half of the sample to another clean, labeled 1.5-mL microcentrifuge tube.

5. Proceed to **step 1** of DNA Isolation Procedure using QIAamp DNA Micro Kit (or equivalent) of the manufacturer's instructions.

3.2. Primer Design

Because DNA extracted from isolated tumor cells is often limited, it may be necessary to design a nested PCR to robustly sequence the region of interest (**Fig. 1**, *see* **Note 2**). DNA extracted from fixed tissue may be sheared; it is therefore recommended that small amplicons, less than 500 base pairs, be defined.

1. Determine reference sequence of gene of interest from public databases: http://www.ncbi.nlm.nih.gov/; http://genome.ucsc.edu/; http://www.ensembl.org/index.html

2. Design primers

3. Many commercial software or freeware programs are available. We have had success with Primer 3 (http://frodo.wi.mit.edu/) *(3)*. In addition, the Wellcome Trust Sanger Institute has designed primers that can be used to amplify all coding regions of the human genome (http://www.sanger.ac.uk/cgi-bin/humgen/exoseq/search)

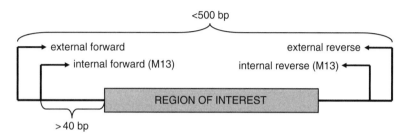

Fig. 1. Ideal primer placement for a nested PCR reaction. The largest amplicon should be less than 500 base pairs. Primers should be no closer than 40 base pairs from the region of interest. The internal primer pairs are tagged with M13 sequencing primers, as this is the PCR product that will be sequenced.

4. General primer design criteria include (*2*):

   Base composition. Low GC content (40–60%)

   Melting temperature. Similar for each primer, 60–62°C will allow for optimal specificity

   Primer length. 18–22 bases

   Primer position. More than 40 bases from the region of interest

5. Avoid sequence composition that will result in hairpins or primer dimers

6. Avoid homology to other regions of the genome to ensure unique amplification. Two resources to determine whether primers are likely to amplify a unique sequence:

   BLAT. http://genome.ucsc.edu/cgi-bin/hgBlat

   In silico PCR. http://genome.ucsc.edu/cgi-bin/hgPcr?db = hg18

7. Avoid regions of known SNPs to avoid allele dropout if a SNP is present underneath a primer binding site. Two resources to help identify whether a known SNP exists in the primer binding site:

   dbSNP. http://www.ncbi.nlm.nih.gov/entrez/query.fcgi?db = snp

   Diagnostic SNPCheck. http://ngrl.man.ac.uk/SNPCheck/

8. Design amplicon sizes of less than 500 bases pairs. Larger exons may require a series of overlapping primer pairs to obtain complete coverage

9. Consider nested PCR for sequencing small amounts of input template

10. Each primer for an amplicon that will be sequenced is also tagged with a universal primer sequence at the 5′ end of the primer:

    M13 Forward Sequencing Primer (18mer) 5′-TGTAAAAC-GACGGCCAGT-3′

    M13 Reverse Sequencing Primer (16mer) 5′-AACAGCTAT-GACCATG-3′

    It is not necessary for the external PCR primers of a nested PCR reaction to have M13 linkers, as these products will not be sequenced directly. Primers should be ordered from a reputable manufacturer for synthesis

3.3. PCR Amplification

3.3.1. External PCR

1. If necessary, create a plate map by typing in or writing in the sample ID and the corresponding primer identification numbers in each well, remembering to set up the appropriate controls, i.e., one positive reaction per master mix, and one negative reaction per primer pair.

2. Dilute DNA to 25 ng/μL.

3. Thaw the PCR reagents, keeping the Taq on ice. To help reduce contamination, reaction set-up should be performed in a hood (if available) in an area dedicated to pre-PCR reactions.

4. Calculate the master mix volume according to the following formula (*see* **Table 1**).

5. Wipe down the hood and pipettors with 70% ethanol.

6. In the Pre-PCR hood, vortex and spin down all reagents. Combine reagents, keeping DNA and primers separate. Keep master mix on ice.

7. Add 12 μL of master mix to each well or tube.

8. Add 1 μL of each forward and reverse primer at 20 μM.

9. Add 1 μL DNA at 25 ng/μL to each sample well. Add 1 μL dH$_2$O to the negative control well(s), and 1 μL of a high-quality DNA sample to the positive control well(s).

10. Close the caps of tubes or seal the plate tightly with adhesive seal, and spin in centrifuge for 10 s above 2,000 rpm to remove air bubbles. If air bubbles are still present, repeat centrifugation.

11. Put the reactions in the thermocycler, and select the appropriate PCR program: (*see* **Table 2**)

3.3.2. Internal PCR

1. The internal PCR set-up is almost identical to the external PCR with a few exceptions.

Table 1
PCR master mix

Reagents	Per Rxn
dH$_2$O	4.9 μL
5 M Betaine	3 μL
10× Buffer	1.5 μL
MgCl$_2$	1.5 μL
DMSO	0.75 μL
Hot start Taq	0.2 μL
100 μM dNTP	0.15 μL
Master Mix	12.0 μl
F&R Primer (20 μM)	1.0 μl (each)
DNA	1.0 at 25 ng/μL

Table 2
PCR thermal cycler conditions

	Temperature (°C)	Time
1 cycle	95	10:00 min
30 cycle	95	30 s
	60	30 s
	72	30s
1 cycle	72	10:00 min
∞	8	

2. Prepare the internal master mix exactly as the external master mix. Master mix should be prepared in the PCR hood.

3. Aliquot 12 μL of master mix into the reaction tube or plate.

4. Add 1 μL of each forward and reverse internal primers. Temporarily seal tube or plate.

5. Wipe down post-PCR set-up area and pipetter with 10% bleach, and then with 70% ethanol.

6. Remove external PCR tubes or plate from thermocycler, briefly spin down at 1,000 rpm for 10 s, and proceed to post PCR set-up area. Use dedicated pipettes to aliquot 1 μL of external PCR product into each internal reaction.

7. Close the tube or seal the plate with a plate sealer or adhesive PCR film and briefly spin for 10 s above 2,000 rpm to remove air bubbles. If air bubbles are still present, repeat centrifugation.

8. Run same amplification cycle as the external reaction.

9. When the program is finished, remove plate from thermocycler and centrifuge for 10 s at 1,000 rpm.

10. To check the success of the PCR, analyze 3 μL of each reaction on a 1% agarose gel. PCR products should be present and the negative controls should not show evidence of amplification.

3.4. PCR Product Clean-Up

1. Contaminants such as unincorporated nucleotides should be removed from the PCR reaction. We prefer magnetic bead clean-up using AMPure® magnetic beads (Agencourt®, *see* **Note 2**). Follow the manufacturer's instructions summarized here and given now:

http://www.agencourt.com/documents/products/ampure/Agencourt_AMPure_Protocol.pdf

2. Shake the AMPure bead container until all magnetic beads are in solution and are at room temperature.

3. Add AMPure beads according to the following equation:

   Volume of AMPure per reaction = 1.8 × reaction volume.

   Pay attention to the volume capacity of the wells and the reaction volume plus additional reagents to ensure that overflow does not occur.

4. Pipette mix or vortex the AMPure beads with the PCR reaction for 30 s.

5. Separate the beads from the reaction by placing the plate on the SPRIPlate.

6. Discard the supernatant.

7. Add 200 μL (96-well) or 30 μL (384-well) freshly diluted 70% ethanol to each reaction well and incubate for 30 s. Repeat for a total of two washes. Perform these washes while the plate is situated on the SPRIPlate.

8. Air-dry the reaction plate for 10–20 min.

9. Add 40 μL (96-well) or 30 μL (384-well) elution buffer (dH$_2$O or TE). Pipette mix or vortex. The total elution volume may need to be increased/decreased depending on the final concentration of PCR products in the well.

3.5. DNA Sequencing

1. Thaw the Big Dye at room temperature and keep it covered (it is light sensitive) and on ice until it is ready to use.

2. Make two tubes of master mix according to recipe as follows (*see* **Note 3**). For each reaction, add 0.12 μL of Forward M13 primer (10 μM) to the Forward master mix and 0.12 μL of Reverse M13 primer (10 μM) to the Reverse master mix. Add 9 μL of Forward master mix to each tube/well designated a forward reaction and 9 μL of Reverse master mix to each tube/well designated a reverse reaction.

   M13 Forward Sequencing Primer (18mer) 5′-TGTAAAAC-GACGGCCAGT-3′.

   M13 Reverse Sequencing Primer (16mer) 5′-AACAGCTAT-GACCATG-3′ (*see* **Table 3**).

3. Add 1 μL template (1–5 ng of clean PCR product) to each reaction tube/well.

4. Close the tubes or seal the reaction plate with a clear adhesive seal, and centrifuge at 3,300 rpm for 1 min in a centrifuge. When done, check that tubes/wells contain similar volumes and do not have air bubbles. If air bubbles persist, repeat centrifuge step until they no longer remain.

5. Place tubes/plates in the thermal cycler. Run with the conditions detailed in **Table 4**.

6. Remove plates from thermocycler and spin down at 3,300 rpm for 1 min.

Table 3
Sequencing master mix

Reagents	Volume per reaction (µL)
5× Big Dye buffer	3.65
Big Dye 3.1	0.35
DMSO	0.50
H_2O	4.38

Table 4
Sequencing thermal cycler conditions

25 cycles	96°C	10 s
	50°C	5 s
	60°C	4 min
1 cycle	4°C	∞

3.6. Dye Terminator Removal

1. After the cycle sequencing reaction, the products should be removed from contaminants. We use CleanSEQ® magnetic beads (Agencourt®) according to the manufacturer's instructions (*see* **Note 4**). Following is the protocol for use in 96- and 384-well plates.

   http://www.agencourt.com/documents/products/cleanseq/ Agencourt_CleanSEQ_Protocol.pdf

2. Shake CleanSEQ magnetic beads until all beads are in solution and are at room temperature (~20 min).

3. Add 5 µL (384-well) or 10 µL (96-well) µL of CleanSEQ magnetic bead solution per tube/well plus an appropriate volume of 85% ethanol to each sequencing reaction tube/plate. Pipette mix several times or vortex.

4. The volume of ethanol to be added can be determined by the following equation:

   VolEtOH = [(VolB + VolS) × (CF/CE]/[1 − (CF/CE)].

   Where

   VolEtOH = volume of ethanol used per reaction

   VolB = volume of Agencourt CleanSEQ used (10 µL for 96-well format, 5 µL for 384-well format)

   VolS = volume of DNA sample to be cleaned up

CF = final concentration of ethanol (57.4% for 96-well format, 50% for 384-well format)

CE = concentration of ethanol used (85%)

5. The beads are separated from the supernatant using a magnetic field (SPRIPlate). Remove and discard the supernatant. Wash with 30 μL (384-well) or 100 μL (96-well) of 85% ethanol. Remove ethanol and air-dry for 10 min.

6. The purified sequencing products are eluted from the magnetic beads using 15 μL (384-well) or 40 μL (96-well) molecular-biology-grade water. Incubate 5 min, and then, using the magnet, separate and transfer the products to a clean tube/plate. If the signal strength is too high, the products should be further diluted and/or elution should be performed in a larger volume of water.

7. Cleaned cycle-sequencing reactions can be stored at –20°C or directly run on a capillary sequencer. If stored, the reactions should be protected from UV light.

3.7. Data Analysis

There are many commercially available software and freeware options for DNA sequence data analysis. The choice depends on the requirements of the project. Ideally, a reference sequence can be defined, and the chromatogram generated from the capillary sequencer will be compared with that reference sequence. Changes from the reference should be reliably identified. Some programs will define the consequence of nucleotide changes at the amino acid level (if applicable), a feature that is useful in the resequencing of a particular locus. Some programs will allow multiple sequence alignment, whereas others will allow visualization of each sequence trace individually. For somatic mutation detection, appropriate settings should be selected. These parameters should reduce the stringency for mutation detection as the mutant signal may be less than 50% as expected for germline heterozygous mutations.

Selected software/freeware options:

1. Phred, Phrap, Consed *(4–6)*:

   http://www.phrap.org/phredphrapconsed.html

   Free to academic users, commercial users ~$10,000

   Phred. Reads DNA sequencing trace files, calls bases, assigns a quality value

   Phrap. Assembles shotgun DNA sequence data

   Consed. A tool for viewing, editing, and finishing sequence assemblies

2. Mutation Surveyor™ (Softgenetics)

   http://www.softgenetics.com

3. Sequencher™ (Gene Codes)

http://www.softpedia.com/get/Science-CAD/Sequencher.shtml

4. Lasergene® (DNASTAR): 2006 Lasergene 7

http://www.dnastar.com/

3.8. Interpretation of the Significance of DNA Variants

3.8.1. Establish Reproducibility

It is advised that suspected variants that are identified be either confirmed by another methodology or, at a minimum, an independent PCR reaction be resequenced. This is critical as both tissue fixation and PCR amplification error early in the amplification process can lead to amplification artifacts, even when high-fidelity Taq polymerase is used (**Fig. 2a–d**).

3.8.2. Establish Somatic Origin of Variant

Variants that occur uniquely in tumor tissue are more likely to be directly involved in tumorigenesis than those that are constitutively present. In order to determine whether the variant is unique to tumor tissue, DNA sequence analysis of a normal tissue sample from the individual can be analyzed (adjacent normal tissue from the slide, peripheral whole blood, buccal sample, or other, **Fig. 2c, d**).

3.8.3. Search the Literature

Variants may be previously reported as either a recognized cause of disease or benign common variants. Review of the literature, publicly available mutation databases (for example, Human Gene Mutation Database: http://www.hgmd.cf.ac.uk/ac/index.php), or locus-specific databases, as well as dbSNP (http://www.ncbi.nlm.nih.gov/projects/SNP/) should be searched. However, the presence of a variant in these databases must be scrutinized carefully, as variants reported as pathogenic may be incorrectly classified and common variants listed in dbSNP can be clinically significant.

3.8.4. Analyze Functional Significance of the Variant

Variants that are predicted to inactivate known tumor suppressor genes (frameshifts, premature truncation, mutation of initiation codon, alteration of splice site) are likely to be significant. Missense and silent variants can be more difficult to interpret, as their

Fig. 2. Sample DNA sequence chromatograms, as viewed using Mutation Surveyor. The upper chromatogram in each image represents the forward strand and the lower chromatogram represents the reverse strand (**a**, **b**) Comparison of a typical missense mutation observed in a lung tumor tissue sample (**a**, *arrows*) with that of one with weak missense mutation signal detectable (**b**, *arrows*). The mutation observed in both samples, 2573T > G (L858R) in EGFR is observed in approximately 4% of all lung adenocarcinomas. The mutation and level of intensity observed in B was reproducible. (**c**, **d**) Allele amplification bias can result in loss of signal beyond detection. Chromatograms (**c**) and (**d**) represent independent PCR reactions from the same DNA sample. In chromatogram (**c**), the 2573G allele was preferentially amplified (*arrows*) as compared with chromatogram (**d**), where both the 2573G and 2573T alleles were comparatively amplified (*arrows*). (**e**, **f**) Comparison of a chromatogram derived from tumor tissue (**e**) with that of a blood sample (**f**) from the same individual. The missense mutation detected in tumor (**e**, *arrow*) is not detected in the blood sample (**f**, *arrow*); therefore, it is unique to tumor tissue (*See Color Plates*).

a

b

c

d

e

f

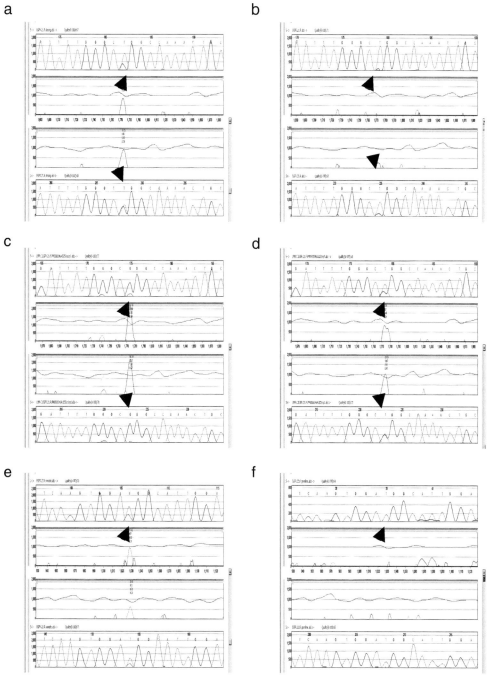

effect on the function of a protein is difficult to predict. A silent variant is one that does not lead to an amino acid change. At the nucleotide level, these variants can create cryptic splice sites, for example, and have deleterious effect on protein function. Additional functional data are required to conclusively determine the significance of variants identified.

4. Notes

1. Tumors are typically a heterogeneous mix of cells. The tumor cells may be difficult to isolate away from normal tissue, inflammatory cells, and necrotic tissue. In addition, tumor cells themselves can be genetically heterogeneous. In our experience, DNA sequencing can reliably detect a heterozygous mutation if it is present in 50% of the cells (25% of the overall signal), but is capable of detecting a heterozygous mutation in 20% of the cells of a sample (i.e., 10% signal overall, unpublished observations). At least three options for tumor cell isolation exist (1) no dissection, (2) manual dissection, (3) laser capture microdissection (LCM). Undissected tumor is the easiest to acquire, as it requires no special treatment and no specific expertise, but contaminating nontumor tissue may dilute the signal of pathogenic mutations beyond detection. Manual dissection is typically performed by comparing a stained reference slide on which tumor cells can be identified with unstained serial sections. Regions of high tumor cellularity can be scraped from the slide and collected. LCM uses a laser beam to cause selected cells to adhere to a substrate which can be removed, leaving unwanted cells behind. LCM can produce a pure tumor cell population, but requires special equipment and expertise. This procedure is time consuming and will produce a low yield of tissue.

2. The tissue fixation procedure is another major consideration in molecular analysis. Tumor is typically available as blocks of tissue that has been fixed (formalin or ethanol) and paraffin embedded, although frozen tissue may also be available. DNA quality extracted from fixed or frozen tissue can vary greatly depending upon both tissue source and fixation protocol used. Bone tumors, for example, can be difficult to analyze as the decalcification process used to remove the bone and isolate cells is extremely harsh. Fixation may result several types of DNA damage. Extracted genomic DNA may be sheared, and PCR amplification of long amplicons may be difficult. In addition, the fixation process itself can cause mutations in the DNA analyzed *(7, 8)*.

3. Alternatives to a nested PCR approach include increasing the amplification cycle number from 30 to 35 or 40 and using the same set of primers in two independent PCR amplification reactions. The advantage of using a nested PCR with two different sets of primers is that specificity of amplification is more likely (the probability that the wrong locus will be amplified twice is lower).

4. Many different procedures can be used to remove reaction contaminants such as unincorporated nucleotides from the PCR reaction. We prefer magnetic bead clean-up; however, other procedures, shrimp alkaline phosphatase, for example, are used successfully by other labs.

5. Some individuals use single-direction sequence rather than bidirectional sequence in order to save on the cost of reagents. This is not recommended as the sequence quality from fixed tissue samples may be low, and bidirectional sequence data can help rule in or out mutation signal.

6. Cycle sequencing products can be precipitated with ethanol or isopropanol with or without sodium acetate or other salt (see protocols http://www.sanger.ac.uk/humgen/exoseq/protocols.shtml), gel filtration (e.g., Sephadex G-50), or magnetic beads. We have had good results with CleanSEQ® magnetic beads (Agencourt®).

7. Limitations of DNA Sequencing Methodology:
Loss of heterozygosity (LOH) is a common occurrence in tumor tissue. Large deletions spanning one or more exons that include primer binding sites will prevent amplification of the region. This may result in PCR failure if homozygous LOH is present, or variants detected may appear to be homozygous.

Poor DNA quality could prevent PCR amplification.

DNA extracted from fixed tissue may be sheared, and amplification of long amplicons may not be possible.

Rare sequence variations or secondary structures of the targeted primer sequences could prevent PCR amplification resulting in allele amplification bias.

References

1. Davies, H., Bignell, G. R., Cox, C., Stephens, P., Edkins, S., Clegg, S., Teague, J., Woffendin, H., Garnett, M. J., Bottomley, W., Davis, N., Dicks, E., Ewing, R., Floyd, Y., Gray, K., Hall, S., Hawes, R., Hughes, J., Kosmidou, V., Menzies, A., Mould, C., Parker, A., Stevens, C., Watt, S., Hooper, S., Wilson, R., Jayatilake, H., Gusterson, B. A., Cooper, C., Shipley, J., Hargrave, D., Pritchard-Jones, K., Maitland, N., Chenevix-Trench, G., Riggins, G. J., Bigner, D. D., Palmieri, G., Cossu, A., Flanagan, A., Nicholson, A., Ho, J. W., Leung, S. Y., Yuen, S. T., Weber, B. L., Seigler, H. F., Darrow, T. L., Paterson, H., Marais, R., Marshall, C. J., Wooster, R., Stratton, M. R., and Futreal, P. A. (2002) Mutations of the BRAF gene in human cancer. Nature 417, 949–54

2. Strachan, T., and Read, A. P. (2004) Human Molecular Genetics 3, Garland Science, London and New York.

3. Rozen, S., and Skaletsky, H. (2000) Primer3 on the WWW for general users and for biologist programmers.

4. Gordon, D., Abajian, C., and Green, P. (1998) Consed: a graphical tool for sequence finishing. Genome Res 8, 195–202.

5. Gordon, D., Desmarais, C., and Green, P. (2001) Automated finishing with autofinish. Genome Res 11, 614–25.

6. Gordon, D. (2004) Viewing and Editing Assembled Sequences Using Consed, Wiley, New York.

7. Greer, C. E., Peterson, S. L., Kiviat, N. B., and Manos, M. M. (1991) PCR amplification from paraffin-embedded tissues. Effects of fixative and fixation time. Am J Clin Pathol 95, 117–24.

8. Quach, N., Goodman, M. F., and Shibata, D. (2004) In vitro mutation artifacts after formalin fixation and error prone translesion synthesis during PCR. BMC Clin Pathol 4, 1.

Chapter 16

Analysis of Loss of Heterozygosity in Circulating DNA

Takeshi Nakamura, Eiji Sunami, Tuny Nguyen and Dave S.B. Hoon

Summary

Analysis of genetic altera tion in circulating DNA can have clinical utility in predicting disease outcome. Loss of heterozygosity (LOH) of DNA microsatellites has been shown to occur commonly among all chromosomes in various cancers, such as melanoma, breast cancer, and lung cancer. In this protocol, we focused on the utility of LOH of microsatellite biomarkers for detection of analyzing circulating DNA. The protocol describes how PCR is performed on each patient's paired DNA samples (normal lymphocyte DNA and serum DNA) using specific microsatellite biomarkers followed by post-PCR product analysis using capillary array electrophoresis (CAE). The utility of CAE is due to its digitalization and accuracy of the post-PCR product results.

Key words: Circulating DNA, Serum, Plasma, Loss of heterozygosity, Allelic imbalance, PCR, Capillary array electrophoresis.

1. Introduction

Among several types of body fluids, plasma and serum are most commonly targeted for research in extracellular DNA of all malignancies. Circulating DNA in plasma/serum has now been demonstrated in multiple types of cancers. Genetic aberrations found in tumors such as loss of heterozygosity (LOH) of microsatellites, mutations, methylation of promoter regions in the genome of tumor cells can also be detected in body fluids of patients. This provides an opportunity to assess tumor genetic biomarkers without assessing the tumor itself. This is highly important when the tumor is not available or for monitoring recurrence of disease in cancer-free patients. The field of assessment of circulating DNA has progressed rapidly in the last

Michael A. Tainsky, *Methods in Molecular Biology, Tumor Biomarker Discovery, Vol. 520*
© Humana Press, a part of Springer Science+Business Media, LLC 2009
DOI: 10.1007/978-1-60327-811-9_16

10 years; however, there are still multiple approaches being applied by different laboratories that make it difficult at times to compare results. After circulating tumor-derived DNA in serum/plasma was discovered, investigators have focused on the clinical utility of these findings in cancer patients.

The inactivation or deletion of tumor-related genes (TRG) is one of the most common molecular events that contribute to tumorigenesis. Microsatellite alterations, such as LOH, are commonly found in tumor cells and are one of mechanisms for TRG inactivation. LOH represents the loss of one or both of the parental alleles present in the patient's normal cells, and this allelic imbalance (AI) can lead to disruption of normal cell function and regulatory mechanisms and may lead to support malignant transformation. LOH can arise via several pathways, including deletions, gene conversion, mitotic recombination, and chromosome loss. LOH is frequently observed in a variety of human cancers and correlated with cancer progression. (1–6) Therefore, LOH of microsatellites can be highly specific biomarkers that can be used to assess disease presence and progression (7, 8). LOH in tumor cells has proven useful in identifying chromosomal regions containing putative TRG (1, 2, 9, 10).

LOH, commonly found in many solid tumors such as melanoma, breast cancer, and lung cancer, can be successfully identified in the plasma of patients and provides valuable prognostic information. LOH in circulating DNA may be a useful predictive marker in cancer patients (3, 10–13). Studies have shown that LOH in circulating DNA may be a useful diagnostic and prognostic biomarker for various cancers (13–17). Detection of circulating LOH by the assessment of multiple microsatellite biomarkers in serum/plasma of cancer patients can have prognostic tool (18, 19). Although LOH can be found frequent in a particular cancer type, often it is not in 100% frequency in the same tumor type of different patients. Therefore, multiple microsatellite biomarkers of different chromosome regions and of any given chromosome site must be assessed to improve sensitivity of an assay when used for detection.

In our studies, we have found LOH to be a useful circulating DNA prognostic biomarker (3, 9–11, 18, 19). In this protocol, we demonstrate our approach of detecting microsatellite biomarkers by assessing for LOH in circulating DNA in serum/plasma using PCR followed by CAE analysis.

2. Materials

2.1. Serum Isolation

1. Serum Filter System, 13 mm × 4in. (Fisher Scientific).
2. 7-mL Red-Top Vacutainer tubes (Fisher Scientific).

3. 2-mL Transfer Pipettes (Fisher Scientific).

4. 2-mL Cryovials (Corning Inc).

2.2. DNA Extraction from Serum

1. Sterile 0.9% NaCl (0.45 g in 50 mL final volume, filter with 0.45-μm syringe).

2. Proteinase K (20 mg/mL) (Qiagen).

3. 10% Sodium Dodecyl Sulfate (SDS) (InVitrogen).

4. 2-mL Eppendorf microcentrifuge tube (Axygen Scientific Inc).

5. Phenol–Chloroform–Isoamyl (PCI) (25:24:1, pH 8).

6. Pellet Paint® NF Co-Precipitant (Novagen).

7. 100% Isopropanol (Fisher Scientific).

8. 90% ethanol, stored at 4°C (200 proof stock) (Pharmco-Aaper).

9. Disposable Plastic Transfer Pipettes, 400 (Fisher Scientific).

10. Molecular-biology-grade H_2O (Fisher Scientific).

2.3. DNA Extraction from PBL

1. 15-mL Falcon tubes (Sarstedt, Inc.).

2. Disposable 10-mL sterile serological pipettes (Fisher Scientific).

3. Disposable sterile pasteur pipettes (Fisher Scientific).

4. Purescript® RBC Lysis Solution (PLS) (Gentra).

5. 1× Phosphate-buffered saline, 7.4 (PBS) (GIBCO).

6. 1.5-mL microcentrifuge tubes (PGC Scientifics Corp.).

7. DNAzol (Molecular Research Center, Inc.).

8. Molecular-biology-grade H_2O (Fisher Scientific).

9. Ethyl alcohol (200 proof, ACS/USP Grade) (Pharmco-Aaper).

2.4. DNA Quantification

1. TE Buffer pH 8 (Sigma).

2. Pico-Green Assay Kit (Molecular Probes).

3. 96-well round- bottom microplate (COSTAR).

2.5. Analysis

1. Capillary array electrophoresis (CEQ 8000XL) (Beckman Coulter).

2. Flat 96-well PCR microplate (VWR).

3. 96-well flat bottom assay plate (COSTAR).

4. GenomeLab Sample loading solution (SLS) (Beckman Coulter).

5. GenomeLab DNA size standard kit-400 (Beckman Coulter).

6. GenomeLab Separation buffer (Beckman Coulter).

7. Mineral oil (Beckman Coulter).

3. Methods

3.1. Serum Isolation

1. Collect 7 mL of blood in a 7 ml Tiger top tube (Kendall) and separate serum from cells by centrifugation at $1,000 \times g$ (PCF) at room temperature for 15 min. Transfer serum to red top tube (7ml).

2. Filter serum through a 13-mm serum filter to a 2-mL cryovial.

3. Cap tightly and store serum temporarily at $-30°C$ (< 30 days). Transfer serum tubes to $-80°C$ for long-term storage.

3.2. DNA Extraction from Serum

1. Thaw serum in $37°C$ oven. Vortex well and then quickly centrifuge for 5 s.

2. Aliquot 0.5 mL plasma or serum into a 2-mL microcentrifuge tube and dilute with 0.3 mL of 0.9% NaCl.

3. Add 95 µL of 10%SDS and 20 µL of Proteinase K.

4. Incubate at $50°C$ for 3 h. Vortex every hour or place on shaker.

5. Add 1 mL of PCI. Vortex for 10 s 3 times.

6. Centrifuge the tube at $15,500 \times g$ (PCF) for 10 min at $22°C$. Do not disturb the layers when removing tubes from the centrifuge.

7. Transfer 75–85% of the aqueous phase to fresh 2-mL Eppendorf tube. Be very careful; this is a critical step: do not touch middle layer.

8. Add 700 µl of isopropanol and 2 µl of pellet paint NF. Vortex well and then quickly centrifuge for 5 s.

9. Precipitate DNA overnight at $-30°C$.

10. Sediment precipitated DNA by centrifugation at $16,000 \times g$ for 30 min at $4°C$.

11. Remove and discard supernatant.

12. Wash out salt from pellet with 1 mL 90% cold ethanol ($4°C$).

13. Centrifuge at $16,000 \times g$ for 10 min at $4°C$ and remove supernatant (excess ethanol) with fine tip transfer pipette.

14. Let air dry or dry pellet in speed vacuum without heat setting.

15. After the samples are completely dry, resuspend DNA in 50 µl H_2O.

3.3. DNA Extraction from PBL

1. Draw 4 ml of blood into sodium citrate (bloctop) tube (4 ml). Obtain one 15-mL Falcon tube for each specimen.

2. First Lysis:

3. Using a sterile 10-mL serological pipette, fill 15-mL Falcon tube with 10 mL PLS.

4. Invert tube several times, and then transfer 4 mL of the blood into the appropriately labeled 15 mL Falcon tube.

5. Gently invert all 15-mL Falcon tubes containing blood and PLS.

6. Allow to incubate on their sides at 22–25°C for 15 min inside the fume hood.

7. Centrifuge at 300 × g and 22–25°C for 10 min.

8. Aspirate the supernatant with sterile Pasteur pipettes. Avoid aspirating any part of the lymphocyte pellet (white). If a white pellet is not clearly visible at the bottom of the 15-mL Falcon tube after centrifugation, leave 2 mL of suspension in the 15-mL Falcon tube.

9. *Second lysis.* (*See* **Note 1**)

10. Use a new 10-mL serological pipette to transfer 10 mL PLS to the 15-mL Falcon tube containing the lymphocyte pellet.

11. Gently pipette up and down to resuspend the pellet.

12. Centrifuge the PLS/Lymphocyte-containing 15-mL Falcon tubes at 300 × g and 22–25°C for 5 min.

13. Aspirate the supernatant as much as possible. Avoid aspirating the lymphocyte pellet.

14. PBS Wash:

15. Use a new 10-mL serological pipette to transfer 10 mL of PBS to the lymphocyte pellet. Resuspend the lymphocyte pellet by gently pipetting up and down.

16. Centrifuge 15-mL Falcon tubes at 300 × g and 22–25°C for 5 min.

17. Aspirate the supernatant as much as possible. Avoid aspirating the lymphocyte pellet.

18. Transfer 1 mL DNAzol to each 15-mL Falcon tube. Lyse the cells by repeated pipetting.

19. Transfer the DNAzol/Lymphocyte content to the labeled 1.5-mL microcentrifuge tube. Cap tightly (*see* **Note 2**). Discard the 15-mL Falcon tube.

20. Add 500 µL of 100% ethanol to the homogenate and invert 5–8 times.

21. Incubate at 22–25°C for 1–3 min.

22. Remove DNA precipitate (clear/cloudy, gel-like substance) by spooling with a P1000 pipette tip and transfer to a new, labeled 1.5-mL microcentrifuge tube. Discard the original DNAzol microcentrifuge tube (*see* **Note 3**).

23. Allow the microcentrifuge tube containing the DNA precipitate by leaving it upright for 1 min at 22–25°C.

24. Use a pipette to remove excess lysate/homogenate from the bottom of the tube.

25. Wash the DNA precipitate with 1 mL of cold 75% ethanol. Invert 3–6 times.

26. Incubate upright at room temperature for 30–60 s to allow the DNA to settle at the bottom, and then pellet the DNA by centrifugation at $1,000 \times g$ for 1 min at 4°C.

27. Remove ethanol by pipetting.

28. Repeat DNA wash (**steps 12–14**).

29. Remove excess ethanol from the bottom of the microcentrifuge tube using a pipette (*see* **Note 4**).

30. Dry the pellet in speed vacuum for 5 min.

31. Add 200–300 µL of 1× TE Buffer. Resuspend the DNA pellet by gentle pipetting (*see* **Notes 5** and **6**).

32. Store DNA samples at –80°C until needed again.

3.4. DNA Quantification

For quantification of double-stranded DNA, reserve 5 µl and mix it with a 95-µl aliquot of TE buffer. Use this diluted sample in the PicoGreen quantification assay, according to the manufacturer's protocol.

3.5. Analysis

1. PCR is performed on each patient's paired samples (normal lymphocyte DNA and serum or plasma DNA). PCR should be carried out after optimizing annealing temperatures for each primer set. Verify the location of microsatellite markers using the current updated National Center for Biotechnology Information (NCBI) database, and use the forward primers labeled with WellRed phosphoramidite-linked dye or active ester-labeled dye.

2. DNA is subjected to PCR amplification in a final reaction volume of 10 µl containing PCR buffer, 2.5–4.5 mM $MgCl_2$, dNTPs, 0.3 µM primers, 0.5 U AmpliTaq gold polymerase, and 50 pmol of each forward and reverse primer. Initial 10-min incubation at 95°C is followed by 40 cycles of denaturation at 95°C for 30 s, annealing for 30 s, extension at 72°C for 30 s, and a final hold of 7 min at 72°C. Molecular-biology-grade H_2O without DNA served is a control for contamination (*see* **Note 7**).

3. Post-PCR product is analyzed using CEQ 8000XL.

4. Mix the sample loading solution (SLS) with a DNA size standard kit-400 (*see* **Note 8**).

5. Put 40 μl of mixed SLS to each well. Add 1 μl post-PCR product to each assigned well.

6. Add one drop of mineral oil to each well.

7. Access the plate to CEQ machine and run the program according to the user's guide.

8. Peak signal intensity and relative size of PCR product are generated by CEQ8000XL genetic analysis system software (*see* **Fig. 1**, **Notes 9** and **10**).

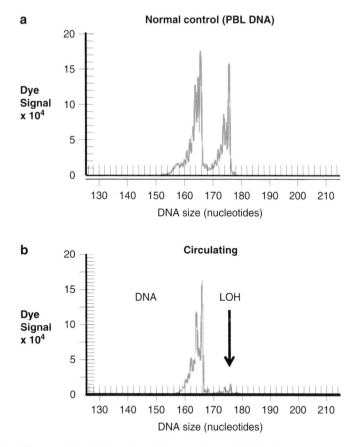

Fig. 1. Representative CAE results of (**a**) normal control PBL DNA and (**b**) circulating DNA of a patient demonstrating a reduction of peak ratio intensity, loss of heterozygosity (LOH), at a specific microsatellite marker (D9S171 at 9p22-p21).

4. Notes

1. If the patient's blood has 2 × 4 mL, divide blood volume among a few tubes at first lysis and combine them at second lysis by transferring the entire volume of PLS/lymphocytes solution to the next tube containing the lymphocyte pellet.

2. The DNA sample can remain at 4°C or –20°C storage for up to 10 months as a DNAzol/lymphocyte suspension.

3. If you cannot see the DNA precipitate or the sample contains degraded DNA or small quantities of DNA (< 15 μg), do not spool onto a pipette tip. In this case, pellet the precipitated DNA via centrifugation at 5,000 × g for 5 min at 4°C.

4. During centrifuge washes, DNA can be stored in 1 mL of 95% ethanol for at least one week at room temperature, 3 months at 4°C, or long term at –80°C.

5. Alternatively, dissolve DNA (without drying) in 200–300 μL of 8 mM NaOH by slowly passing the pellet through the pipette tip. Using NaOH will ensure more rapid and complete solubilization of the DNA precipitate.

6. A fresh working solution of 8 mM NaOH must be prepared monthly using a 2–3 M NaOH stock solution that is < 6 months old.

7. PCR product is light sensitive. Keep away from the light until loading.

8. After mixed with a DNA standard kit, sample is light sensitive. Keep away from light while preparing the procedure, and store in a freezer.

9. Serum DNA is scored as exhibiting LOH if there is an absence or > 40% reduction in the intensity ratio of one allele compared with the respective allele in the normal matched lymphocytes. The percent reduction can be increased for genetic specificity.

10. If a certain microsatellite marker shows homozygosity in the normal matched lymphocytes DNA, it is scored as a noninformative sample, and we cannot get any further information from this marker for this sample; this is the limitation of this method for detecting LOH. Therefore, it will help to use multiple microsatellite markers, which lowers the chance of noninformative results. The AI status of a sample can be determined according to the nearest informative markers. All AIs should be confirmed by repeating the assay.

References

1. van der Riet P., Nawroz H., Hruban R. H., Corio R., Tokino K., Koch W., and Sidransky D. (1994) Frequent loss of chromosome 9p21–22 early in head and neck cancer progression. Cancer Res 54, 1156–1158.

2. Fujimoto A., Takeuchi H., Taback B., Hsueh E. C., Elashoff D., Morton D. L., and Hoon D. S. (2004) Allelic imbalance of 12q22–23 associated with APAF-1 locus correlates with poor disease outcome in cutaneous melanoma. Cancer Res 64, 2245–2250.

3. Taback B., Giuliano A. E., Hansen N. M., and Hoon D. S. (2001) Microsatellite alterations detected in the serum of early stage breast cancer patients. Ann N Y Acad Sci 945, 22–30.

4. Umetani N., Fujimoto A., Takeuchi H., Shinozaki M., Bilchik A. J., and Hoon D. S. (2004) Allelic imbalance of APAF-1 locus at 12q23 is related to progression of colorectal carcinoma. Oncogene 23, 8292–8300.

5. So C. K., Nie Y., Song Y., Yang G. Y., Chen S., Wei C., Wang L. D., Doggett N. A., and Yang C. S. (2004) Loss of heterozygosity and internal tandem duplication mutations of the CBP gene are frequent events in human esophageal squamous cell carcinoma. Clin Cancer Res 10, 19–27.

6. Mihaila D., Jankowski M., Gutierrez J. A., Rosenblum M. L., Newsham I. F., Bogler O., and Rempel S. A. (2003) Meningiomas: loss of heterozygosity on chromosome 10 and marker-specific correlations with grade, recurrence, and survival. Clin Cancer Res 9, 4443–4451.

7. Califano J., Westra W. H., Meininger G., Corio R., Koch W. M., and Sidransky D. (2000) Genetic progression and clonal relationship of recurrent premalignant head and neck lesions. Clin Cancer Res 6, 347–352.

8. Nakayama T., Taback B., Turner R., Morton D. L., and Hoon D. S. (2001) Molecular clonality of in-transit melanoma metastasis. Am J Pathol 158, 1371–1378.

9. Fujiwara Y., Chi D. D., Wang H., Keleman P., Morton D. L., Turner R., and Hoon D. S. (1999) Plasma DNA microsatellites as tumor-specific markers and indicators of tumor progression in melanoma patients. Cancer Res 59, 1567–1571.

10. Fujimoto A., O'Day S. J., Taback B., Elashoff D., and Hoon D. S. (2004) Allelic imbalance on 12q22–23 in serum circulating DNA of melanoma patients predicts disease outcome. Cancer Res 64, 4085–4088.

11. Taback B., Fujiwara Y., Wang H. J., Foshag L. J., Morton D. L., and Hoon D. S. (2001) Prognostic significance of circulating microsatellite markers in the plasma of melanoma patients. Cancer Res 61, 5723–5726.

12. Taback B., Saha S., and Hoon D. S. (2006) Comparative analysis of mesenteric and peripheral blood circulating tumor DNA in colorectal cancer patients. Ann N Y Acad Sci 1075, 197–203.

13. Chen X., Bonnefoi H., Diebold-Berger S., Lyautey J., Lederrey C., Faltin-Traub E., Stroun M., and Anker P. (1999) Detecting tumor-related alterations in plasma or serum DNA of patients diagnosed with breast cancer. Clin Cancer Res 5, 2297–2303.

14. Gonzalgo M. L., Eisenberger C. F., Lee S. M., Trock B. J., Marshall F. F., Hortopan S., Sidransky D., and Schoenberg M. P. (2002) Prognostic significance of preoperative molecular serum analysis in renal cancer. Clin Cancer Res 8, 1878–1881.

15. Sozzi G., Conte D., Mariani L., Lo Vullo S., Roz L., Lombardo C., Pierotti M. A., and Tavecchio L. (2001) Analysis of circulating tumor DNA in plasma at diagnosis and during follow-up of lung cancer patients. Cancer Res 61, 4675–4678.

16. Utting M., Werner W., Dahse R., Schubert J., and Junker K. (2002) Microsatellite analysis of free tumor DNA in urine, serum, and plasma of patients: a minimally invasive method for the detection of bladder cancer. Clin Cancer Res 8, 35–40.

17. Eisenberger C. F., Knoefel W. T., Peiper M., Merkert P., Yekebas E. F., Scheunemann P., Steffani K., Stoecklein N. H., Hosch S. B., and Izbicki J. R. (2003) Squamous cell carcinoma of the esophagus can be detected by microsatellite analysis in tumor and serum. Clin Cancer Res 9, 4178–4183.

18. Nakayama T., Taback B., Nguyen D. H., Chi D. D., Morton D. L., Fujiwara Y., and Hoon D. S. (2000) Clinical significance of circulating DNA microsatellite markers in plasma of melanoma patients. Ann N Y Acad Sci 906, 87–98.

19. Taback B., O'Day S. J., Boasberg P. D., Shu S., Fournier P., Elashoff R., Wang H. J., and Hoon D. S. (2004) Circulating DNA microsatellites: molecular determinants of response to biochemotherapy in patients with metastatic melanoma. J Natl Cancer Inst 96, 152–156.

Chapter 17

Pharmacogenomics

Shilong Zhong and Marjorie Romkes

Summary

Pharmacogenomics encompasses several major areas including the identification and analysis of variations of DNA and RNA that affect the efficacy and toxicity of drug therapy. It represents an integration of analytical approaches including DNA and RNA detection and quantitation which may be applied to either candidate genes or a global genome analysis.

Key words: Pharmacogenomics, Pharmacogenetics, SNP detection, mRNA expression profiling, Individualized medicine.

1. Introduction

With the recent advances in the human genome sequencing project and the International HapMap Project, the initial applications include the emerging fields of pharmacogenetics and pharmacogenomics *(1, 2)*. Pharmacogenetic studies evaluate the influence of variations in DNA sequence on drug response, while pharmacogenomic studies focus on the identification and analysis of variations of both DNA and RNA that affect the efficacy and toxicity of drug therapy. The identification and screening of pharmacogenomic biomarkers typically involves both DNA and RNA detection approaches for either single gene loci, a targeted gene panel, or a genome-wide scan depending on the research or clinical application. The foremost objectives of pharmacogenomic analyses are the development of individualized drug therapy regimens, facilitation of advances in novel approaches in drug discovery, and to improve the understanding of the disease

Michael A. Tainsky, *Methods in Molecular Biology, Tumor Biomarker Discovery*, Vol. 520
© Humana Press, a part of Springer Science + Business Media, LLC 2009
DOI: 10.1007/978-1-60327-811-9_17

pathogenesis to develop strategies for early diagnosis and disease prevention.

Several of the first US Food and Drug Administration (FDA)-approved pharmacogenomic tests are assays to screen for specific DNA polymorphisms. In August 2005, the FDA approved a test marketed by Third Wave, the Invader *UGT1A1* Molecular Assay, to screen for polymorphisms in the UDP-glucuronosyltransferase enzyme. This phase II metabolic enzyme is involved in the metabolism of a number of drugs, including irinotecan, a drug used in colorectal cancer treatment. *UGT1A1* genetic variations can modulate a patient's ability to metabolize irinotecan, which may lead to increased blood levels of the drug and a higher risk of adverse side effects. For patients with specific *UGT1A1* genetic polymorphisms, a dose of irinotecan that is safe for the majority of other patients, might be too high and increases the risk of certain known side effects. The Invader assay joins a growing list of genetic tests used by clinicians to personalize treatment decisions used to individualize dosage of antidepressants, antipsychotics, beta-blockers, and some chemotherapy drugs *(3)*.

In this chapter, several research-based techniques which are commonly used for the characterization of DNA and RNA markers are described. In addition, two approaches for the application of pharmacogenomic endpoints in combination with drug response and disease biomarkers are summarized.

2. Genomic Markers

2.1. DNA Markers

Genetic diversity of variation is a consequence of differences in DNA sequences. There are multiple types of genetic variation including single nucleotide polymorphisms (SNPs), copy-number variations (CNVs), insertions/deletions (Indels), including microsatellite polymorphisms, and cytogenetic rearrangements.

2.1.1. DNA Sequencing and Molecular Techniques

DNA sequencing is the process of determining the nucleotide order within a genome. Because of the essential nature of DNA to living things, knowledge of DNA sequence is useful in practically any biological research. DNA sequencing can be used to identify, diagnose, and potentially develop treatments for genetic diseases.

There are several approaches to DNA sequencing (1) dideoxy sequencing, such as Sanger-based sequencing methods, (2) cyclic array sequencing, (3) sequencing by hybridization, (4) microelectrophoresis, (5) mass spectrometry, and (6) nanopore sequencing. Among these, cyclic array sequencing is a new generation of non-Sanger-based sequencing technologies and holds promise for sequencing DNA at unprecedented coverage, throughput, and low cost, thereby enabling many new applications including the characterization of novel pharmacogenomic markers *(4, 5)*. These next-generation high-throughput strategies include the Solexa sequencing technology using the Illumina Genome Analyzer, 454 Sequencing with the Roche Genome Sequencer, and the SOLiD™ System by Applied Biosystems.

2.1.2. Single Nucleotide Polymorphisms and Molecular Techniques

There are many types of genetic variation in the genome and SNPs are the most abundant. SNPs can greatly affect how humans develop diseases and respond to pathogens, environmental insults, and drugs. In pharmacogenomic studies, genetic polymorphisms in genes encoding drug-metabolizing enzymes, drug transporters, and receptors contribute, at least in part, to the interindividual variability in drug response and efficacy. These pathways influence drug absorption, distribution, metabolism, and excretion. SNP-genotyping technologies are used to identify genetic polymorphisms affecting drug response and to understand the mechanisms of interindividual differences in drug response. By establishing the association between the genetic make-up of an individual and drug response, it may be possible to develop genome-based medicines *(6)*.

There is a vast variety of SNP-genotyping methods. Basically, genotyping methods are divided into three main groups: low-throughput, medium-throughput, and genome-wide genotyping methods.

Low-throughput methods include Restriction Fragment Length Polymorphism (RFLP)-Polymerase Chain Reaction (PCR), Single-strand conformation polymorphism (SSCP) assays, the TaqMan assay based on allele discrimination using Fluorescence Resonance Energy Transfer detection, and denaturing HPLC. These methods are useful for the specific gene association study involving a few SNPs, but they are labor intensive and difficult to apply to high-throughput genotyping in pharmacogenomic studies.

Medium-throughput methods include many DNA microarray assays, fluorescence polarization methods, PCR-free genotyping methods such as the Invader method, mass spectrometric methods, and the Pyrosequencing method. These methods are suitable for large-scale genotyping analysis.

At present, the two most commonly used systems for genome-wide SNP detection are the Affymetrix GeneChip assays and the Illumina Infinium assays. The GeneChip assays are based on direct hybridization of genomic DNA to arrays containing locus-specific oligonucleotides (25mers) capable of distinguishing between the two alleles. The Illumina assays are based on the ordered arraying of oligo-coated beads. In the Infinium assay each oligonucleotide (bead type) represents a specific SNP. Both systems can now be used to screen one million SNPs in a single sample array.

234   Zhong and Romkes

2.1.3. Copy-Number
Variation and Molecular
Techniques

CNV refers to a DNA segment of at least 1 kb in size, with a variable copy number compared with a reference genome. CNV carries no implication of relative frequency or phenotypic effect. These quantitative variants can be genomic copy-number gains (insertions or duplications) or losses (deletions or null genotypes) relative to a designated reference genome sequence. A copy-number polymorphism (CNP) is a CNV that occurs in more than 1% of the population (7). By disrupting genes and altering gene dosage, CNVs influence gene expression, phenotypic variation, and adaptation and therefore can contribute significantly to differential drug response and specific genetic disorders (8).

Real-time PCR, multiplex amplifiable probe hybridization (MAPH) (9), and multiplex ligation-dependent probe amplification (MLPA) are low-throughput technologies that have been used to determine or confirm copy-number changes associated with genomic disorders. Fluorescence in situ hybridization (FISH) is a higher-resolution technique, but prohibitively labor intensive on a genomic scale.

Comparative genomic hybridization (CGH) was developed to survey DNA copy-number variations across a whole genome. With CGH, differentially labeled test and reference genomic DNAs are cohybridized to normal metaphase chromosomes, and fluorescence ratios along the length of chromosomes provide a cytogenetic representation of DNA copy-number variation. CGH, however, has a limited (approximately 20 Mb) mapping resolution.

Microarray-based formats for CGH analysis, i.e., array CGH (assembly of microarrays for genome-wide measurement of DNA copy number) with higher resolutions and alternative methods such as multiplex ligation-dependent probe amplification (MLPA) (10), multiplex amplification, and probe hybridization (MAPH) (11) or quantitative multiplex PCR of short fluorescent fragment (QMPSF) (12) for selected regions of the genome, allow for the detection of small CNVs while providing precise quantitative estimates of copy numbers (13).

Recently, commercially available platforms such as those developed by Affymetrix, Inc. and Illumina, Inc. that typically utilize oligonucleotides representing from tens of thousands to more than one million SNPs distributed across the genome are now frequently being used to also assess genome-wide copy number.

2.1.4. Insertion/Deletion
(Indel) and Molecular
Techniques

The term indel is used to describe relative gain or loss of a segment of one or more nucleotides in a genomic sequence. It has typically been used to denote relatively small-scale variants (particularly those smaller than 1 kb). Indels are important both because of their relative abundance and their functional significance. They are the second most frequent type of polymorphism in humans after SNPs. Mechanistically, small Indels tend to affect gene function in a similar fashion as SNPs, although because bases are being added or removed rather than being substituted, there is a higher likelihood of a functional effect compared with a simple substitution. Indels can be of substantial pharmacogenomic importance.

There are several ways to detect Indels: these methods include PCR-gel electrophoresis and TaqMan technology for low-throughput detection. For moderate throughput, temperature gradient capillary electrophoresis (TGCE) can be used to distinguish heteroduplex from homoduplex DNA molecules and can therefore be applied to the detection of various types of DNA polymorphisms. TGCE can be used even in the absence of prior knowledge of the sequences of the underlying polymorphisms. TGCE is both sensitive and reliable in detecting SNPs, small Indel polymorphisms, and simple sequence repeats, and when using this technique, it is possible to detect a single SNP in amplicons of over 800 bp and 1-bp Indels in amplicons of approximately 500 bp. Multiplexing can increase TGCE throughput to 12 markers on 94 samples per day *(14)*.

The tagged microarray marker (TAM) method allows high-throughput differentiation between predicted alternative PCR products. Typically, the method is used as a molecular marker approach to determining the allelic states of SNPs or Indel alleles at genomic loci in multiple individuals. The complete approach involves the following subprocedures (a) PCR setup, (b) sample arraying, (c) detector hybridization, (d) posthybridization washing, (e) fluorescence scanning and (f) data acquisition and analysis *(15)*.

2.1.5. Microsatellite Polymorphisms and Molecular Techniques

One specific type of Indels are microsatellite polymorphisms (also known as nucleotide repeats) and are regions of DNA containing canonical repetitive sequences including mononucleotide repeats (e.g., "tttttttttt"), dinucleotide repeats (e.g., "tatatatata"), trinucleotide (e.g., "tactactactac") repeats, and even higher forms. These repeat regions are common sites for additional DNA polymorphisms leading to further expansion of the repeat, possibly related to errors generated by the DNA polymerases as it passes through.

The most common way to detect microsatellites is to design PCR primers that are unique to one locus in the genome and that base pair on either side of the repeated portion. Then microsatellites are amplified by PCR and the PCR products are separated by either gel electrophoresis or capillary electrophoresis.

2.1.6. Cytogenetic Rearrangements and Molecular Techniques

Cytogenetic rearrangements are structural variants at the largest end of the scale in genome. Cytogenetic rearrangements comprise chromosome translocations, amplifications, inversions, deletion of whole chromosome arms, and interstitial deletions. These large-scale variants are often the basis for dysfunction owing to dosage imbalance and may also be part of normal functional variation. The identification of the chromosome rearrangements can help to understand disease pathogenesis, improve diagnosis, and stratify patients for risk. The identification of chromosomal rearrangements also can help to predict drug response *(16)*.

G-banding coupled with other techniques such as fluorescence in situ hybridization (FISH), has been the standard approach to detect cytogenetic rearrangements. Spectral karyotyping (SKY) *(17)* and multicolor FISH (M-FISH) *(18)* are whole-genome painting approaches and can help to detect chromosomal aberrations precisely and effectively. Array CGH has been widely used in the detection of chromosomal imbalances. Comparative genomic hybridization (CGH) is also a FISH-based technique which can detect gains and losses of whole chromosomes and subchromosomal regions.

2.2 RNA Markers

2.2.1. RNA Expression Levels and Molecular Techniques

Gene expression is the entire process that turns information contained in genes into RNA or protein. It plays a critical role in the biology of both normal and malignant cells. The determination of gene expression patterns can provide significant insights into biological responses and mechanisms of disease initiation and progression. Gene expression profiling involves the measurement of the levels of thousands of genes at once, creating a global picture of cellular function. In the field of pharmacogenomics, gene expression profiling technology can be used to identify novel molecular drug targets and to elucidate mechanisms of drug action. Gene expression profiling can also be used to predict and monitor the nature of the response of an individual to drugs within a target organ or cell line, and to accelerate drug discovery and testing.

There are multiple strategies available to measure mRNA levels. Northern blots, in situ hybridization, RT-PCR, and ribonuclease protection assays (RPA) are classical techniques for the study of gene expression, and typically allow investigators to study only one or a few genes at a time. Among these methods, quantitative or real-time RT-PCR is the most commonly used.

Microarray technology is a high-throughput approach for differential gene expression studies and can efficiently generate massive amount of gene regulation data, which facilitates the identification of gene candidates for subsequent functional characterization studies. There are two main classes of microarrays, the cDNA array and the oligonucleotide array. cDNA microarrays use approximately 200–500-bp fragments, usually produced by polymerase chain reaction (PCR), and oligonucleotide microarrays use 30–70-bp length oligonucleotides. For example, total RNA is extracted from disease and control tissue/cells and reverse transcribed to make cDNA, which is either directly or indirectly labeled with a fluorophore (such as Cy3/Cy5). Both cDNA and oligonucleotide DNA fragments are incubated on the microarray slide for a prescribed period of time, the unbound probe is washed off, and the microarray slide is then scanned at the particular laser intensity for the fluorophore to be excited and emit a quantifiable light. These quantified-light emissions are then analyzed as a representation of the expression of the message transcript for that gene to be compared with the respective genes on the control *(19)*.

Serial Analysis of Gene Expression (SAGE) *(20)* and Massively Parallel Signature Sequencing (MPSS) *(21)* are also considered high-throughput technologies. An advantage of SAGE and MPSS over DNA microarrays is that expression of unknown genes can be observed, since no sequence-specific nucleic acid probes are required for detection. SAGE and MPSS use type IIS restriction endonucleases, i.e., tagging enzymes, to collect short tags (typically 10–22 bases) from each mRNA molecule, provided a relevant recognition site exists for an anchoring enzyme. Then, SAGE and MPSS identify transcripts by sequencing long concatamers of tags using conventional sequencer and by performing iterative parallel sequencing using a proprietary technique, respectively.

2.2.2. RNA Processing and Molecular Techniques

RNA processing is to generate a mature mRNA (for protein genes) or a functional tRNA or rRNA from the primary transcript. Splicing and editing are essential steps of RNA processing.

RNA splicing is a critical, precisely regulated process that occurs after gene transcription and before mRNA translation. During this process, intros regions are removed from the pre-mRNA and exons are retained within the mature mRNA. Alternative splicing is a RNA splicing variation mechanism in which pre-mRNAs can be spliced in multiple ways to produce different mature mRNAs that encode different protein sequences. This process allows for the production of a large variety of proteins from a limited amount of DNA. There is increasing evidence that alternative splicing impacts drug efficacy or toxicity. Alternative splicing has been observed within cytochrome P450 family members (phase I metabolic enzymes) with an observable effect on drug metabolism or substrate specificity. For example, alternative splice variants play a critical role with several cancer chemotherapeutic agents, resulting in the failure of some patients to activate the administered prodrug, or leading to high toxicity due to inappropriate metabolism and variability of the apoptotic thresholds necessary to trigger cell death. Alternative splicing can be considered, therefore, to represent a class of pharmacogenomic biomarkers *(22)*.

There are several methods available to detect RNA splicing variants. The reverse transcriptase (RT)-PCR-based technique is a traditional gene-by-gene based method to analyze the presence of alternative splicing. High-throughput analysis of expressed sequence tags (ESTs) is a method used to assess alternative splicing on a genome-wide level *(23)*. The drawback to this type of approach is that EST coverage in the protein-coding sequence of many genes is inadequate to predict splice events to a large extent, and that this type of genome-wide screen for alternative splicing is unable to relate the splice event directly to drug efficacy or adverse drug response *(24)*.

mRNA expression arrays are low-cost and high-throughput strategies for the identification of alternative splice events related to drug efficacy, but they are not accurate enough for splicing profiling. A specific microarray application has been developed to monitor splice variants on a genome-wide scale. These arrays contain oligonucleotide probes that span exon–exon junctions, and probes positioned within exons to calculate individual exon levels and overall transcript expression *(25)*.

Differential analysis of transcripts with alternative splicing (DATAS) is a gene expression profiling technology that has been developed to capture mRNA splice variants that distinguish different pathological or cellular conditions. It has a major advantage over other techniques described in that it allows the systematic generation of libraries of alternative RNA splicing events without prior knowledge of the splice events *(26)*. DATAS is performed by hybridizing cDNA from one population with mRNA from the second. The reciprocal experiment (mRNA from the first population with cDNA from the second) is also performed to allow qualitative changes in both conditions to be isolated. The cDNA is generated using a biotinylated oligo-dT primer, which allows subsequent isolation of the double-stranded molecules by magnetic streptavidin beads. These hybrids are then treated with RNase H to release mRNA that does not hybridize to the heteroduplex. These released mRNAs, which encode qualitative differences between the two conditions, can then be isolated, reverse transcribed, cloned, and collected into libraries.

RNA Editing

RNA editing is a site-specific modification of RNA molecules, occurring by nucleotide insertion/deletion, nucleotide substitution, or nucleotide modification, usually by deamination of A to I or C to U. RNA editing alters the sequence of mRNAs, tRNAs, rRNAs, and small regulatory RNAs *(25)*. RNA editing in mRNAs effectively alters the amino acid sequence of the encoded protein so that it differs from that predicted by the genomic DNA sequence.

There are several methods used to determine RNA editing. A quantitative PCR (qPCR) method is a traditional method for determine the A-to-I RNA editing frequencies at specific sites. cDNA sequencing and pyrosequencing are also used for high-throughput investigation of RNA editing, but these are relatively expensive, and are too labor intensive and not sensitive enough for high-throughput screens.

High-resolution melting (HRM) of PCR amplicons is a one-step, high-throughput method that allows both the scanning of transcripts for new editing sites and the quantification of RNA editing *(27)*. In this method, PCR is performed using a fluorescent double-stranded DNA dye at high concentrations. Then four duplexes are formed: two homoduplexes and two heteroduplexes. Each duplex has a characteristic melting temperature, and the sum of all transitions can be observed by melting curve analysis. This method is used as a closed-tube method for mutation scanning and genotyping that does not require probes or labeled oligonucleotides, and no purification step is needed *(28)*.

2.2.3. MicroRNA Levels and Molecular Techniques

MicroRNAs (miRNAs) are single-stranded RNA molecules of about 19–25 nucleotides in length and are crucial regulators of gene expression. miRNAs are encoded by genes that are transcribed from DNA, but not translated into protein. They are processed from long primary transcripts (pri-miRNAs) to short stem-loop structures called pre-miRNA and finally to functional miRNA. Mature miRNA molecules are partially complementary to one or more messenger RNA (mRNA) molecules. microRNAs control the activity of approximately 30% of all protein-coding genes and affect a wide variety of cellular functions *(29)*.

Pharmacogenomic studies of miRNA are a novel and promising field of research that holds new possibilities for tailor-made medical therapy. miRNA polymorphisms affecting the expression of genes involved in pathways of drug absorption, metabolism, and disposition, and target receptors that participate in the overall clinical effect of a drug may contribute to drug resistance *(30)*.

A variety of methods have been developed for detecting and quantifying miRNA. These techniques can be mainly divided into three categories: The cloning of miRNA, PCR-based detection, and hybridization with selective probes *(31)*. The cloning of miRNA such as miRAGE *(32)* was the main tool initially used to identify miRNAs. Cloning offers the advantage for discovery of new miRNAs not predicted using computational biology tools and for the sequencing of miRNAs. However, there are limitations for quantitation of miRNA using the cloning approach. A PCR-based technique such as real-time PCR is able to detect low copy number with high sensitivity and specificity on both the precursor and the mature form of miRNAs. It is relatively inexpensive and it can be used for clinical samples with minute amounts of available RNA. The hybridization techniques include Northern blotting, in situ hybridization, bead-based flow cytometry, and microarrays. Northern blotting was the first method used to detect miRNAs and can also be used for miRNA discovery. Owing to the adaptability and high throughput, microarrays may prove to be the preferred platform for whole-genome miRNA expression analysis.

2.2.4. Epigenomics and Molecular Techniques

Epigenetic alterations are heritable changes in gene function without an accompanying change in the nuclear DNA sequence. Unlike genetic changes in cancer, epigenetic changes are potentially reversible. Two major mechanisms that cause epigenetic changes are post-translational histone modifications and DNA methylation at cytosine bases within a CpG dinucleotide.

DNA Methylation

DNA methylation in vertebrates typically occurs at CpG sites (cytosine-phosphate-guanine sites; that is, where a cytosine is directly followed by a guanine in the DNA sequence); this methylation results in the conversion of the cytosine to 5-methylcytosine. The formation of Me-CpG is catalyzed by the enzyme DNA methyltransferase. CpG sites are relatively uncommon in vertebrate genomes but are often found at higher density near vertebrate gene promoters where they are collectively referred to as CpG islands. The methylation state of these CpG sites can have a major impact on gene activity/expression. Aberrant methylation of CpG islands represents an ideal candidate for both diagnostic and prognostic drug response and disease biomarkers. For example in cancer, DNA hypermethylation is highly prevalent, is tumor specific, and potentially far more readily detectable than most genetic alterations *(33)*.

Molecular techniques used in a candidate gene level: Traditionally, DNA methylation has been studied by digesting genomic DNA with ethylation-sensitive restriction enzymes, followed by Southern blot analysis or PCR. Bisulfite reaction-based methods such as methylation-specific PCR (MSP) have become a very popular method to study DNA methylation at candidate genes. This assay entails initial modification of DNA by sodium bisulfite, converting all unmethylated, but not methylated, cytosines to uracil, and subsequent amplification with primers specific for methylated vs. unmethylated DNA *(34)*.

High-performance liquid chromatography (HPLC) and high-performance capillary electrophoresis (HPCE) are alternative methods to study DNA methylation of particular sequences and measure the total amount of 5-methylcytosine after being cut by methylation-sensitive restriction enzymes. However, these methods involve incomplete restriction-enzyme cutting and thus limit which regions can be studied.

Molecular techniques used in a genome-wide level: Restriction landmark genomic scanning (RLGS) was one of the earliest methods to be adapted for genome-wide methylation analysis *(35)*. With this technique, DNA is first radioactively labeled at unmethylated sites within methylation-sensitive restriction enzyme targets and is then size-fractionated in one dimension. The digestion products are digested with a second restriction endonuclease that is specific for high-frequency targets, and the fragments are separated in the second dimension, yielding a number of scattered hot spots of DNA methylation. When normal and tumor tissues are compared, the position and strength of a spot reveals its location and the copy number of the corresponding restriction site, respectively. Methylation-sensitive arbitrary primed PCR *(36)*, methylated CpG-island amplification (MCA) *(37)*, and amplification of intermethylated sites (AIMS) *(38)* are additional methods for the detection of altered patterns of DNA methylation across the genome. However, all of these techniques require further validation by bisulfite genomic sequencing, and a background of PCR 'noise' from repetitive sequences must be taken into account.

CpG-island and promoter microarrays are the most efficient means of studying CpG-island methylation at a genome-wide scale. A widely used example of such an approach is differential methylation hybridization (DMH), which allows the simultaneous determination of the methylation levels of a large number of CpG-island loci *(39)*. The CpG-island library DNA fragments are gridded on high-density arrays, genomic DNA from the tissues of interest is digested with methylation-sensitive enzymes, and digestion products are used as templates for PCR after ligation to linkers. The resulting oligonucleotides are used as probes to screen for hypermethylated sequences within the CpG-island library to identify sequences that are hypermethylated. The HELP assay (HpaII tiny fragment enrichment by ligation-mediated PCR) is a recently developed method. it involves cohybridization of the DNA samples to a genomic DNA microarray after cutting with a methylation-sensitive restriction enzyme or its methylation-insensitive isoschizomer *(40)*. Recently, Illumina, Inc. has also developed several methylation array applications including both a genome-wide infinium assay and a candidate gene array.

Techniques based on chromatin immunoprecipitation using the ChIP-on-chip approach have provided another important recent advance in the epigenomic profiling of cancer cells. Finally, another means of assessing genome-wide DNA-methylation patterns is gene-expression profiling using microarrays, which is now becoming widely used and has the potential to be particularly useful in cancer epigenomics. This method involves comparing mRNA levels from cancer cell lines before and after treatment with a demethylating drug, and has proved successful in identifying hypermethylated genes, avoiding the cloning step that is required when other technologies are used *(33)*.

Histone Modifications

Chromatin modification has emerged as a new fundamental mechanism for gene transcriptional activity control associated with many cellular processes like proliferation, growth, and differentiation. Mass spectrometry *(41)* or single-gene chromatin immunoprecipitation (ChIP) *(42)* uses antibodies against specific histone modifications to detect markers at candidate genes. These are the most accurate techniques for identifying histone modifications. ChIP is combined with DNA arrays (ChIP-on-chip) can be used to detect patterns across the genome.

3. Pharmacogenomic Study Approaches

An essential first step in pharmacogenomic studies is the availability of precisely defining phenotypic markers of drug response and efficacy. Failure in this effort ensures failure for any subsequent genetic analysis. Phenotypic markers include well-defined clinical endpoints, and biomarkers and surrogate endpoints, such as altered tumor size, change in blood pressure, or altered serum concentrations of a specific disease-related protein. Because both biomarkers and surrogate endpoints can serve as relevant intermediate phenotypes that define important subgroups of disease or drug responses, their definition is a critical component of minimizing confounding variables in genetic-based analysis *(43)*.

3.1. Candidate Gene Approach

With the candidate gene approach, there is a prerequisite for a basic understanding of the most likely molecular mechanisms underlying altered response to the particular drug being studied. Genes encoding proteins potentially involved in these mechanisms are then scanned for the presence of genetic variants that are predictive of outcome response. Typically, the genes analyzed would include those encoding drug-metabolizing enzymes, uptake and efflux transporters, and drug target receptors or enzymes. Phenotype–genotype correlative analyses are then conducted using statistical methods to identify genetic variants that are most predictive of altered drug response. Such analyses should also account for potentially important covariates such as race and ethnicity, age, and gender.

3.2. Whole Genome Approach

With this approach, there is no *a priori* need to understand the mechanisms responsible for altered drug response. Consequently, this approach tends to be somewhat exploratory in nature with the potential for identifying genes not previously associated with the drug of interest. Until recently, the approach has been iterative. Initially, a well-characterized set of genetic markers, usually microsatellite polymorphisms and SNPs that are distributed across the genome, are assayed and the genotype results are correlated with the drug phenotype. Genomic regions that show the highest correlation with phenotype are then scanned with a higher density set of known genetic markers until a particular gene is identified, which may then be sequenced directly to identify novel genetic variants that are most highly predictive of drug phenotype.

4. Notes

There are clearly a variety of technologies and analytical strategies for the development of novel pharmacogenomic markers and translation to clinical practice. The selection of any of these methods will necessarily depend on the application, for example, whether the objective of the testing is pharmacogenomic endpoint discovery in a research laboratory or the screening of an individual patient sample to predict drug response in a clinical molecular diagnostics testing facility. In addition to this basic question about the rationale for the analysis, there are several key features to also consider in the selection of a particular method. These factors include cost; throughput needs; accuracy, sensitivity, specificity, and reproducibility of the assay, feasibility for automation of the assay; ease of data analysis; and robustness of the assay with less than ideal sample quality.

References

1. International HapMap Consortium. (2003) The International HapMap Project. Nature 426, 789–796.

2. International HapMap Consortium. (2005) A haplotype map of the human genome. Nature 437, 1299–1320.

3. http://www.fda.gov/bbs/topics/NEWS/2005/NEW01220.html.

4. Shendure, J.A., G.J. Porreca, and G.M. Church, Overview of DNA sequencing strategies. Curr Protoc Mol Biol, 2008. Chapter 7: p. Unit 7 1

5. Schuster, S. C. (2008) Next-generation sequencing transforms today's biology. Nat Methods 5, 16–18.

6. Shastry, B. S. (2007) SNPs in disease gene mapping, medicinal drug development and evolution. J Hum Genet. 52, 871–880.

7. Scherer, S. W., Lee, C., Birney, E., Altshuler, D. M., Eichler, E. E., Carter, N. P., Hurles, M. E., and Feuk, L. (2007) Challenges and standards in integrating surveys of structural variation. Nat Genet. 39, S7–15.

8. Lee, C., Iafrate, A. J., and Brothman, A. R. (2007) Copy number variations and clinical cytogenetic diagnosis of constitutional disorders. Nat Genet. 39, S48–54.

9. Armour, J. A., Sismani, C., Patsalis, P. C., and Cross, G. (2000) Measurement of locus copy number by hybridisation with amplifiable probes. Nucleic Acids Res. 28, 605–609.

10. Schouten, J. P., McElgunn, C. J., Waaijer, R., Zwijnenburg, D., Diepvens, F., and Pals, G. (2002) Relative quantification of 40 nucleic acid sequences by multiplex ligation-dependent probe amplification. Nucleic Acids Res. 30, e57.

11. Sellner, L. N., and Taylor, G. R. (2004) MLPA and MAPH: new techniques for detection of gene deletions. Hum Mutat. 23, 413–419.

12. Saugier-Veber, P., Goldenberg, A., Drouin-Garraud, V., de La Rochebrochard, C., Layet, V., Drouot, N., Le Meur, N., Gilbert-Dussardier, B., Joly-Helas, G., Moirot, H., Rossi, A., Tosi, M., and Frebourg, T. (2006) Simple detection of genomic microdeletions and microduplications using QMPSF in patients with idiopathic mental retardation. Eur J Hum Genet. 14, 1009–1017.

13. Beckmann, J. S., Estivill, X., and Antonarakis, S. E. (2007) Copy number variants and genetic traits: closer to the resolution of phenotypic to genotypic variability. Nat Rev Genet. 8, 639–646.

14. Hsia, A. P., Wen, T. J., Chen, H. D., Liu, Z., Yandeau-Nelson, M. D., Wei, Y., Guo, L., and Schnable, P. S. (2005) Temperature gradient capillary electrophoresis (TGCE)--a tool for the high-throughput discovery and mapping of SNPs and IDPs. Theor Appl Genet. 111, 218–225.

15. Jing, R., Bolshakov, V., and Flavell, A. J. (2007) The tagged microarray marker (TAM) method for high-throughput detection of single nucleotide and indel polymorphisms. Nat Protoc. 2, 168–177.

16. Terpos, E., Eleutherakis-Papaiakovou, V., and Dimopoulos, M. A. (2006) Clinical implications of chromosomal abnormalities in multiple myeloma. Leuk Lymphoma. 47, 803–814.

17. Schrock, E., du Manoir, S., Veldman, T., Schoell, B., Wienberg, J., Ferguson-Smith, M. A., Ning, Y., Ledbetter, D. H., Bar-Am, I., Soenksen, D., Garini, Y., and Ried, T. (1996) Multicolor spectral karyotyping of human chromosomes. Science 273, 494–497.

18. Chudoba, I., Plesch, A., Lorch, T., Lemke, J., Claussen, U., and Senger, G. (1999) High resolution multicolor-banding: a new technique for refined FISH analysis of human chromosomes. Cytogenet Cell Genet. 84, 156–160.

19. Peeters, J. K., and Van der Spek, P. J. (2005) Growing applications and advancements in microarray technology and analysis tools. Cell Biochem Biophys. 43, 149–166.

20. Velculescu, V. E., Zhang, L., Vogelstein, B., and Kinzler, K. W. (1995) Serial analysis of gene expression. Science. 270, 484–487.

21. Brenner, S., Johnson, M., Bridgham, J., Golda, G., Lloyd, D. H., Johnson, D., Luo, S., McCurdy, S., Foy, M., Ewan, M., Roth, R., George, D., Eletr, S., Albrecht, G., Vermaas, E., Williams, S. R., Moon, K., Burcham, T., Pallas, M., DuBridge, R. B., Kirchner, J., Fearon, K., Mao, J., and Corcoran, K. (2000) Gene expression analysis by massively parallel signature sequencing (MPSS) on microbead arrays. Nat Biotechnol. 18, 630–634.

22. Bracco, L., and Kearsey, J. (2003) The relevance of alternative RNA splicing to pharmacogenomics. Trends Biotechnol 21, 346–353.

23. Chan, E. Y. (2005) Advances in sequencing technology. Mutat Res. 573, 13–40.

24. Black, D. L. (2000) Protein diversity from alternative splicing: a challenge for bioinformatics and post-genome biology. Cell 103, 367–370.

25. Pajares, M. J., Ezponda, T., Catena, R., Calvo, A., Pio, R., and Montuenga, L. M. (2007) Alternative splicing: an emerging topic in molecular and clinical oncology. Lancet Oncol. 8, 349–357.

26. Schweighoffer, F., Ait-Ikhlef, A., Resink, A. L., Brinkman, B., Melle-Milovanovic, D., Laurent-Puig, P., Kearsey, J., and Bracco, L. (2000) Qualitative gene profiling: a novel tool in genomics and in pharmacogenomics that deciphers messenger RNA isoforms diversity. Pharmacogenomics 1, 187–197.

27. Herrmann, M. G., Durtschi, J. D., Bromley, L. K., Wittwer, C. T., and Voelkerding, K. V. (2006) Amplicon DNA melting analysis for mutation scanning and genotyping: cross-platform comparison of instruments and dyes. Clin Chem. 52, 494–503.

28. Chateigner-Boutin, A. L., and Small, I. (2007) A rapid high-throughput method for the detection and quantification of RNA editing based on high-resolution melting of amplicons. Nucleic Acids Res. 35, e114.

29. Filipowicz, W., Bhattacharyya, S. N., and Sonenberg, N. (2008) Mechanisms of post-transcriptional regulation by microRNAs: are the answers in sight? Nat Rev Genet. 9, 102–114.

30. Bertino, J. R., Banerjee, D., and Mishra, P. J. (2007) Pharmacogenomics of microRNA: a miRSNP towards individualized therapy. Pharmacogenomics. 8, 1625–1627.

31. Liu, C. G., Spizzo, R., Calin, G. A., and Croce, C. M. (2008) Expression profiling of microRNA using oligo DNA arrays. Methods 44, 22–30.

32. Cummins, J. M., He, Y., Leary, R. J., Pagliarini, R., Diaz, L. A. Jr., , Sjoblom, T., Barad, O., Bentwich, Z., Szafranska, A. E., Labourier, E., Raymond, C. K., Roberts, B. S., Juhl, H., Kinzler, K. W., Vogelstein, B., and Velculescu, V. E. (2006) The colorectal microRNAome. Proc Natl Acad Sci U S A. 103, 3687–3692.

33. Esteller, M. (2007) Cancer epigenomics: DNA methylomes and histone-modification maps. Nat Rev Genet. 8, 286–298.

34. Gitan, R. S., Shi, H., Chen, C. M., Yan, P. S., and Huang, T. H. (2002) Methylation-specific oligonucleotide microarray: a new potential for high-throughput methylation analysis. Genome Res. 12, 158–164.

35. Costello, J. F., Fruhwald, M. C., Smiraglia, D. J., Rush, L. J., Robertson, G. P., Gao, X., Wright, F. A., Feramisco, J. D., Peltomaki, P., Lang, J. C., Schuller, D. E., Yu, L., Bloomfield, C. D., Caligiuri, M. A., Yates, A., Nishikawa, R., Su Huang, H., Petrelli, N. J., Zhang, X., O'Dorisio, M. S., Held, W. A., Cavenee, W. K., and Plass, C. (2000) Aberrant CpG-island methylation has non-random and tumour-type-specific patterns. Nat Genet. 24, 132–138.

36. Gonzalgo, M. L., Liang, G., Spruck, C. H. III, Zingg, J. M., Rideout, W. M. 3rd, and Jones, P. A. (1997) Identification and characterization of differentially methylated regions of genomic DNA by methylation-sensitive arbitrarily primed PCR. Cancer Res. 57, 594–599.

37. Toyota, M., Ho, C., Ahuja, N., Jair, K. W., Li, Q., Ohe-Toyota, M., Baylin, S. B., and Issa, J. P. (1999) Identification of differentially methylated sequences in colorectal cancer by methylated CpG island amplification. Cancer Res. 59, 2307–2312.

38. Frigola, J., Ribas, M., Risques, R. A., and Peinado, M. A. (2002) Methylome profiling of cancer cells by amplification of inter-methylated sites (AIMS). Nucleic Acids Res. 30, e28.

39. Huang, T. H., Perry, M. R., and Laux, D. E. (1999) Methylation profiling of CpG islands in human breast cancer cells. Hum Mol Genet. 8, 459–470.

40. Khulan, B., Thompson, R. F., Ye, K., Fazzari, M. J., Suzuki, M., Stasiek, E., Figueroa, M. E., Glass, J. L., Chen, Q., Montagna, C., Hatchwell, E., Selzer, R. R., Richmond, T. A., Green, R. D., Melnick, A., and Greally, J. M. (2006) Comparative isoschizomer profiling of cytosine methylation: the HELP assay. Genome Res. 16, 1046–1055.

41. Fraga, M. F., Ballestar, E., Villar-Garea, A., Boix-Chornet, M., Espada, J., Schotta, G., Bonaldi, T., Haydon, C., Ropero, S., Petrie, K., Iyer, N. G., Perez-Rosado, A., Calvo, E., Lopez, J. A., Cano, A., Calasanz, M. J., Colomer, D., Piris, M. A., Ahn, N., Imhof, A., Caldas, C., Jenuwein, T., and Esteller, M. (2005) Loss of acetylation at Lys16 and tri-methylation at Lys20 of histone H4 is a common hallmark of human cancer. Nat Genet. 37, 391–400.

42. Kurdistani, S. K., Tavazoie, S., and Grunstein, M. (2004) Mapping global histone acetylation patterns to gene expression. Cell 117, 721–33.

43. Court, M. H. (2007) A pharmacogenomics primer. J Clin Pharmacol. 47, 1087–1103.

Chapter 18

Study Designs in Genetic Epidemiology

Michele L. Cote

Summary

Identification of germline mutations that may modulate individual risk of developing cancer is a rapidly developing field. Over the last few decades, germline mutations in *p53, BRCA1, BRCA2, APC, MLH1, MSH2,* and *MSH6* have been identified in families with a large number of relatives who have been diagnosed with particular types of cancer. These mutations are rare but substantially increase the risk of cancer in carriers, and account for a small fraction of cancer cases diagnosed in the general population. The search for common mutations that correlate with a very modest increased risk of developing cancer is ongoing. With the completion of the Human Genome Project, a large array of methods to identify these genes and their variants are under development. The following chapter describes methods to provide evidence of a genetic component associated with disease risk, how to identify chromosomal regions of interest to identify rare but highly penetrant genetic variants, and methods used to identify more common mutations which modulate cancer development.

Key words: Genetic epidemiology, Familial aggregation, Linkage analyses, Segregation analyses, Association studies.

1. Introduction

Most complex traits such as cancer or cardiovascular disease are attributed to genetics, environmental factors, or some combination of both of these factors. With an estimated 30,000 genes in the human genome, the question of where to begin searching for disease-associated variants is of great interest and relevance to cancer biologists. The process of identifying germline mutations in cancer predisposition genes has involved epidemiologists, geneticists, biologists, statisticians, and more recently, individuals with expertise in bioinformatics, computational and systems biology.

Michael A. Tainsky, *Methods in Molecular Biology, Tumor Biomarker Discovery, Vol. 520*
© Humana Press, a part of Springer Science + Business Media, LLC 2009
DOI: 10.1007/978-1-60327-811-9_18

Molecular studies can inform the search for germline mutations, but it should be recognized that the way the study subjects are identified and recruited into the study, and how other factors may modulate risk can greatly influence the findings. These "genetic epidemiology" studies take a variety of approaches, and often combine both personal interview and molecular data from individuals, their relatives, and/or unrelated controls. Epidemiologic approaches to gene identification rely on sampling schemes (e.g., family-based, population) which vary depending on the analytical approach taken to test the main hypothesis. The following chapter describes methods to provide evidence of a genetic component associated with disease risk, how to identify chromosomal regions of interest to identify rare but highly penetrant genetic variants, and methods used to identify more common mutations which modulate cancer development.

2. Identifying a Genetic Component to Disease Risk

2.1. Evidence of Disease Clustering in Families

While it is now more commonly accepted that the development of the majority of cancers is due, at least in part, to an individual's underlying genetic makeup, it is often necessary to first provide statistical evidence that cancer risk is elevated in relatives of affected individuals before embarking on molecular studies. Three types of family studies that do not require DNA or tissue for analysis are described: twin studies, familial aggregation, and segregation analyses.

2.2. Twin Studies

Twins have long been studied to provide estimates of the proportion of disease that favors a genetic versus environmental component. Studies of monozygotic twins (who are genetically identical) and same-sex dizygotic twins (who share, on average, half of their genes) provide insight to the underlying etiology of the disease. If both twins of a pair are affected, they are said to be concordant for the disease. Rates of concordance can be compared between monozygotic twins (MZ) and dizygotic twins (DZ) to estimate what proportion of disease is due to genetic versus environmental factors. If monozygotic twins are 100% concordant for disease, and dizygotic twins are only 50% concordant, this suggests that the disease is purely (100%) genetic. Rarely is it so clear cut, and the fundamental assumption that the environmental component is the same for each twin may not be valid. An example of twin studies comes from the Nordic twin study, which combined cohorts of twins from Sweden, Denmark, and Finland, resulting in 44,788 pairs of twins (1). Approximately 21% of the twin pairs had at least once cancer reported, with the strongest statistical evidence supporting a heritable component for prostate, colorectal, and breast cancers *(1)*. Even with this large study population, there was not sufficient statistical power to examine a wider variety of cancers, and no adjustments could be made for exposure to environmental risk factors. Thus, twin studies may not be the ideal way to establish a genetic component to cancer risk, as cancer is relatively rare compared to other common, chronic diseases.

2.3. Familial Aggregation

Another way to establish whether or not a genetic component to cancer development exists is through the use of nuclear or extended families. Familial aggregation is the tendency for disease to cluster in families, above what would be expected in the population as a whole. A simple approach to assess aggregation in families is to identify a group of affected case subjects and corresponding control subjects, and compare the proportion of case subjects who report a positive family history of disease to control subjects who report a positive family history of disease. Thus, an odds ratio can be estimated in the following manner:

$$OR = \frac{Pr(D|FH)/Pr(ND|FH)}{Pr(D|NFH)/Pr(ND|NFH)},$$

where Pr is the probability, D the Disease (a case), FH the positive family history, ND the no disease (a control), and NFH is the no family history.

While this approach is straightforward, it is also imprecise, as the probability of a positive family history of disease increases with the ages and number of relatives considered. In addition, there is no way to control for individual risk factors for each relative, which may be driving the aggregation (e.g., smoking aggregates in families and is also a contributing factor to many cancers). A second approach that allows for adjustment of individual risk factors among the relatives, for relatives' ages and family size, is the family-based case-control design. In this type of study, the disease risk among the relatives of cases is compared to the disease risk in relatives of the controls. A more detailed family history with enumeration of each relative (and potential risk factors such as age, sex, smoking, etc.) allows for the incorporation of environmental exposures that may also aggregate in families. Familial aggregation can then be assessed in the relatives in the following manner *(2)*:

$$\frac{Pr(D \text{ in a relative of a case} \mid \text{affected case})}{Pr(D \text{ in a relative of control} \mid \text{unaffected control})}.$$

Thus, a ratio greater than 1 provides evidence of familial aggregation of disease. One way to adjust for variables which may be confounding the degree of familial aggregation that is associated with environmental factors is through the use of logistic regression modeling. The major assumption in logistic regression, i.e., the observations are independent, is not met in family studies. Because correlations between family members exist, they need to be accounted for during analysis. Familial aggregation of cancer risk can be measured using generalized estimating equations (GEE). The GEE method proposed by Liang and Zeger is an extension of generalized linear models that provides estimates of the regression parameters and their sampling variances with limited assumptions about the joint distribution *(3)*. This method corrects for correlated relative data and can be used to measure the association of each relative's phenotype (disease status) with case or control status of each subject. Use of GEE modeling is especially appropriate when environmental risk factors have been strongly associated with disease development or have been shown to aggregate in families. For example, an approximate twofold increase in risk of lung cancer has been identified in relatives related to early-onset lung cancer cases, after adjusting for age, sex, race, pack-years of cigarette smoking, and personal history of COPD for each relative *(4)*. Providing evidence of familial aggregation is often a precursor to further exploring the genetic component of a disease.

2.4. Segregation Analyses

Another method to examine familial aggregation that uses family data but does not require biospecimens is complex segregation analysis. Generally speaking, in segregation analyses involving cancer, data collection is similar to the case-control family design, and families should not be selected based on the number of family members affected. Segregation analysis evaluates the statistical evidence to determine whether the transmission pattern of a disease within a family is consistent with the existence of a major gene responsible for influencing age at onset of disease or susceptibility to the disease *(5)*. Segregation analysis has been expanded to include environmental and other types of models, in addition to examining evidence supporting a Mendelian inheritance model. It is a reliable and robust method in the assessment of both qualitative and quantitative traits *(6)*. In cancer, segregation analysis results have contributed to the identification of susceptibility genes for breast cancer *(7–9)*. An early study by Williams et al. reported that segregation analysis of 200 pedigrees suggested that an allele transmitted in the autosomal dominant pattern, with a frequency of 0.00756, increased risk of breast cancer in these families *(7)*. A second study of 1,579 nuclear pedigrees also reported the same transmission pattern, and a slightly lower population frequency of the segregating allele (0.0006) *(8)*. A third study by Claus et al., including 4,730 earlier-onset breast cancer case families and 4,688 age and geography-matched control families, also reported evidence for autosomal dominant transmission, with a higher allele frequency (0.0033) *(9)*. These studies provided a foundation for model-based linkage analyses that lead to the eventual localization of breast cancer susceptibility genes. Pedigree analysis remains the only way to ascertain the mode of inheritance of most human traits *(10)*.

3. Identifying a Chromosomal Region Linked with Disease Risk

Once a genetic component to a disease is established, identifying a chromosomal region(s) linked with increased risk of disease is a logical next step. Linkage analysis refers to a group of methods to analyze the distribution of DNA markers within families to identify a particular region (or regions) of the genome related to the disease of interest. It is the first step in positional cloning and provides a region to search for potential candidate genes. Typically, linkage analyses have been more successful at identifying variations in genes that are relatively rare in the general population, and have high penetrance (the probability of displaying a certain phenotype given you carry the "risk" genotype). Linkage analysis has been a powerful method for detecting genetic loci in single gene disorders, but is less powerful in common, complex diseases such as cancer. Linkage analysis helped identify the region containing the *BRCA1* gene, located on chromosome 17q21, which contributes to risk of familial breast cancer *(11)*.

Two broad types of linkage analysis exist: parametric and nonparametric. Both rely on concepts of Mendel's second law, namely the idea that alleles at different loci segregate independently during meiosis. During meiosis, crossovers occur between pairs of homologous chromosomes. The smaller the distance between two loci, the smaller the probability that crossover will occur between these regions. Thus, alleles on loci near each other are more likely to remain, or segregate, together. A measure of the probability that a crossover event occurs is the recombination fraction, theta (θ). Two loci that are unlinked would have $\theta = 0.5$, evidence for some degree of linkage if $\theta < 0.5$, and complete linkage if $\theta = 0$. Both types of linkage analyses described here have their strengths, but there are significant differences between the methods, which are described as follows.

3.1. Parametric Linkage Analysis

Parametric linkage analysis, also known as "model-based" or "classical" linkage analysis, requires DNA from multiple members of informative families (i.e., families with multiple affected members) and a known (or at least strongly suspected based on segregation analyses) mode of inheritance. Larger, extended families, with multiple generations of affected individuals (particularly those with early-onset disease), are generally considered superior for parametric linkage analyses compared to less extensive pedigrees with fewer affected members. After numerous markers have been genotyped (generally hundreds or thousands of microsatellite or single nucleotide polymorphisms (SNPs) for each individual, both affected and unaffected, in a family), the likelihood (L) of θ is estimated for different values of θ, and a likelihood ratio is calculated by dividing L(θ) by the probability of no linkage (i.e., L(θ) = 0.5) across a range of values from 0 to 0.5 for each family (12):

$$LR(\theta) = L(\theta)/L(\theta) = 0.5.$$

A lod score is created by summing the log of LR (θ) across all families, which represents the $\log_{10}$ of the odds for linkage ($Z(\theta) = \log_{10}LR(\theta)$) (13, 14). Generally, a lod score of 3.0 or more is considered evidence of linkage (15). Two-point analyses, where $Z(\theta)$ is calculated one marker at a time, and multipoint analysis, which calculates $Z(\theta)$ across each possible point along a map of genetic markers, are two different types of analyses possible.

Parametric linkage analyses can be challenging, from the time and cost associated with collecting DNA from the families, to determining the correct underlying genetic model. If the assumed genetic model is wrong, false-negative and false-positive results are possible. Additionally, incomplete penetrance, genetic heterogeneity (if more than one locus confers disease susceptibility), and phenocopies (where the disease is actually associated with an environmental factor, not a gene) can all result in linkage findings which are incorrect. Thus, care must be taken to comprehensively consider all linkage findings, both positive and negative.

3.2. Nonparametric Linkage Analysis

A second category of linkage analysis is "model-free" or nonparametric linkage analysis. While somewhat less robust than parametric linkage analysis when the genetic model underlying disease is known, it offers more flexibility when the genetic model is unknown. Nonparametric linkage focuses on affected individuals, such as affected sibling-pairs in nuclear families with two or more children (unaffected relatives may be used to determine common ancestry of an allele but don't directly impact the analysis).

A concept important in nonparametric linkage analysis is "identity by descent" (IBD). IBD occurs when it can be determined that two individuals (e.g., affected siblings) share a marker allele at a particular locus that was derived from the same common ancestor. If a marker is linked to a susceptibility gene, affected relatives will share more alleles IBD than expected by chance. Determining IBD can be difficult if there are missing individuals in the pedigree, and often only "identity by state" (IBS) can be concluded. IBS occurs when the alleles are identical, but common origin cannot be adequately assessed. There are a wide variety on nonparametric linkage analyses that can be performed, including those developed by Weeks et al. in 1988 and Kruglyak et al. in 1996 *(16, 17)*. These methods are advantageous in that fewer individuals per family are genotyped, reducing the overall cost of the study.

4. Identifying Common Alleles Associated with Disease Risk

While linkage studies have been most successful at identifying polymorphisms in genes that are relatively rare and highly penetrant, association studies are used to find more common genetic variations that are highly prevalent in the general population, but low in penetrance. These genes would be difficult to identify via linkage analyses and are likely responsible for a greater proportion of disease seen in the general population. Association studies use statistical methods to determine if a polymorphism occurs more commonly among affected individuals compared to unaffected individuals. The study subjects may be unrelated cases and controls identified from a specified population (i.e., cases identified from a hospital and healthy controls from the region surrounding the hospital, cases identified from a health care organization and unaffected controls that are also members of the same health care organization) or affected and unaffected members of a family. Two types of analyses will be described, direct and indirect.

4.1. Direct Association Analyses

To date, candidate-gene studies are perhaps the most common type of genetic association study performed in the search for cancer susceptibility genes. A gene is selected based on a prior knowledge of the function the gene product(s) plays in the disease process (e.g., candidate genes in the tobacco-metabolism pathway are often considered for lung cancer association studies). Polymorphisms that may affect the function of the gene are then identified, and cases and controls are genotyped at that locus. Odds ratios (OR) to estimate the relative risk of the association between the genotype and disease can be calculated as follows:

$$OR = \frac{\text{Affected with risk genotype}}{\text{Affected without risk genotype}} \times \frac{\text{Unaffected without risk genotype}}{\text{Unaffected with risk genotype}}$$

with an OR = 1 describing no association between the genotype and disease, an OR greater than 1 describing a positive association between the genotype and disease, and an OR less than 1 describing a negative, or protective, association between the genotype and disease. Other methods, such as logistic regression models to incorporate the effects of other important disease-specific risk factors (such as age, gender, and smoking in lung cancer) should be implemented to better establish the association between the genotype and disease. Unfortunately, there has been limited success in identifying common disease-susceptibility variants through the use of the candidate-gene approach. This failure is due to a number of reasons, including small studies with inadequate sample sizes and power, the variation of allele frequencies between different populations, discrepancies between studies in adjustment for suspected confounders, and limited knowledge regarding the underlying processes involved in cancer initiation and progression.

4.2. Indirect Association Analyses

The overall failure to replicate studies of particular candidate genes that increase susceptibility to cancer has increased the interest in other methods to identify common susceptibility genes. The completion of the Human Genome Project and the availability of SNP information in publicly available databases, coupled with decreasing costs associated with large-scale, high-throughput genotyping, and the development of the HapMap has allowed for the conduct of genome-wide association studies (18–20). Similar to the candidate-gene approach in design, these studies genotype both affected and unaffected individuals, but instead of looking at a handful of variants in candidate genes, individuals are genotyped across a dense set of thousands, or hundreds of thousands of SNPs that cover the whole genome. These studies then compare the genotypes or allele frequencies at a particular locus between the cases and controls. With millions of SNPs identified in humans (as of June 2007, 11.8 million reported to dbSNP, a database maintained by the National Center for Biotechnology Information (http://www.ncbi.nlm.nih.gov/SNP/), it is unlikely that the genotyped SNP is the cause of increased risk of disease, but instead is in linkage disequilibrium with the causal allele. The HapMap project provides estimates of linkage disequilibrium (LD), a measure of the correlation between SNPs, where the neighboring alleles on the same chromosome are associated within a population more frequently than would be expected. In regions of strong LD, which are common across the genome, one SNP can be typed to serve as a proxy for the other SNPs in the region. Thus, these genotyped "marker" SNPs can be selected to serve as a "tag" for a number of SNPs in the surrounding region. This tag SNP approach has also been used in candidate-gene studies. An example of the genome-wide approach to susceptibility gene identification was recently performed by a large consortium, which examined 227,876 SNPs in 4,398 breast cancer cases and 4,316 controls, then followed up their most significant findings in an additional 21,860 cases and 22,578 controls (21). Using this approach, the researchers identified four plausible candidate genes involved in modulating risk of breast cancer that had not been identified through any other methods (21). While the number of women genotyped in this study may appear to be cost prohibitive, the development of international consortiums, comprising independent researchers with banked DNA samples from previous studies, makes this sort of collaborative research feasible.

5. Materials

Twin studies, familial aggregation analyses and segregation analyses, require only the ascertainment of pedigree information (i.e., family history). For twin studies, the minimum amount of information collected should include whether the twins are identical or fraternal, disease status, age of onset (current age or age at death for unaffected individuals), and any information regarding exposure to known risk factors for each twin. Depending on the cancer type of interest, this may include smoking status, body mass index, exposures to certain chemicals, other cancers, etc. For studies of familial aggregation and segregation analyses, this type of information should be collected for all blood-related relatives, regardless of affection status, for individuals in as many generations back as possible.

Linkage analyses, both parametric and model-free, require information similar to familial aggregation studies and segregation analyses, but also require DNA. There are a variety of types of linkage analyses that require different information, but generally speaking, DNA on affected members is especially critical to success of the analysis. Additionally, collecting DNA from unaffected members, including individuals who have "married in" to the pedigree (are not blood-related) may be necessary to recreate the genotypes of individuals for whom DNA is unavailable, or may be used in other types of analyses, such as in association studies. Both direct and indirect traditional association studies using cases and unrelated controls also require DNA from the participants, as well as risk factor information. Blood should be collected from participants using standard methods (22). In the event that a blood sample is unavailable, a DNA sample should be obtained by buccal sample (23), or permission to access archived tissue should be requested from the next of kin.

6. Notes

Traditional genetic epidemiology approaches are still relevant today as investigators attempt to describe the impact of germline polymorphisms in carcinogenesis. In families where a great proportion of relatives are affected, linkage analyses can be used to identify rare variants that profoundly increase disease risk. For individuals who carry the risk variant, increased screening and clinical surveillance is warranted. However, these cases account for a small proportion of cancers in the total population. Genetic association studies are a better approach to identify common mutations with modest increases in disease risk. While the candidate-gene approach has not been as successful as hoped, the advent of whole genome association studies offers investigators another avenue to identify cancer susceptibility genes.

References

1. Lichtenstein, P., Holm, N. V., Verkasalo, P. K., Iliadou, A., Kaprio, J., Koskenvuo, M., Pukkala, E., Skytthe, A. and Hemminki, K. (2000). Environmental and heritable factors in the causation of cancer-analyses of cohorts of twins from Sweden, Denmark, and Finland. *N Engl J Med* 343, 78–85.

2. Majumder, P. P., Chakraborty, R. and Weiss, K. M. (1983). Relative risks of diseases in the presence of incomplete penetrance and sporadics. *Stat Med* 2, 13–24.

3. Zeger, S. L. and Liang, K. Y. (1986). Longitudinal data analysis for discrete and continuous outcomes. *Biometrics* 42, 121–130.

4. Cote, M. L., Kardia, S. L., Wenzlaff, A. S., Ruckdeschel, J. C. and Schwartz, A. G. (2005). Risk of lung cancer among white and black relatives of individuals with early-onset lung cancer. *JAMA* 293, 3036–3042.

5. Elston, R. C. (1981). Segregation analysis. *Adv Hum Genet* 11, 63–120, 372–723.

6. Jarvik, G. P. (1998). Complex segregation analyses: uses and limitations. *Am J Hum Genet* 63, 942–946.

7. Williams, W. R. and Anderson, D. E. (1984). Genetic epidemiology of breast cancer: segregation analysis of 200 Danish pedigrees. *Genet Epidemiol* 1, 7–20.

8. Newman, B., Austin, M. A., Lee, M. and King, M. C. (1988). Inheritance of human breast cancer: evidence for autosomal dominant transmission in high-risk families. *Proc Natl Acad Sci U S A* 85, 3044–3048.

9. Claus, E. B., Risch, N. and Thompson, W. D. (1991). Genetic analysis of breast cancer in the cancer and steroid hormone study. *Am J Hum Genet* 48, 232–242.

10. Ginsburg, E. and Livshits, G. (1999). Segregation analysis of quantitative traits. *Ann Hum Biol* 26, 103–129.

11. Hall, J. M., Lee, M. K., Newman, B., Morrow, J. E., Anderson, L. A., Huey, B. and King, M. C. (1990). Linkage of early-onset familial breast cancer to chromosome 17q21. *Science* 250, 1684–1689.

12. Haldane, J. and Smith, C. (1947). A new estimate of the linkage between the genes for colour-blindness and hemophilia in man. *Ann Eugen* 14, 10–31.

13. Morton, N. (1955). Sequential tests for the detection of linkage. *Am J Hum Genet* 7, 277–318.

14. Barnard, G. (1949). Statistical inference. *J R Stat Soc* B11, 115–135.

15. Lander, E. and Kruglyak, L. (1995). Genetic dissection of complex traits: guidelines for interpreting and reporting linkage results. *Nat Genet* 11, 241–247.

16. Kruglyak, L., Daly, M., Reeve-Daly, M. and Lander, E. (1996). Parametric and nonparametric linkage analysis: A unified multipoint approach. *Am J Hum Genet* 58, 1347–1363.

17. Weeks, D. and Lang, K. (1988). The affected-pedigree-member method of linkage analysis. *Am J Hum Genet* 42, 315–326.

18. Lander, E. S., Linton, L. M., Birren, B., Nusbaum, C., Zody, M. C., Baldwin, J., Devon, K., Dewar, K., Doyle, M., FitzHugh, W., Funke, R., Gage, D., Harris, K., Heaford, A., Howland, J., Kann, L., Lehoczky, J., LeVine, R., McEwan, P., McKernan, K., Meldrim, J., Mesirov, J. P., Miranda, C., Morris, W., Naylor, J., Raymond, C., Rosetti, M., Santos, R., Sheridan, A., Sougnez, C., Stange-Thomann, N., Stojanovic, N., Subramanian, A., Wyman, D., Rogers, J., Sulston, J., Ainscough, R., Beck, S., Bentley, D., Burton, J., Clee, C., Carter, N., Coulson, A., Deadman, R., Deloukas, P., Dunham, A., Dunham, I., Durbin, R., French, L., Grafham, D., Gregory, S., Hubbard, T.,

Humphray, S., Hunt, A., Jones, M., Lloyd, C., McMurray, A., Matthews, L., Mercer, S., Milne, S., Mullikin, J. C., Mungall, A., Plumb, R., Ross, M., Shownkeen, R., Sims, S., Waterston, R. H., Wilson, R. K., Hillier, L. W., McPherson, J. D., Marra, M. A., Mardis, E. R., Fulton, L. A., Chinwalla, A. T., Pepin, K. H., Gish, W. R., Chissoe, S. L., Wendl, M. C., Delehaunty, K. D., Miner, T. L., Delehaunty, A., Kramer, J. B., Cook, L. L., Fulton, R. S., Johnson, D. L., Minx, P. J., Clifton, S. W., Hawkins, T., Branscomb, E., Predki, P., Richardson, P., Wenning, S., Slezak, T., Doggett, N., Cheng, J. F., Olsen, A., Lucas, S., Elkin, C., Uberbacher, E., Frazier, M., et-al. (2001). Initial sequencing and analysis of the human genome. *Nature* 409, 860–921.

19. Sachidanandam, R., Weissman, D., Schmidt, S. C., Kakol, J. M., Stein, L. D., Marth, G., Sherry, S., Mullikin, J. C., Mortimore, B. J., Willey, D. L., Hunt, S. E., Cole, C. G., Coggill, P. C., Rice, C. M., Ning, Z., Rogers, J., Bentley, D. R., Kwok, P. Y., Mardis, E. R., Yeh, R. T., Schultz, B., Cook, L., Davenport, R., Dante, M., Fulton, L., Hillier, L., Waterston, R. H., McPherson, J. D., Gilman, B., Schaffner, S., Van Etten, W. J., Reich, D., Higgins, J., Daly, M. J., Blumenstiel, B., Baldwin, J., Stange-Thomann, N., Zody, M. C., Linton, L., Lander, E. S. and Altshuler, D. (2001). A map of human genome sequence variation containing 1.42 million single nucleotide polymorphisms. *Nature* 409, 928–933.

20. The International HapMap Consortium (2005). A haplotype map of the human genome. *Nature* 437, 1299–1320.

21. Easton, D. F., Pooley, K. A., Dunning, A. M., Pharoah, P. D., Thompson, D., Ballinger, D. G., Struewing, J. P., Morrison, J., Field, H., Luben, R., Wareham, N., Ahmed, S., Healey, C. S., Bowman, R., Luccarini, C., Conroy, D., Shah, M., Munday, H., Jordan, C., Perkins, B., West, J., Redman, K., Meyer, K. B., Haiman, C. A., Kolonel, L. K., Henderson, B. E., Le Marchand, L., Brennan, P., Sangrajrang, S., Gaborieau, V., Odefrey, F., Shen, C. Y., Wu, P. E., Wang, H. C., Eccles, D., Evans, D. G., Peto, J., Fletcher, O., Johnson, N., Seal, S., Stratton, M. R., Rahman, N., Chenevix-Trench, G., Bojesen, S. E., Nordestgaard, B. G., Axelsson, C. K., Garcia-Closas, M., Brinton, L., Chanock, S., Lissowska, J., Peplonska, B., Nevanlinna, H., Fagerholm, R., Eerola, H., Kang, D., Yoo, K. Y., Noh, D. Y., Ahn, S. H., Hunter, D. J., Hankinson, S. E., Cox, D. G., Hall, P., Wedren, S., Liu, J., Low, Y. L., Bogdanova, N., Schurmann, P., Dork, T., Tollenaar, R. A., Jacobi, C. E., Devilee, P., Klijn, J. G., Sigurdson, A. J., Doody, M. M., Alexander, B. H., Zhang, J., Cox, A., Brock, I. W., Macpherson, G., Reed, M. W., Couch, F. J., Goode, E. L., Olson, J. E., Meijers-Heijboer, H., van den Ouweland, A., Uitterlinden, A., Rivadeneira, F., Milne, R. L., Ribas, G., Gonzalez-Neira, A., Benitez, J., Hopper, J. L., McCredie, M., Southey, M., Giles, G. G., Schroen, C., Justenhoven, C., Brauch, H., Hamann, U., Ko, Y. D., et al. (2007). Genome-wide association study identifies novel breast cancer susceptibility loci. *Nature* 447, 1087–1093.

22. Austin, M. A., Ordovas, J. M., Eckfeldt, J. H., et al. (1996). Guidelines of the National Heart, Lung and Blood Institute Working Group on blood drawing, processing, and storage for genetic studies. *Am J Epidemiol* 144, 437–441.

23. Feigelson, H. S., Rodriguez, C., Robertson, A. S., et al. (2001). Determinants of DNA yield and quality from buccal cell samples collected with mouthwash. *Cancer Epidemiol Biomarkers Prev Sep*;10(9) , 1005–1008.

Chapter 19

Developing Classifiers for the Detection of Cancer Using Multianalytes

Adi Laurentiu Tarca, Sorin Draghici, and Roberto Romero

Summary

The development of a successful classifier from multiple predictors (analytes) is a multistage process complicated typically by the paucity of the data samples when compared to the number of available predictors. Choosing an adequate validation strategy is key for drawing sound conclusions about the usefulness of the classifier. Other important decisions have to be made regarding the type of prediction model to be used and training algorithm, as well as the way in which the markers are selected. This chapter describes the principles of the classifier development and underlines the most common pitfalls. A simulated dataset is used to illustrate the main concepts involved in supervised classification.

Key words: Multiple predictors, Supervised classification, Feature/marker selection.

1. Introduction

Current high-throughput technologies empowered life scientists with the ability of measuring the level of thousands of analytes (genes, proteins, antibodies, etc.) in a given biological sample. One of the major goals in these types of studies is to accurately classify a group of samples based on the measured expression profiles *(1–4)*. This type of application is also known as *class prediction*, *classification* or *supervised learning*.

The classification process starts with a collection of samples with known outcome for which the expression level of several analytes is available. Let $x_{i,j}$ denote the expression level of the *j*th analyte (feature) in the *i*th sample and y_i the outcome. Even though the following discussion will imply that the outcome is a two-level factor, i.e., $y_i = 1$ for disease and $y_i = 0$ for healthy samples,

Michael A. Tainsky, *Methods in Molecular Biology, Tumor Biomarker Discovery, Vol. 520*
© Humana Press, a part of Springer Science+Business Media, LLC 2009
DOI: 10.1007/978-1-60327-811-9_19

most of the principles to be described further can be used when the outcome is a continuous variable (e.g., a survival time) or a multiclass problem (e.g., disease 1, disease 2, ..., disease k). After suitable data preprocessing, the next step is to decide which validation strategy will be used to assess the classifier's performance in an unbiased way. A straightforward strategy for instance is to randomly split the samples into two disjunct sets called *training* and *test* sets. The training data will be used to learn the association between expression levels and the outcome, while the test data will be used to assess the classifier's generalization ability. The next step is to choose a type of prediction model, e.g., a logistic regression model or a neural network model. Then, a reduced set of most predictive analytes must be selected. Using the selected predictors, the model's internal parameters are then tuned (optimized) so that the predicted outcome matches as much as possible the desired outcome for the samples in the training set. This process is called learning or training. The classifier development is illustrated in **Fig. 1**.

Later in this chapter, we will use the term *model* to denote the mathematical equation that associates the analyte expression profile of the ith sample, $\mathbf{x}_i$, to a predicted outcome $\hat{y}_i$, and the term of *classification* to the entire procedure used to select markers, train the model, and compute the predicted outcome.

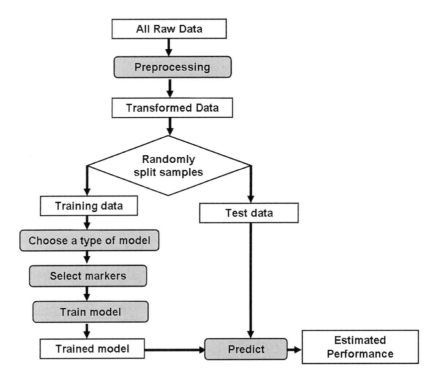

Fig. 1. Multianalyte classifier development. Data are preprocessed and then split into a training and a testing set. Using the training data, the most predictive analytes are identified and a model is trained. The resulting model is used to predict the samples membership in the test dataset and compute an unbiased estimate of the classifier's performance.

The rest of this chapter is organized as follows: First we briefly discuss issues related to data preprocessing and then we introduce classifier performance measures (e.g., accuracy) as well as practical methods to estimate them. Then, a brief introduction to various types of classification models will be given, followed by an introduction to methods for marker selection.

2. Data Preprocessing

Regardless of the way they are measured, the analyte concentration levels cover usually a wide range of values, showing typically a skewed distribution. A simple method to improve the normality of the distribution in such cases is to use a logarithmic transformation. Most of the classifiers would benefit from such data transformation resulting by improving the prediction accuracy. In addition, when using a high-throughput platform to measure analyte expression levels, the resulting data may contain systematic biases. Hence the measured levels of the analytes have to be normalized in some way in order to make them comparable between the samples. For example, the probe intensities for a particular microarray can be much higher on average that those of the other arrays. More details about the most common normalization procedures related to microarrays, which are probably the most common current multianalyte platform, can be found in the literature *(5, 6)*. Caution should be taken not to choose any preprocessing method that makes use of the sample outcome since the group information may be either unavailable or prohibited to use.

3. Classifier Figures of Merit

The result of a classification process can be summarized in a contingency table, also called *confusion matrix*. The confusion matrix contrasts the predicted class labels of the samples $\hat{y}_i$ with the true class labels y_i, as shown in **Table 1**. An example confusion matrix computed for a set of 60 healthy and 40 diseased samples is shown in **Table 2**.

The *classification rate* or *accuracy* of the prediction is defined as the average number of successfully classified samples, i.e., the sum of diagonal elements of the confusion matrix, divided by the total number of samples. In the example mentioned earlier, $Acc = (30 + 40)/(40 + 60) = 70\%$. The *sensitivity* of the classifier is defined as the fraction of positive (disease) samples correctly

Table 1
A generic confusion matrix for a 2-class problem

		True	
		Disease	Healthy
Predicted	Disease	True positives	False positives
	Healthy	False negatives	True negatives

Table 2
An example of a confusion matrix in a 2-class classification problem

		True	
		Disease	Healthy
Predicted	Disease	30	20
	Healthy	10	40

classified: $Sen = (30)/(30 + 10) = 75\%$, while the *specificity* is the fraction of negative (healthy) samples correctly classified: $Spec = (40)/(40 + 20) = 66.7\%$. The sensitivity characterizes the ability of the classifier to classify the diseased samples as such, while the specificity characterizes the ability to classify the healthy samples as such. Both are needed in a real-world application. For instance a classifier that predicts disease all the time will have a sensitivity of 100%, but zero specificity. Such a classifier would of course be useless in any application. Similarly, a high specificity can be obtained by biasing the classifiers prediction toward a healthy outcome which will in turn reduce the sensitivity. High sensitivity and specificity together imply high accuracy. The reverse is not true, however. For instance, a classifier that predicts disease all the time can yield an accuracy of 100% if there are no healthy samples in the set used to evaluate its performance. Other useful performance indices are the *positive predicted value* (PPV) and *negative predicted values* (NPV). The PPV represents the fraction of true positives among all positive predicted samples, while the NPV represents the fraction of true negatives among all negative predicted samples.

Most of the classification models do not produce directly the class label $\hat{y}_i$ from the vector of input values $\mathbf{x}_i$, but rather a continuous output Ψ_i which ranges in a certain interval, e.g., from 0 to 1. When Ψ_i is less than a given threshold, e.g., $T = 0.5$, then the sample i is classified as healthy ($\hat{y}_i = 0$), otherwise as disease ($\hat{y}_i = 1$). For a given dataset, using a threshold T lower than 0.5 will cause the prediction to be biased toward the disease class, and therefore improve the sensitivity to the detriment of specificity. The sensitivity and the specificity obtained when applying a trained model on a set of samples depend therefore on the choice of the threshold T. A receiver-operating characteristic (ROC) curve can be obtained by plotting sensitivity against 1-specificity values obtained by varying T from 0 to 1. The area under the resulting ROC curve (AUC) gives a complete picture of the performance of a trained classifier on a given dataset. The AUC ranges from 0 to 1, with 1 being the most fortunate situation when maximum sensitivity is obtained for all values of specificity.

4. Validation Strategies

In the following discussion, we will use the term performance index to refer any of the aforementioned goodness measures: accuracy, sensitivity and specificity, AUC, or other. As shown in **Fig. 1** the classifier performance should be evaluated by applying the trained model on a set of samples that were not used in the training procedure. Using the training data themselves to compute the performance indices would result in an optimistically biased estimate (7). This is because the model may *overfit* the training samples and recall them perfectly without necessarily being able to generalize well on new samples. A straightforward approach to avoid this common pitfall is to use a *hold-out* procedure in which all available samples are split at random into two parts. The first half is used to train the classifier (the *training set*), while the remaining half is used to assess the error (the *test set*). It is important that the training and the test set receive amounts of samples from each of the two classes (healthy or disease) that are proportional with the ratio between the classes in the expected application. This property is called stratification. A dataset split that respects the proportion is said to be well stratified or balanced.

The hold-out procedure is simple and easily understood as a correct method to use when it comes to validating a classifier. However, it is has the disadvantage of using the data in a suboptimal way. This is because the classifier was neither trained nor tested on all available samples, but only a subset of them. The more samples used in training, the better the model will be; while the more samples used for testing, the more accurate is the performance estimate. An alternative classifier

Fig. 2. A 3-fold crossvalidation procedure applied on six healthy and six diseased samples dataset.

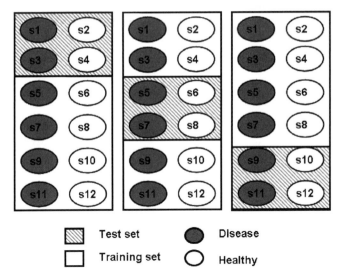

Test set   Disease
Training set   Healthy

validation strategy is the use of *leave-one-out* crossvalidation method (LOO) in which the classifier is developed n times using $(n–1)$ samples and tested on the remaining sample. The n test results obtained in this way can be arranged into a confusion matrix, and the performance indices computed as described earlier. Although the estimate of the error obtained with the LOO procedure gives low bias, it may show high variance *(8)*. A good trade-off between bias and variance may be obtained by using *N-fold crossvalidation* in which the dataset is split into $(n–m)$ training samples and m test samples $(N = n/m)$. A threefold crossvalidation procedure is illustrated in **Fig. 2**.

5. Prediction Models

At the core of the classification process there is a prediction model M. This can usually be expressed as a set of mathematical expressions. The model takes as input the levels of d analytes observed for a given sample i, $\mathbf{x}_i$, and produces an output Ψ_i. The model M has typically a series of internal parameters $\mathbf{w}$ that are determined during the training process. The general prediction relation can be written as:

$$M(\mathbf{x}_i, \mathbf{w}) = \psi \tag{1}$$

The class to which the sample i will be assigned depends on the magnitude of the output Ψ_i and a custom threshold T:

$$\hat{y}_i = \begin{cases} \text{Disease} & \text{if } \psi_i > T \\ \text{Healthy} & \text{otherwise} \end{cases} \qquad (2)$$

The classifiers used in real applications include logistic regression and linear discriminants *(9)*, weighted voting methods *(10)*, support vector machines *(11)*, and neural networks *(12, 13)*. The differences among these types of classifiers include their complexity and ability to handle nonlinear class boundaries, as well as the way in which the parameters in the models are estimated. It is outside of the scope of this chapter to provide full details about various types of classifiers. More details about can be found in the literature *(14)*. However, in order to illustrate important concepts we will briefly introduce the logistic regression model. This model can be written as:

$$M(\mathbf{x}_i, \mathbf{w}) = \frac{1}{1 + \exp(-(w_0 + w_1 x_{i,1} + w_2 x_{i,2} + \cdots + w_d x_{i,d}))}. \qquad (3)$$

It basically computes the weighted sum of the features plus an off-set (w_0) and transforms the result via the logistic function $f(z)$ = $1/[1 + \exp(-z)]$. The training of this classifier involves the estimation of the parameters $\mathbf{w}$ on the set of training samples. Once this step is completed via a sum of squared errors minimization, the model can be used to predict the class of any new sample. The prediction involves applying **Eq. 2** with a threshold value, for instance, $T = 0.5$. Actually the value of ψ_i for the logistic regression model is equivalent with the probability that the sample *i* belongs to the disease group. This interpretation holds if the class labels for diseased samples in the training set were set to 1, while those of the healthy samples were set to 0. The remainder of this chapter will illustrate the use of this classifier using a simulated dataset. In this simulation we consider we have 100 samples in each of the two groups (disease and healthy) and that we have measured ten analytes for each sample. We design the first two analytes to be somehow useful in predicting the class of samples, while the other eight to play the role of noise, i.e., no predictive value. The values of the predictor x_1 in the healthy group are drawn from a normal distribution with mean 0 and standard deviation of 1, while for the disease group the mean is set to 2. The values of the predictor x_2 in the healthy group are drawn from a normal distribution with mean –1 and standard deviation of 1, while for the disease group the mean is set to 0. The values of the remaining eight analytes in both groups are drawn from a normal distribution with mean 0 and standard deviation of 1, therefore deeming them not useful in the classification process. This dataset is shown in **Fig. 3**.

We split at random the simulated dataset into two equal and balanced parts simulating a hold-out validation strategy. Both the

Fig. 3. A simulated dataset of 100 samples per group and ten analytes. The first two analytes are deemed predictive about the class, while the remaining eight are noise.

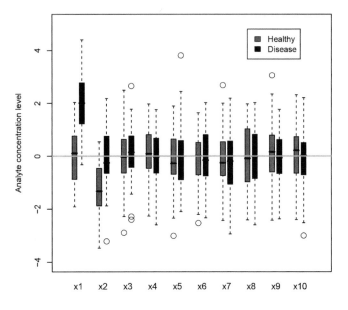

training and the test set have therefore 50 healthy and 50 diseased samples. Using the training dataset we train a logistic regression model, i.e., we estimate the coefficients $\mathbf{w}$ in **Eq. 3** using the *glm* function in the R statistical language (http://www.r-project.org). These resulting coefficients are shown in **Table 3** along with their significance p-value. The analyte x_1 appears to be the most significant followed by x_2. This is exactly what we would have expected given the design of the simulated dataset. To test the ability of the trained model to generalize on unseen data, we apply the classifier to the simulated test set. The resulting confusion matrix is shown in **Table 4**. The performance indices on the test samples are: Acc = 86%, Sen = 88%, Spec = 84%, and AUC = 91.3%. However, if we estimate the same performance indices of the trained model on the training data themselves, slightly optimistic values are obtained: Acc = 88%, Sen = 88%, Spec = 90%, AUC = 94.5%. The ROC curves for the training and test sets are shown in **Fig. 4.** These performance indices show that, as expected, evaluating the performance of the classifier on the training data will provide an optimistic view of its capabilities. Some readers might think that the differences between the two series of performance estimates are not too large. This is only because there were enough samples to train well the model (ten samples per analyte), and because the logistic regression model is robust to overfitting. With fewer data samples and more complex models the differences would have been much larger. **Figure 5** shows the decision regions produced by the logistic regression model trained on the simulated dataset

Table 3
Coefficients of the logistic regression model for the dataset illustrated in Fig. 3

	Estimate	Std. error	z value	$Pr(>|z|)$
Intercept	−1.08	0.544	−1.989	0.0467
x_1	2.02	0.466	4.338	0.0000
x_2	0.95	0.363	2.609	0.0091
x_3	−0.02	0.362	−0.048	0.9615
x_4	−0.29	0.384	−0.757	0.4492
x_5	0.14	0.306	0.460	0.6458
x_6	−0.10	0.353	−0.281	0.7785
x_7	−0.04	0.314	−0.123	0.9019
x_8	−0.04	0.276	−0.150	0.8807
x_9	0.52	0.359	1.448	0.1476
x_{10}	−0.57	0.340	−1.673	0.0943

Table 4
Confusion matrix obtained with the logistic regression model on the simulated test set

		True	
		Disease	Healthy
Predicted	Disease	44	8
	Healthy	6	42

based only on the predictive features x_1 and x_2. For comparison, the decision boundary of a three-layered neural network model with two hidden units is shown there, as well. It can be seen in this figure that two different prediction models produce different decision boundaries. However, since the number of data samples is not very large, both models produced the same accuracy on the test set. The same neural network model type, trained using a regularization procedure, provided 2% better accuracy than the logistic regression model on the same test dataset.

Fig. 4. ROC curves for a 10-analyte logistic regression classifier.

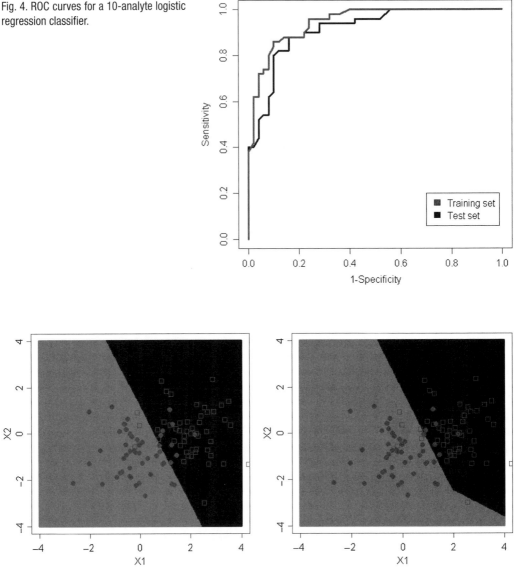

Fig. 5. Decision boundaries for two two-analyte classifiers. A logistic regression model (*left panel*) and a neural network model (*right panel*) are trained on the same data. The decision region for the simulated disease and healthy samples is shown in black and red, respectively. The simulated test data samples used to compute the classifier's performance are shown in *blue* (*filled circles* = healthy, *empty rectangles* = diseased).

6. Biomarker/
Feature Selection

Feature selection is a process in which one selects a subset containing ideally the most predictive features among all the measured ones. The feature selection step is very important in the classifier development because of several reasons, as follows. Firstly, several classifiers models (e.g., the logistic regression used earlier) cannot be trained when the number of samples is less than the number of features. Even though there are classification models, such as neural networks or support vector machines, that do not require more samples than features, it is always a good idea to have the number of features at least comparable if not lower than the number of available samples. Ideally, a ratio of ten samples per feature would provide solid and trustworthy models. Secondly, using uninformative features in the model together with the useful ones introduces noise and may, in fact, reduce the accuracy of the classifier. In the simulated dataset shown in **Fig. 3**, dropping the eight noisy features would increase the AUC on the test set from 91.3 to 94.7%. This is possible because the more the number of features there are in the model, the fewer degrees of freedom are needed in order to estimate the parameters in the model. As a literature example, a classifier able to distinguish between two types of leukemia (ALL and AML) was built by Golub et al. *(10)* using 50 marker genes. Subsequently, it was shown that the same prediction accuracy can be obtained with only two or three of them *(15)*. A third reason why few is better than more when it comes to inputs in a model is that a reduced number of features are easier to interpret in conjunction with the biology of the experiment under the study. Also, a simpler model reduced costs in a clinical setting *(16)* and the prediction time. However, the dimensionality reduction is not a goal per se, but only a means to improve the chances of obtaining a robust predictor that has good generalization ability.

In the context of the overall strategy for classifier development illustrated in **Fig. 1**, the feature selection step brings two challenges. The first challenge is to decide how to assess (measure) the goodness of a given subset of features, and the second challenge is how to search for the best subset of features in the explosive combinatorial space. A handy solution to the first challenge is to use the accuracy or AUC of the classifier using the given subset of features when trained and tested on the training set. The advantage of doing this is that no additional data are required and the model is trained with the full training set. The disadvantage of this is that there is no independent validation that the features are useful, and the truly best features may not necessarily be found. Nevertheless, the classifier development strategy as a whole is validated because the final test is done on an independent dataset (*see* **Fig. 1**). A second possibility to address the first challenge above is to use a hold-out or crossvalidation procedure and to internally validate the choice of markers on the training data itself. The disadvantages of this are that there are less data to train the model (and therefore it may not predict well on the test dataset) and that the procedure is time consuming.

Given that a choice has been made on how to measure the goodness of a given subset of features, the second challenge, i.e., how to search for the best combination of them has to be addressed. The only way to find the optimal combination that maximizes the goodness measure is to test all possibilities. For example, searching the best subset of markers out of ten available features would require to train all ten models of one inputs, all 45 models of two inputs,..., 1 model of ten inputs, for a total of 1,023 models. However if the number of available features is 100, this would require testing all 1.26×10^{30} possible combinations which is not feasible in the lifetime of any scientist, using any available computer. Even if one would know in advance which is the optimal subset size, for example knowing that the best set contains 20 markers, finding the best set of 20 marker out of 100 is not tractable either.

A straightforward but clearly suboptimal solution to finding the best combination of d markers out of p available ones is to select the best single d features. This can be done by ranking the features based on a measure of the distribution dissimilarity among the sample groups. In this category of *filter* methods we can include the t-statistic *(10)* and Wilcoxon-rank-based U statistic. Another simple and informative measure of the predictive power of a single feature is the area under the ROC curve constructed in this case using a threshold classifier. We have applied these three filter methods to our simulated dataset given in **Fig. 3.** The results are shown in Table 5. It can be seen that all three filter methods ranked the features as expected: x_1 comes first followed by x_2, and the remaining eight noisy features received much worse scores than the first 2.

A second feasible suboptimal solution to finding the best combination of d markers out of p available ones is to firstly reduce

Table 5
Ranking of the features in the simulated dataset shown in Fig. 1

Feature	P(t-test)	P (U-test)	AUC
x_1	4.07–16	8.11e-13	0.914
x_2	4.52e–07	1.03e–06	0.783
x_3	0.5581	0.6969	0.523
x_4	0.5622	0.6566	0.474
x_5	0.4849	0.8442	0.509
x_6	0.8651	0.9917	0.501
x_7	0.6414	0.7801	0.485
x_8	0.7564	0.8227	0.487
x_9	0.6936	0.6666	0.473
x_{10}	0.2291	0.3574	0.446

drastically the value of p by a filtering approach, to as low as a few hundred potentially interesting features. Then a *forward inclusion* or a *backward deletion* can be applied. With the forward inclusion the best single feature is selected first, then all combinations of the selected feature with the remaining ones are tested and the best one is retained. The procedure continues until d features are selected. The backward deletion starts with a large model of p inputs. One feature is removed at the time from the model, and the one that produced the minimum loss or the maximum gain in accuracy (compared with the full model) is definitely removed. The procedure is reiterated until there are only d features left in the model. More details on feature selection methods and classification can be found in the literature *(9, 17, 18)*.

---

7. Conclusion

Developing a successful classifier requires an appropriate number of samples, ideally larger than the number of features used in the prediction model. Array-based technologies typically screen tens of thousands of analytes; therefore, selection of a reduced number of markers is required. The marker selection process together with the model training should be done on a separate dataset than the set on which the performance is measured. Crossvalidation methods provide a good compromise between the amount of data used to train the classifier and the reliability of the performance estimates.

References

1. A. A. Alizadeh et al.Distinct type of diffuse large B-cell lymphoma identified by gene expression profiling. *Nature*, 403:503–510, 2000.
2. C. Perou, S. Jeffrey, M. van der Rijni, C. Rees, M. Eisen, D. Ross, A. Pergamenschikov, C. Williams, S. Zhu, et al. Distinctive gene expression patterns in human mammary epithelial cells and breast cancers. *Proc. Natl. Acad. Sci. USA*, 96(16):9212–9217, 1999.
3. U. Alon, N. Barkai, D. A. Notterman, K. Gish, S. Ybarra, D. Mack, and A. J. Levine. Broad patterns of gene expression revealed by clustering of tumor and normal colon tissues probed by nucleotide arrays. *Proc. Natl. Acad. Sci.*, 96:6745–6750, 1999.
4. D. T. Ross, U. Scherf, M. B. Eisen, C. M. Perou, C. Rees, P. Spellman, V. Iyer, S. S. Jeffrey, M. V. de Rijn, M. Waltham, A. Pergamenschikov, J. C. Lee, D. Lashkari, D.

Shalon, T. G. Myers, J. N. Weinstein, D. Botstein, and P. O. Brown. Systematic variation in gene expression patterns in human cancer cell lines. *Nat. Genet.*, 24(3):227–235, 2000.
5. S. Drăghici. *Data Analysis Tools for DNA Microarrays.* Chapman and Hall/CRC, Boca Raton, FL, 2003.
6. A. L. Tarca, R. Romero, and S. Draghici. Analysis of microarray experiments of gene expression profiling. *Am. J. Obstet. Gynecol.*, 195(2):373–88, 2006.
7. E. Bradley. Estimating the error rate of a prediction rule: improvement on cross-validation. *J. Am. Stat. Assoc.*, 78:316–331, 1983.
8. T. Hastie, R. Tibshirani, and J. Friedman. *The Elements of Statistical Learning.* Springer, 2001.
9. S. Dudoit, J. Fridlyand, and T. Speed. Comparison of discrimination methods for the

classification of tumors using gene expression data. *J. Am. Stat. Assoc.*, 97(457):77–87, 2002.

10. T. R. Golub, D. K. Slonim, P. Tamayo, C. Huard, M. Gaasenbeek, J. P. Mesirov, H. Coller, H. Lo, J. R. Downing, M. A. Caligiuri, C. Bloomfield, and E. Lander. Molecular classification of cancer: class discovery and class predication by gene expression monitoring. *Science*, 286:531–537, 1999.

11. S. Ramaswamy, P. Tamayo, R. Rifkin, S. Mukherjee, C. Yeang, M. Angelo, C. Ladd, M. Reich, E. Latulippe, J. Mesirov, T. Poggio, W. Gerald, M. Loda, E. Lander, and T. Golub. Multiclass cancer diagnosis using tumor gene expression signatures. *Proc. Natl. Acad. Sci. USA*, 98(26):15149–15154, 2001.

12. M. Chatterjee, S. Mohapatra, A. Ionan, G. Bawa, R. Ali-Fehmi, X. Wang, J. Nowak, B. Ye, F. A. Nahhas, K. Lu, S. S. Witkin, D. Fishman, A. Munkarah, R. Morris, N. K. Levin, N. N. Shirley, G. Tromp, J. Abrams, S. Draghici, and M. A. Tainsky. Diagnostic markers of ovarian cancer by high-throughput antigen cloning and detection on arrays. *Cancer Res.*, 66(2):1181–1190, 2006.

13. H. -S. Lin, H. S. Talwar, A. L. Tarca, A. Ionan, M. Chatterjee, B. Ye, J. Wojciechowski, S. Mohapatra, M. D. Basson, G. H. Yoo, B. Peshek, F. Lonardo, C. -J. G. Pan, A. J. Folbe, S. Draghici, J. Abrams, and M. A. Tainsky. Autoantibody approach for serum-based detection of head and neck cancer. *Cancer Epidemiol. Biomarkers Prev.*, 16(11):2396–405, 2007.

14. A. L. Tarca, V. J. Carey, X. wen Chen, R. Romero, and S. Draghici Machine learning and its applications to biology. *PLoS Comput. Biol.*, 3(6):e116, 2007.

15. R. L. Somorjai, B. Dolenko, and R. Baumgartner. Class prediction and discovery using gene microarray and proteomics mass spectroscopy data: curses, caveats, cautions. *Bioinformatics*, 19(12):1484–1491, 2003.

16. Y. Wang, F. Makedon, J. Ford, and J. Pearlman. Hykgene: a hybrid approach for selecting marker genes for phenotype classification using microarray gene expression data. *Bioinformatics*, 21(8):1530–1537, 2005.

17. S. Rogers, R. Williams, and C. Campbell. *Bioinformatics Using Computational Intelligence Paradigms*, chapter Class Prediction with Microarray Datasets, pages 119–142. Springer, Berlin, 2005.

18. L. A. Tarca, B. P. A. Grandjean, and F. Larachi. Feature selection methods for multiphase reactors data classification. *Ind. Eng. Chem. Res.*, 44(4):1073–1084, 2005.

Chapter 20

Metabolomics of Cancer

Natalie J. Serkova and Kristine Glunde

Summary

Metabolomics, one of the "omic" sciences in systems biology, is the global assessment and validation of endogenous small-molecule biochemicals (metabolites) within a biologic system. Initially, putative quantitative metabolic biomarkers for cancer detection and/or assessment of efficacy of anticancer treatment are usually discovered in a preclinical setting (using animal and human cell cultures), followed by translational validation of these biomarkers in biofluid or tumor tissue. Based on the tumor origin, various biofluids, such as blood, urine, and expressed prostatic secretions, can be used for validating metabolic biomarkers noninvasively in cancer patients. Metabolite detection and quantification is usually carried out by nuclear magnetic resonance (NMR) spectroscopy, while mass spectrometry (MS) provides another highly sensitive metabolomics technology. Usually, sophisticated statistical analyses are carried out either on spectroscopic or on quantitative metabolic data sets to provide meaningful information about the metabolic makeup of the sample. Various metabolic biomarkers, related to glycolysis, mitochondrial citric cycle acid, choline and fatty acid metabolism, were recently reported to play important roles in cancer development and responsiveness to anticancer treatment using NMR-based metabolic profiling.

Carefully designed and validated protocols for sample handling and sample extraction followed by appropriate NMR techniques and statistical analyses, which are required to establish quantitative ^{1}H-NMR-based metabolomics as a reliable analytical tool in the area of cancer biomarker discovery, are discussed in the present chapter.

Key words: Endogenous metabolites, Blood extraction, Magic angle spinning NMR, Principal component analysis, Glycolysis, Choline metabolism, Quantitative metabolomics.

1. Introduction

The concept of a biomarker can comprise anything from a single molecular species (gene, protein, metabolite) to a complex fingerprint of molecular changes (genomics, proteomics, metabolomics) indicative of human pathology, for example, cancer (**Fig. 1a**). In conjunction with significant aberrations in

Michael A. Tainsky, *Methods in Molecular Biology, Tumor Biomarker Discovery, Vol. 520*
© Humana Press, a part of Springer Science + Business Media, LLC 2009
DOI: 10.1007/978-1-60327-811-9_20

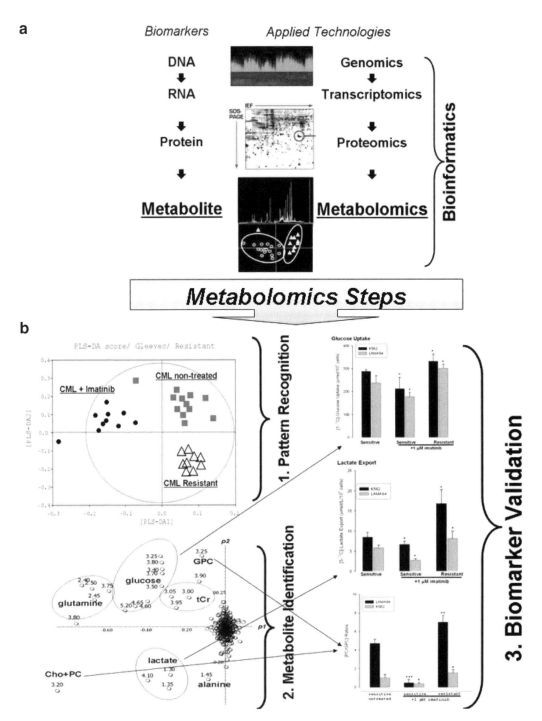

Fig. 1. (**a**) Potential applications of genomics, proteomics, and metabolomics technologies in cancer research; (**b**) Three steps of NMR-based metabolomics analysis (as an example for imatinib treatment in chronic myeloid leukemia cells) using principal component analysis: pattern recognition ("black box" using PCA scores) → metabolite identification ("biomarker" using PCA plot) → metabolite quantification ("validation") (*See Color Plates*).

genome and proteome, cancer cells possess a highly unique metabolic phenotype which is characterized by high glucose uptake,
increased glycolytic activity, decreased mitochondrial activity,
low bioenergetic status, and aberrant phospholipid metabolism
(1–4). In addition to these general metabolic markers of malignancy, specific endogenous metabolites are implicated in particular tumors, such as *N*-acetyl aspartate and *myo*-inositol in brain
cancers, citrate in prostate cancer, or triglycerides in liposarco-
mas, based on tissue-specific biochemistry *(4–6)*. Finally, using
modern analytical technologies in combination with statistical
approaches, known as "metabolomics," a global metabolic profile on study samples can also be established and validated for
early cancer detection as well as for therapeutic efficacy (responders vs. nonresponders) *(5, 7–9)*.

In general, nuclear magnetic resonance spectroscopy (mostly
^{1}H-NMR) and mass spectrometry (especially liquid chromatography (LC)-MS and Fourier-transform (FT) ion cyclotron resonance FT-MS) are two major spectroscopic techniques applied
for metabolic profiling analysis *(10, 11)*. Each technique has
distinct advantages and disadvantages. Compared to MS, NMR
offers a relatively low sensitivity, a low level of automation, and
higher costs. In addition, ^{1}H-NMR spectra are sensitive to pH,
ionic content, and temperature and sometimes require solvent
suppression (*see* **Note 1**). However, MS is very sensitive to salt
content, pH, and highly selective for detected metabolites as
well. In contrast, the major advantage of ^{1}H-NMR is its nonselec-
tivity in metabolite detection and its ability to quantify multiple
metabolites (*see* **Note 2**). In addition, ^{1}H-NMR is robust and can
be used for liquid and solid samples with minimal sample preparation. Another significant advantage of NMR is that metabolic
markers that were discovered in vitro by NMR can often be translated into in vivo protocols using localized magnetic resonance
spectroscopy (MRS, *see* **Chap. 22**).

In the past decade, an increasing number of studies have
applied high-resolution NMR spectroscopy to the study of biological systems, especially in body fluids. The application of Fourier transformation in NMR spectroscopy, multipulse sequences
(e.g., for water suppression), and the great improvement in sensitivity due to the availability of high-field magnets enabled the
detection and identification based on chemical shifts (*see* **Note 3**)
as well as quantification of hundreds of endogenous small-molecule metabolites simultaneously in biological tissues and fluids.
The most widely used NMR active isotope in the study of tissues
and body fluids is proton (^{1}H-NMR), which allows for detection of all proton-containing low molecular weight metabolites
< 1,000 Da in concentration ranges above 10 μM. Since ^{1}H-NMR
spectra from biofluids contain hundreds of NMR signals from

endogenous metabolites and are highly convoluted, spectral data sets (reduced to the 100–500 spectral intervals with respective signal intensities) are usually loaded into statistical programs (**Fig. 1b**) *(10)*. This is the first step of a metabolomics analysis, and it allows for pattern recognition (or group clustering) – such as normal versus cancer or responders versus nonresponders - based on spectral pattern differences. In the next step of a metabolomics statistical analysis, the specific spectral regions, which are responsible for group clustering in **step 1**, are identified and linked to a specific metabolite based on its NMR chemical shifts and a database search, for example, at the Human Metabolome Database *(12)*. The final, third step includes quantitation and validation of putative biomarkers with respect to tumor grade or response to therapy (**Fig. 1b**). It is very important to link the spectral pattern (**step 1**) back to biological mechanisms (**steps 2 and 3**), because only understanding a metabolite's biological role can determine its relevance in cancer and link it to genomics and proteomics data *(13)*. In addition to ^{1}H-NMR, ^{31}P-NMR of extracted or live perfused tissue specimens and cultured cells can provide additional information on biomarkers from energy or phospholipid metabolism *(3, 14, 15)*. Moreover, ^{13}C-NMR on tissues and cell extracts following incubation with a ^{13}C-labeled precursor can provide dynamic carbon fluxes such as glucose metabolism *(3, 14, 15)*. The ^{31}P- and ^{13}C-NMR spectra are usually quantified manually before statistical data analysis is performed because they contain a rather limited amount of endogenous metabolites compared to high-resolution ^{1}H-NMR spectra.

Since the majority of metabolomics work in cell models, biofluids, and biopsy specimens has been performed with NMR, this chapter will address only NMR-related metabolomics protocols. Indeed, ^{31}P-, ^{13}C-, and ^{1}H-NMR spectroscopy on cell and tissue extracts, cell suspensions, and perfused cells has been applied for decades *(15)*. Metabolic markers of cancer (increased glucose uptake, increased lactate production, and altered phospholipid metabolism) have been reported for various tumor cell lines *(16, 17)* and were monitored for their response to anticancer therapies *(14, 18, 19)*. Based on the cell size, 10^7–10^8 cells, resulting in 100–200 mg of wet cell weight, are usually required per cell extract or cell perfusion studies for conventional NMR analyses (**Fig. 2b**)

Furthermore, the use of cell perfusion studies with NMR spectroscopy provides an experimental system that can close the gap between high-resolution cell extract studies and corresponding studies in animal models or patients. The NMR spectra obtained from such studies exhibit less highly resolved NMR spectra as compared to high-resolution cell extract studies (**Fig. 2c**). The advantage of cell perfusion studies is that live cells are being studied. Therefore, time-course experiments can be

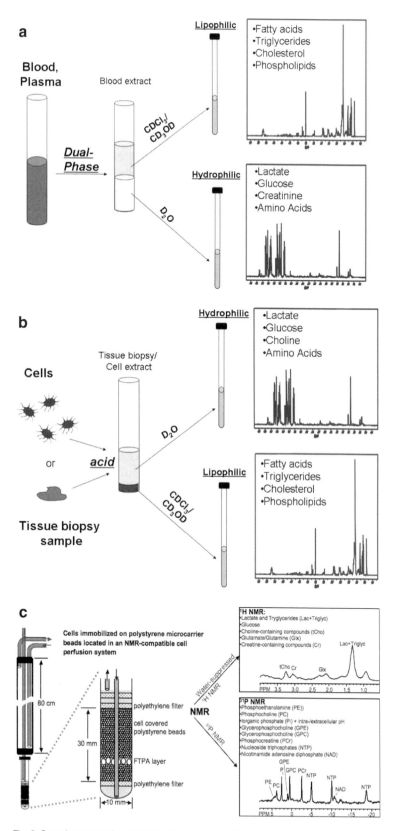

a

Blood, Plasma

Blood extract

Dual-Phase

CDCl₃/CD₃OD

D₂O

Lipophilic
•Fatty acids
•Triglycerides
•Cholesterol
•Phospholipids

Hydrophilic
•Lactate
•Glucose
•Creatinine
•Amino Acids

b

Cells

or

Tissue biopsy sample

acid

Tissue biopsy/Cell extract

D₂O

CDCl₃/CD₃OD

Hydrophilic
•Lactate
•Glucose
•Choline
•Amino Acids

Lipophilic
•Fatty acids
•Triglycerides
•Cholesterol
•Phospholipids

c

Cells immobilized on polystyrene microcarrier beads located in an NMR-compatible cell perfusion system

80 cm

30 mm

10 mm

polyethylene filter
cell covered polystyrene beads
FTPA layer
polyethylene filter

NMR

Water-suppressed ¹H NMR

³¹P NMR

¹H NMR:
•Lactate and Tryglycerides (Lac+Triglyc)
•Glucose
•Choline-containing compounds (tCho)
•Glutamate/Glutamine (Glx)
•Creatine-containing compounds (Cr)

tCho Cr   Glx   Lac+Triglyc

PPM 3.5   3.0   2.5   2.0   1.5   1.0

³¹P NMR:
•Phosphoethanolamine (PE))
•Phosphocholine (PC)
•Inorganic phosphate (Pi) + intra-/extracellular pH
•Glycerophosphocholine (GPE)
•Glycerophosphocholine (GPC)
•Phosphocreatine (PCr)
•Nucleoside triphosphates (NTP)
•Nicotinamide adenosine diphosphate (NAD)

GPE
Pi GPC PCr
PE PC   NTP   NTP   NTP
                     NAD

PPM 5   0   -5   -10   -15   -20

Fig. 2. Sample preparation charts for (**a**) dual-phase blood extraction; (**b**) acidic tissue or cell extraction; (**c**) perfused cells (*See Color Plates*).

performed in which dynamic, real-time changes in the perfused cells can be observed, such as for example in drug treatment studies (20). The extracellular conditions can be tightly controlled in such a system. Moreover, several parameters that can only be observed in live cells can be assessed noninvasively with NMR in cell perfusion studies. Such parameters include intra- and extracellular pH, cell swelling and shrinkage, time-dependent increases and decreases of metabolites (20, 21)(see **Note 4**). Proton NMR spectroscopy in cell perfusion studies requires water suppression because of the high water content of living cells, which results in a large water signal that overlaps with the much smaller metabolite signals. Water suppression can be achieved by CHESS or VAPOR water suppression (see **Note 1**). Phosphor NMR spectroscopy and ^{13}C NMR spectroscopy following administration of ^{13}C-labeled substrates to the perfusion medium have the advantage of not requiring any suppression techniques in cell perfusion studies.

Metabolic changes, observed in cell models, can then be compared and validated with NMR analyses of tissue biopsies. Since conventional high-resolution NMR is a liquid-phase based technique, the tissue specimens – either from tumor-bearing animals or directly from cancer patients - typically undergo various extraction protocols (22–24) (**Fig. 2b**). In the past few years, intact tissue specimens (e.g., biopsies, fine needle aspirates) are increasingly being used for metabolic analysis with the introduction of high-resolution magic angle spinning (hr-MAS) NMR spectroscopy (see **Note 5**). Using this unique solid-state NMR technique, metabolic patterns and marker identification for tumor staging and classification were performed on breast cancer (25–27), prostate cancer (28–30), brain tumor (31, 32), cervical carcinoma (33, 34), renal cell carcinoma (35), liposarcoma (6), and melanoma specimens (36). Conventional high-resolution NMR is generally based on the use of 3–5-mm probes. These probes deal with a total sample volume of 0.5 mL (after addition of deuterated solvents) which requires a rather large volume for sampling (above 100 µL for body fluids or homogenized tissues). Hr-MAS probes for solid-state NMR, as well as cryoprobes and microprobes for liquid NMR, allow for quantitative NMR metabolic analysis on samples as small as 3 µL with significantly improved signal-to-noise ratios and solvent suppression.

The notion that the development and growth of solid tumors can be identified by using statistical approaches from NMR spectra in biofluids is very attractive but needs to be handled with precaution. Whole blood samples provide a "metabolic window" of the overall global metabolic response of an organism, and not only the cancer-bearing organ. Nevertheless, promising results were obtained in clinical pilot studies with ovarian cancer (9), renal cell carcinomas (37), and other cancers (38) using NMR-based metabolomics on blood products. Blood samples contain a complex mixture of low- and high-molecular weight metabolites (e.g., fatty acids and lipoproteins) which can compromise spectral quality and require special NMR pulse sequences or, alternatively, sample extractions. Usually 0.5–1.0 mL of blood samples (whole blood, plasma, serum) is required for NMR metabolomics analysis (**Fig. 2a**).

Table 1
Summary on biofluids used for ¹H-NMR metabolic analysis in various areas of biomedical research

Sample	Required sample handling	References
Cell cultures	Oxygenated perfused samples	(14–21, 44)
	Perchloric acid extraction on 10^7–10^8 cells (100–200 mg)	
	Methanol/chloroform extraction on 10^7–10^8 cells (100–200 mg)	
Tissue	Add 0.01 mL deuterium oxide to 3–10 × *g* tissue in MAS rotor	(6, 8, 22–36)
	Perchloric acid extraction on 20–200 × *g* frozen tissue	
	Methanol/chloroform extraction on 20–200 × *g* frozen tissue	
Blood	For 0.5 mL of heparinized blood product:	(9, 37, 38)
Plasma	Only deuterium oxide addition (lock)	
Serum	Acetonitrile addition (protein precipitation)	
	Methanol/chloroform extraction (lipid separation)	
Urine	Add deuterated phosphate buffer to 0.4–3 mL urine	(39)
CSF	Addition of deuterium oxide to 0.5 mL CSF	(42)
EPS	Add deuterium oxide to 0.03–0.10 mL EPS	(40, 41)
Semen fluids	Add deuterium oxide to 0.25–0.5 mL fluids	(41)
Ovarian fluids	Deproteinization, then freeze drying of 10–40 mL fluids and addition of 0.5 mL deuterium oxide to the extract	(43)

Although urine is the most frequently used biofluid for preclinical toxicological application of metabolomics, very limited experience exists with urinary metabolic markers for cancer diagnosis. A recent study on a combined NMR and MS approach has reported different metabolic patterns in urine between lung cancer-bearing and healthy mice *(39)*. One of the biggest challenges for global urine metabolic profiling in the clinic is its high variability depending on life style, diet, and therapy regimens, just to mention a few. From a methodological point of view, however, urine represents an ideal biofluid for NMR metabolomics analysis because it contains the highest number of water-soluble metabolites, is produced continuously (such that it can be sampled unlimitedly and noninvasively), and requires minimal sample preparation. A half mL of urine is usually required for NMR analysis.

Other more specific biofluids, such as expressed prostatic and semen fluids for prostate cancer *(40, 41)*, cerebrospinal fluids (CSF) for subarachnoid hemorrhage *(42)*, and ovarian cyst fluids for cystadenocarcinomas *(43)*, were used in clinical pilot studies. The amount of sample size for NMR analysis depends on the specific clinical question asked (**Table 1**).

2. Materials

2.1. Sample Collection

1. Ice container.
2. Heparin-coated glass tubes.
3. Tissue crasher.
4. Liquid nitrogen.

2.2. Cell Cultures

1. Dulbecco's Modified Eagle's Medium (DMEM) (Gibco) without glucose.
2. [1-^{13}C]-labeled glucose or other [^{13}C]-labeled substrates (Cambridge Isotopes Laboratories).
3. Phosphate-Buffered Solution (PBS) (Gibco).
4. 0.9% sodium chloride (NaCl).
5. Teflon cell scrapers (Fisher).
6. Cell perfusion system consisting of an 8-mm or 10-mm NMR tube (Wilmad) attached to an NMR-compatible perfusion system (*see* **Fig. 2c**).
7. Viton, Noprene, and/or Tygon tubing for the NMR-compatible perfusion system (Masterflex).
8. Water bath to preheat the perfusion medium (Fisher).

9. Perfusion pumps to reperfuse the cell culture medium through the NMR tube (Masterflex, Cole-Parmer).

10. 5% CO_2/95% O_2 gas cylinder to presaturate perfusion medium with gas.

11. Perfluorotripropylamine trapped in alginate beads to measure the oxygen content of the perfused sample *(19)*.

12. Biosilon microcarrier beads to immobilize cells (Nunc).

13. Heating unit inside of the NMR magnet to maintain physiological temperature of 37°C (Bruker or Varian).

2.3. Sample Extraction

1. Methanol.
2. Chloroform.
3. Perchloric acid ($HClO_4$).
4. Potassium hydroxide (KOH).

2.4. NMR Run

1. Deuterium oxide (D_2O) (Cambridge Isotope Laboratories).
2. Deuterated chloroform ($CDCl_3$) (Cambridge Isotope Laboratories).
3. Deuterated methanol (CD_3OD) (Cambridge Isotope Laboratories).
4. Deuterated DCl and NaoD (Cambridge Isotope Laboratories).
5. Trimethylsilyl propionic-2,2,3,3,-d_4 acid (TSP) (Cambridge Isotope Laboratories or Sigma-Aldrich).
6. Tetramethylsilane (TMS, Sigma-Aldrich or Cambridge Isotope Laboratories).
7. Methyl diphosphoric acid (MDP, Sigma-Aldrich).
8. Ethylene diamine tetraacetic acid (EDTA, Sigma-Aldrich).
9. 5-mm NMR tube (Wilmad).
10. 1-mm NMR capillaries (Bruker Medical).
11. Zirconium oxide MAS rotor (Bruker Medical).

3. Methods

It is important to remember that during sample collection, sample handling and extraction, biochemical degradation, due to enzyme activities, occurs very rapidly. Therefore it is important to maintain low temperature for all samples, solvents, and materials until extraction is completed.

3.1. Dual-Phase Blood Extraction (Fig. 2a)

1. Collect 1 mL of whole blood in a heparin-coated glass tube. Shake well and put on ice. For plasma separation, centrifuge at $800 \times g$ for 15 min at 8°C. Store the whole blood or plasma at −20°C.

2. Slowly unfreeze blood samples at 4°C.

3. Precool methanol/ chloroform in an ice bath. Set and precool the centrifuge at 8°C.

4. Transfer 0.5 mL of blood into a glass centrifuge tube.

5. Add 1 mL of ice-cold methanol/ chloroform (1:1). Vortex well. Centrifuge at $1,300 \times g$ for 20 min at 8°C.

6. Transfer the supernatant into a new glass tube (organic phase) and keep it cold.

7. Resuspend the pellet in 0.5 mL of ice-cold methanol/ chloroform (1:1). Vortex. Centrifuge at $1,300 \times g$ for 20 min at 8°C.

8. Collect the supernatant in the same glass tube as before (organic phase).

9. The pellet is put into the refrigerator for later water-soluble metabolite extraction.

10. *Organic phase (lipophilic)*.

11. Add 0.5 mL of ice-cold bidistilled water to the organic phase. Vortex.

12. Cool for 15 min at −20°C. Two phases should be discernible.

13. Add the top "water" layer to the pellet (from the refrigerator).

14. Evaporate the bottom dark residue, containing lipids, under the jet of nitrogen in the basement lab. Or, alternatively, use the vacuum speed centrifuge to evaporate the solvents.

15. Wrap with parafilm and store at −20°C until NMR analysis.

16. *Water-soluble phase (hydrophilic)*.

17. Add additional 0.5 mL of bidest water to the pellet (containing the water rest from the previous steps). Resuspend the pellet with a spatula.

18. Vortex well. Centrifuge at $1,300 \times g$ for 20 min at 8°C.

19. Collect the supernatant in a lyophilizer glass.

20. Resuspend the pellet with 1 mL of ice-cold bidest. Water using a spatula.

21. Vortex well. Centrifuge at $1,300 \times g$ for 20 min at 8°C.

22. Collect the supernatant in the same lyophilizer glass.

23. Freeze in liquid nitrogen. Lyophilize over 2 days.

24. The lyophilized water-soluble metabolites will be redissolved in 0.5 mL of D_2O, centrifuged at $1,300 \times g$ for 10 min, and transferred into a 5-mm NMR tube.

25. The dried lipids will be redissolved in 0.6 mL deuterium methanol/chloroform (1:2) solution, centrifuged at 1,300 × g for 10 min, and transferred into a 5-mm NMR tube.

3.2. Biofluid Preparation without Extraction (Urine, EPS)

1. For urine, collect 1–3 mL of urine in a plastic tube and put immediately on ice.

2. For expressed prostatic fluids and other low-abundance biofluids, collect as much as possible (but no less than 10 µL).

3. Add deuterated phosphate buffer to urine or deuterium oxide to all other biofluids (10–30% of the sample volume). The deuterated solvent should contain TSP. If no TSP is added to D_2O, use a thin sealed glass capillary with a defined concentration of TSP for ¹H-NMR experiments (*see* **Subheading 3.8**) when using 5-mm tubes.

4. Centrifuge at 4,000 × g for 15 min at 4°C to remove macromolecules.

5. Transfer the supernatant into a 5-mm NMR tube (for sample volumes above 0.45 mL) or, using a fine-needle syringe, into a 1-mm microtube (for sample volume below 0.05 mL).

6. Adjust pH if needed.

3.3. Acidic Tissue Extraction (Fig. 2b)

1. Quickly remove 100–300 mg tissue and immediately snap freeze it using precooled tissue crasher (liquid nitrogen to be used for precooling). Wrap frozen crashed tissue in precooled aluminum foil and immediately place in liquid nitrogen. Store all frozen tissue samples at –80°C.

2. Precool 8% PCA in an ice bath. Precool a mortar, pestle, and spatula by immersing them in a liquid N_2 bath. Set and precool the centrifuge at 4°C. Take 4 mL of 8% PCA in a 50 mL centrifuge tube and precool it in an ice bath.

3. Place 100–200 mg of frozen tissue (check for tissue weight!) in the precooled pestle and powdered by crushing with the mortar, while periodically cooling the pestle and mortar in liquid N_2.

4. Using the precooled spatula, the powdered tissue is transferred to the tube containing 4 mL of 8% PCA (ice cold). Add an additional 2 mL of 8% PCA (ice cold). Mix well using a vortex mixer, then homogenize using an electric tissue homogenizer (always precool the knife in the ice-cold water bath between the samples).

5. Place the tube containing tissue/PCA extract in an ultrasound ice bath for approximately 5 min.

6. Centrifuge at 1,300 × g for 20 min at 4°C. Transfer the supernatant into a new 50-mL tube.

7. Resuspend the pellet in 2-mL ice-cold 8% PCA in the old 50-mL tube. Vortex well to resuspend the pellet. Centrifuge the resulting suspension under the same conditions as in **step 6**. Collect the supernatant in the same 50-mL tube as before, and save the pellet for **step 12**.

8. Neutralize the supernatant with KOH (first using 8 M, then 1 M and 0.1 M) so that it is at pH 7.0.

9. Centrifuge at $1,300 \times g$ for 10 min at 4°C.

10. Collect the supernatant in a lyophilizer glass, freeze in liquid nitrogen, and lyophilize it in the freeze-dry system overnight.

11. The lyophilized sample will be redissolved in 0.5 mL D_2O, centrifuged at $1,300 \times g$ for 10 min, transferred into a 5-mm NMR glass and its pH adjusted to 7.2 using DCl and NaOD, for NMR analysis.

12. Redissolve the tissue pellet (which remains after centrifugation in **step 7**) in 4-mL ice-cold water, vortex well, and put it in an ultrasound ice bath for 10 min.

13. Neutralize the pellet suspension (containing tissue lipids) with KOH so that it is at pH 7.0, transfer it into a lyophilizer glass (do not centrifuge!), freeze in liquid nitrogen, and lyophilize it in the freeze-dry system overnight.

14. The lyophilized lipids will be redissolved in 1 mL deuterium methanol/chloroform (1:2) solution, centrifuged at $1,300 \times g$ for 10 min, and transferred into a 5-mm NMR glass for NMR analysis.

3.4. Tissue Preparation for Hr-MAS NMR (see Note 4)

1. Freeze collected tissues immediately in liquid nitrogen and store at −80°C until NMR analysis.

2. Cut frozen sample into 50-μL sections (mean sample weight: 10 mg) to fit a zirconium oxide MAS rotor.

3. Add ice-cold 10 μL deuterated phosphate-buffered saline containing TSP.

4. Place the MAS rotor in an NMR magnet equipped with a MAS probe and maintain at +4°C.

3.5. Acidic Cell Extraction (Fig. 2b)

1. This protocol describes a 4-h incubation with 5 mmol/L [1-^{13}C]-labeled glucose for glucose uptake and metabolism studies by ^{13}C-NMR. However, glucose can be replaced with other labeled precursors (carbohydrates, amino acids, fatty acids, ketone bodies, etc.) based on the study focus.

2. Use 3–4 confluently grown Petri dishes (15-cm diameters). Remove culture medium, wash each dish with 5 mL sterile PBS, add 15 mL of glucose-free serum-free medium

supplemented with 13.7 mg of [1-^{13}C]labeled glucose (5 mmol/L).

3. Incubate for 4 h at 37°C and 5%CO$_2$.

4. Precool NaCl in an ice bath. Precool 8% PCA. Precool bidestilled water. Precool the centrifuge to 4°C.

5. Collect 5 mL of [1–^{13}C] labeled medium from each Petri dish in a 50-mL tube (ice bath).

6. Remove the rest of the medium.

7. Wash cells with 6 mL of ice-cold NaCl; remove NaCl.

8. Place the dish in liquid nitrogen for 30–60 s (until all cells are frozen).

9. Add 2 mL ice-cold 8% PCA to the frozen cells.

10. Scratch the cells from the dish surface and transfer cell suspension into a 50-mL tube (ice-bath).

11. Add 2 mL of ice-cold water into the dish and place the rest of the cells from the dish in the same tube.

12. Repeat with all four dishes.

13. Place the tube containing cell PCA extract in an ultrasound ice bath for 5 min.

14. Centrifuge at 1,300 × g for 20 min at 4°C.

15. Transfer the supernatant into a new 50-mL tube (ice bath).

16. Resuspend the pellet in 2 mL ice-cold 8% PCA in the old 50-mL tube. Vortex well to resuspend the pellet.

17. Place the tube in an ultrasound ice bath for 5 min.

18. Centrifuge the resulting suspension at 1,300 × g for 20 min at 4°C.

19. Collect the supernatant in the same 50-mL tube as before, and save the pellet for **step 24** (ice bath).

20. Neutralize the supernatant with KOH (first using 8 M, then 1 M and 0.1 M) so that it is at pH 7.0.

21. Centrifuge at 1,300 × g for 10 min at 4°C.

22. Collect the supernatant, transfer into a lyophilizer glass, freeze in liquid nitrogen, and lyophilize it in the freeze-dry system overnight.

23. The lyophilized sample will be redissolved in 0.5 mL D$_2$O, centrifuged at 1,300 × g for 10 min, transferred into a 5-mm NMR tube, and its pH adjusted to 7.2 using DCl and NaOD, for NMR analysis.

24. Redissolve the tissue pellet (which remains after centrifugation in **step 19**) in 4 mL ice-cold water, vortex well, and put it in an ultrasound ice bath for 10 min.

25. Neutralize the pellet suspension (containing tissue lipids) with KOH so that it is at pH 7.0, transfer it into a lyophilizer glass (do not centrifuge!), freeze in liquid nitrogen, and lyophilize it in the freeze-dry system overnight.

26. The lyophilized lipids will be redissolved in 0.6 mL deuterium methanol/chloroform (1:2) solution, centrifuged at $1,300 \times g$ for 10 min, and transferred into a 5-mm NMR glass for NMR analysis.

27. The collected 20 mL of ^{13}C-labeled medium will be centrifuged at $1,300 \times g$ for 5 min at 4°C (to remove cell debris).

28. Ten mL of medium will be lyophilized overnight.

29. The lyophilized media will be redissolved in 1 mL of D_2O, centrifuged at $1,300 \times g$ for 10 min, and transferred into a 5-mm NMR glass for NMR analysis.

3.6. Cell Perfusion (Fig. 2c)

1. Cell perfusion studies require an NMR-compatible system that can maintain cells at 37°C, keep them well oxygenated, and continuously provide fresh or reperfused media as shown in Fig. 2c. The entire perfusion system needs to be cleaned and autoclaved to provide sterile conditions for long-term cell perfusion experiments of more than 3 h. In short-term experiments that are run for less than 3 h, no sterile technique is required. In the following, the set-up of an experiment will be described.

2. Grow cells adherently grown on 2.5 mL of polystyrene microcarriers (Biosilon®, Nunc, Denmark) up to a density of approximately 35×10^7 cells/mL beads as outlined in the following:

3. To achieve this cell density, first culture cells in 175-cm² tissue culture flasks to 80% confluency.

4. Then harvest cells by trypsinization, and seed 1.5×10^7 cells onto 2.5 mL of polystyrene microcarriers and keep them in petri dishes in cell culture medium, which needs to be changed daily, for three days prior to the NMR experiment.

5. For the NMR studies, transfer 2 mL of cell-covered beads, under sterile conditions, into a 10-mm screw cap NMR tube connected to a perfusion system *(44)*.

6. Once the cell transfer is complete, circulate preheated, gas-equilibrated cell culture medium (400 mL) through the system at a rate of 1 mL/min.

7. Determine the temperature of the cells from the chemical shift of the intracellular water signal and maintain it at 37°C.

8. Equilibrate the perfusion medium as well as water in the jacket above the NMR tube with 5% CO_2/95% O_2 to maintain a physiological pH_e and to ensure sufficient oxygenation.

9. Determine the oxygen concentration in the sample from localized ^{19}F T_1 measurements of perfluorotripropylamine trapped in alginate beads, which should be layered between the microcarriers. Measure the oxygen tension 2–3 times per experiment throughout the experiment. The localized ^{19}F inversion recovery experiments should result in a value indicative of good oxygenation of the cells (e.g., close to $T_1 = 0.65$ s corresponding to an oxygen tension of 67.1 ± 2.7 [%] O_2 obtained with a calibration curve).

10. Use appropriate buffer systems in your reperfusion medium, e.g., the physiological mixture of bicarbonate (23.8 mM) combined with 5% CO_2.

11. Before and after each NMR experiment, release nuclei from a 0.5-mL aliquot of cell-covered beads, stain with crystal violet, and count the cells to verify the cell density on the microcarrier beads.

12. To measure pH, a medium composition with no more than 1 mM inorganic phosphate (P_i) should be used because otherwise the intracellular P_i will be masked by the extracellular P_i signal.

13. Acquire diffusion-weighted ^1H NMR and/or ^{31}P NMR and/or ^{13}C NMR spectra of cells perfused with medium. With the careful use of sterile technique, NMR cell perfusion studies can be performed for up to 5 days depending on the proliferation rate of the cells (which will eventually lead to an overgrowth of the cells in the perfusion system). Drugs to be tested can be added to the perfusion medium (under sterile conditions) as required.

3.7. NMR Acquisition Parameters

These instructions require the use of superconductive high-resolution NMR spectrometers with the proton resonance frequency of 300–600 MHz (magnetic field strength: 7.0–14.0 T) equipped with inverse (for proton detection) or QNP (for multinuclear detection) 5-mm probes. The X, Y, Z gradients are required for some solvent suppression sequences (*see* **Note 1**), as well as for two-dimensional NMR. For ultrasmall volume samples the use of 1-mm micro- or cryoprobes is recommended. The following protocols describe only experimental parameters for one-dimensional NMR for metabolite quantification. If metabolite identification is required by 2D-NMR, conventional NMR parameters for 2D-NMR sequences (such as COSY, HSQC) should be used.

Proton acquisition parameters (^1H-NMR) for body fluid, cell and tissue extract studies. The following are possible acquisition parameters for fully relaxed ^1H-NMR spectra, which are free of saturation effects and provide a linear correlation of metabolite concentration and signal integral. To be able to calculated metabolite concentrations it is necessary to add concentration standards TSP into D_2O or TMS in $CDCl_3/CD_3OD$ (1) directly into deuterated solvents before preparing samples; or (2) into thin sealed glass capillaries, which can be placed in the 5-mm NMR tube as external concentration standards. Fully relaxed ^{1}H-NMR spectra (without saturation effects) of water-soluble metabolites and lipids can be obtained at 500 MHz (11.7 T) using a 5-mm HX (or TXI) inverse probe using solvent presaturation pulses (such as "zgpr" for Bruker) and the following acquisition parameters: 30° flip angle, 6,000 Hz sweep width, 12.8 s repetition time, time-domain data points of 32 K, power level for solvent presaturation of 59 dB and 128 transients (can vary).

^{1}H-NMR parameters for cell perfusion studies. Record diffusion-weighted chemical shift selective (CHESS) water-suppressed ^{1}H-NMR and diffusion-weighted ^{1}H-NMR spectra without water suppression should be recorded per time point at intervals that are suitable for the time resolution of the performed study. Acquire diffusion-weighted ^{1}H-NMR spectra using, for example, the stimulated echo pulse sequence (STEAM) with an echo time TE = 11 ms and a repetition time TR = 2 s. Other acquisition parameters can be as follows: gradient ramp time of 0.3 s, *x* and *y* diffusion gradient strength of 180 mT/m each, diffusion gradient duration of 3 ms, mixing time TM = 100 ms, TM crusher gradient along the z axis of 65 mT/m, 5,000 Hz sweep width, 128 scans (two scans for spectra of intracellular water), and a data block size of 1 K. Water suppression using CHESS pulses can be achieved with 5-ms single-lobe sinc radio frequency (rf) pulses followed by gradient dephasing before the first and third rf pulses of the STEAM sequence (*see* **Note 1**). Lactate-edited ^{1}H-NMR spectra can be acquired.

Carbon acquisition parameters (^{13}C-NMR). For ^{13}C-NMR measurements, composite pulse (WALTZ-16) proton decoupling is required for the acquisition of ^{13}C-NMR spectra. The use of QNP or broad-band probes is recommended. Water-soluble and lipid ^{13}C-NMR spectra can be recorded with 30° flip angle, 29,411 Hz sweep width, 3 s repetition time, time-domain data points of 16 K (zero filled to 32 K before Fourier transform), and 20,000 transients for water-soluble metabolites or 6,000 transients for lipids. For quantification of ^{13}C-NMR spectra *see* **Note 6**.

Phosphor acquisition parameters (^{31}P-NMR) for cell and tissue extracts. Addition of 100 mmol/L EDTA can be helpful for cell extract studies to chelate divalent cations which otherwise would cause signal broadening of the nucleoside tri- and diphosphate signals. A thin sealed capillary, containing methyl diphosphoric acid (MDP), can be placed in NMR tubes for ^{31}P-metabolite quantification. The following acquisition parameters can be used to acquire fully relaxed ^{31}P-NMR spectra (without saturation effects) of water-soluble metabolites and lipids using the following acquisition parameters: 30° flip angle, 10,000 Hz sweep width, 3.7 s repetition time, time-domain data points of 16 K (zero filled to 32 K before Fourier transform), and 4,000–8,000 transients.

^{31}P-NMR for cell perfusion studies. Record ^{31}P-NMR spectra per time point with intervals that are suited for the time resolution required in the study. For ^{31}P-NMR measurements, 2,000 scans were acquired using a 45° pulse, 10,000 Hz sweep width, and a data block size of 1 or 8 K with a 1 or 2 s repetition time. Assuming [31]P T_1 relaxation times of 0.5–1.5 s for the signals typically detected in ^{31}P NMR spectra of perfused cells, such as NTP/NDP, GPC, and PC potential errors due to partial saturation of the signals would be <15% using the acquisition parameters described. For assessment of intracellular pH by ^{31}P-NMR please refer to **Note 4**.

3.8. Postprocessing Data Analysis (Fig. 3)

For NMR data processing, various NMR software can be used such as TopSpin, XWINNMR, 1D- and 2D-WINNMR. For statistical packages commercially available software (such as SIMCA, MatLab) or free software (such as Bioconductor 2.00 Package) can be utilized.

Perform exponential multiplication and Fourier transformation on acquired spectral FID (free induction decay) with following line broadening: LB = 0.2 Hz (^{1}H-NMR on biofluids and extract samples), 5 Hz (^{1}H-NMR on perfused cells), 2 Hz (^{13}C-NMR on extracts); 1 Hz (^{31}P-NMR on extracts), and 10 Hz (^{31}P-NMR on perfused cells). Proceed further with phase and baseline correction.

For calibration, set TSP or TMS to 0 ppm (^{1}H-NMR), C3-lactate to 21 ppm (^{13}C-NMR), and α-NTP signal to –10 ppm or MDP signal to 18.6 ppm (^{31}P-NMR).

Perform pe ak identification based on internal and web-based metabolite chemical shift database (for example, http://www.hmdb.ca/).

Perform peak integration and metabolite quantification using an NMR postprocessing software (quantitative database approach). The absolute concentrations of single metabolites will be referred to the TSP, integrals and calculated according to the equation:

$$C_x = \frac{I_x : N_x \times C}{I : N} \times V : M,$$

where C_x is the etabolite concentration, I_x the integral of metabolite ^{1}H or ^{31}P peak, N_x the number of protons (or phosphors) in metabolite peak, C the TSP, TMS, or MDP concentration, I the integral of TSP or TMS ^{1}H peak at 0 ppm, or of MDP ^{31}P peak at 18.6 ppm, N the number of protons (or phosphors) in TSP,

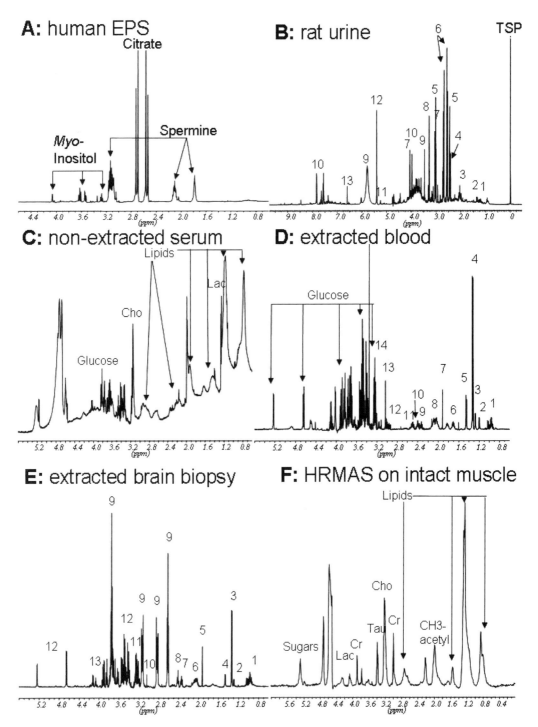

Fig. 3. Representative high-resolution ¹H-NMR spectra obtained at a Bruker 500 MHz spectrometer on (a) human expressed prostatic secretions (EPS); (b) rat urine; (c) nonextracted human serum; (d) hydrophilic fraction of the whole rat blood after dual methanol/ chloroform extraction; (e) hydrophilic fraction of a human brain biopsy (9 mg) after dual acid extraction using a 1-mm Bruker microprobe; (f) intact rat muscle by HR-MAS. *Selected peak assignments:* (b) rat urine: 1, valine, leucine, isoleucine; 2, lactate; 3, CH3-acetyl groups; 4, succinate; 5, 2-oxoglutarate; 6, citrate; 7, creatinine

TMS, or MDP, V the volume of the extract, M is the weight of cell and tissue or volume of blood sample

Alternatively, perform spectral segmentation (interval buckets) for loading into a statistical software (spectral data approach). Divide each ^{1}H-NMR spectral set into 175–400 segments (i.e., "buckets," based on spectral width). Perform Fourier transformation, phase and cubic splines base corrections of each ^{1}H-NMR spectrum prior to reduction to bucket histograms. Each bucket width should be 0.05 ppm to provide the optimal group separation in statistical analysis. Exclude the region of 4.65–5.05 ppm from segmentation and data analysis due to water presaturation and water residue. Bucket values can be scaled to the total integral or to the TSP signal region at –0.05–0.05 ppm.

Load quantitative or spectral data sets into a statistical software (such as MatLab, SIMCA, 2.00 R Package) to perform principal component analysis (PCA), partial least square discriminate analysis (PLS-DA), logistic regression, etc.

4. Notes

1. *Solvent suppression*. Solvent suppression such as water suppression is necessary for performing NMR spectroscopy of perfused cells. Water suppression can be achieved by NMR pulse sequences such as CHESS pulses in the STEAM sequence or VAPOR suppression.

2. *Area of an NMR peak*. Peak area (or integral) is measured in arbitrary units and is often called the integral or intensity of the resonance signal. The value is conveniently obtained by computer integration (using NMR software) and is proportional to the number of nuclei contributing to the resonance (such that for example the intensity ratios of –CH$_3$ to –CH peaks in lactate will be 3:1). Note that normalized integral values (divided by the number of nuclei) are proportional to the metabolite concentration.

Fig. 3. (continued) (and creatine); 8, trimethylamine-N-oxide (TMAO with betaine and taurine); 9, trans-aconitate; 10, hippurate; 11, alantoin; 12, urea; 13, trans-aconitate. (**d**) extracted blood: 1, valine, leucine, isoleucine; 2, hydroxybutyrate; 3, threonine; 4, lactate; 5, alanine; 6, arginine and lysine; 7, acetate; 8, CH3-acetyl groups; 9, glutamate and hydroxybutyrate; 10, glutamine; 11, total glutathione; 12, reduced glutathione (GSH); 13, creatine and creatinine; 14, trimethylamine-N-oxide (TMAO with betaine, taurine, glucose, and arginine). (**e**) extracted brain biopsy: 1, valine, leucine, isoleucine; 2, threonine; 3, lactate; 4, alanine; 5, N-acetyl aspartate (NAA); 6, CH3-acetyl groups; 7, glutamate; 8, glutamine; 9, xenobiotics; 10, phosphocreatine and creatine; 11, cholines and taurine; 12, glucose; 13, *myo*-inositol. *Cho* Cholines, *Cr* Creatine, *Lac* Lactate, *Tau* Taurine.

3. *Chemical shift.* All metabolites are characterized by their NMR chemical shift. The chemical shift (δ) is the normalized absorption frequency, which is expressed in parts per million (ppm) and is independent of the applied magnetic field. Because of the possibility of overlapping chemical shifts of various metabolites in one-dimensional NMR spectra, two-dimensional NMR techniques (such as $^1H/^{13}C$-HSQC) can be used for precise metabolite identification, which can serve as unique metabolite NMR fingerprints.

4. *Assessment of pH using ^{31}P-NMR of perfused cells.* To analyze intra- and extracellular inorganic phosphate in 31P-NMR of perfused cells, process ^{31}P NMR spectra with a line broadening of 2 Hz. Analyze all spectra with an algorithm for NMR data analysis that uses a combination of linear and nonlinear least-square fitting of the free induction decays, assuming a Lorentzian line shape. The signal intensities resulting from this time-domain fitting can be normalized to the corresponding intracellular water signal intensity (acquired at the same time point) that reflects the actual cell density of the sample. This is necessary to account for cell proliferation taking part during the experiment. The inorganic phosphate (P_i) signal will consist of two partially overlapping signals that can be fitted as two Lorentzian signals assuming that the signal at lower field originated from extracellular P_i and the signal at higher field from intracellular P_i. Values of pH_i and pH_e can be calculated from the chemical shift of the respective P_i signal (δP_i) as described before according to the equation $pH = 6.66 + \log[(\delta P_i - 0.729)/(3.22 - \delta P_i)]$.

5. *hr-MAS NMR parameters.* Intact tissues in the MAS rotor need to be spun at 5 kHz at the "magic" angle (54.7° to the magnetic field B) at an instrumental temperature setting of 4°C. Special NMR sequences need to be applied in order to suppress water (such as a three-pulse NOESY presaturation) and to remove the broad NMR signals from macromolecules (such as Carr-Purcell-Meiboom-Gill spin-echo sequence with appropriate T_2 relaxation delays).

6. *Quantification of ^{13}C-NMR spectra.* The ^{13}C-NMR spectra of water-soluble metabolites, as well as lipid samples, need to be corrected for saturation effects and Nuclear Overhauser effect (NOE). Partially saturated spectra of control cells acquired with NOE can be compared to spectra of identical samples acquired under fully relaxed conditions (6 s repetition time) without NOE using inverse-gated decoupling. This will provide correction factors for each signal, which can be applied to the partially saturated spectra.

Acknowledgments

The authors would like to thank Jaimi L. Brown, B.S., for her continuous help in developing and validating sample preparation protocols, as well as Dr. Eduard J. Gamito for his help with statistical methods. This work was supported by the National Institutes of Health grants R21 CA112216 (KG), P50 CA103175 (JHU ICMIC Program, KG), R21 CA108624 (NJS) and P30 CA046934 (NJS).

References

1. Griffin, J.L., and Shockcor, J.P. (2004) Metabolic profiles of cancer cells. *Nat. Rev.* 4, 551–560.

2. Griffin, J.L., and Kauppinen, R.A. (2007) Tumour metabolomics in animal models of human cancer. *J. Proteome Res.* 6, 498–505.

3. Glunde, K., and Serkova, N.J. (2006) Therapeutic targets and biomarkers identified in cancer choline phospholipid metabolism. *Pharmacogenomics.* 7, 1109–1123.

4. Costello, L.C., and Franklin, R.B. (2005) "Why do tumour cells glycolyse?": from glycolysis through citrate to lipogenesis. *Mol. Cell Biochem.* 280, 1–8.

5. Griffin, J.L., and Kauppinen, R.A. (2007) A metabolomics perspective of human brain tumours. *FEBS J.* 274, 1132–1139.

6. Millis, K., Weybright, P., Campbell, N., Fletcher, J.A., Fletcher, C.D., Cory, D.G., et-al. (1999) Classification of human liposarcoma and lipoma using ex vivo proton NMR spectroscopy. *Magn. Reson. Med.* 41, 257–267.

7. Nicholson, J.K., and Wilson, I.D. (2003) Understanding "global" systems biology: metabolomics and the continuum of metabolism. *Nat. Rev.* 2, 668–676.

8. Morvan, D., and Demidem, A. (2007) Metabolomics by proton nuclear magnetic resonance spectroscopy of the response to chloroethylnitrosourea reveals drug efficacy and tumor adaptive metabolic pathways. *Cancer Res.* 67, 2150–2159.

9. Odunsi, K., Wollman, R.M., Ambrosone, C.B., Hutson, A., McCann, S.E., Tammela, J., et al. (2005) Detection of epithelial ovarian cancer using 1H-NMR-based metabolomics. *Int. J. Cancer.* 113, 782–788.

10. Serkova, N.J., and Niemann, C.U. (2006) Pattern recognition and biomarker validation using quantitative 1H-NMR-based metabolomics. *Expert Rev. Mol. Diagn.* 6, 717–731.

11. Weckwerth, W., and Morgenthal, K. (2005) Metabolomics from pattern recognition to biological interpretation. *Drug Disc. Today.* 10, 1551–1558.

12. Wishart, D.S., Tzur, D., Knox, C., Eisner, R., Guo, A.C., Young, N., et al. (2007) HMDB: the human metabolome database. *Nucleic Acids Res.* 35, D521–D526.

13. Schmidt, C. (2004) Metabolomics takes its place as latest up-and-coming "omic" science. *J. Natl. Cancer Inst.* 96, 732–734.

14. Gottschalk, S., Anderson, N., Hainz, C., Eckhardt, G., and Serkova, N.J. (2004) Imatinib (STI571)-mediated changes in glucose metabolism in human leukemia BCR-ABL-positive cells. *Clin. Cancer Res.* 10, 6661–6668.

15. King, G.F., and Kuchel, P.W. (1994) Theoretical and practical aspects of NMR studies of cells. *Immunomethods.* 4, 85–97.

16. Katz-Brull, R., Seger, D., Rivenson-Segal, D., Rushkin, E., and Degani, H. (2002) Metabolic markers of breast cancer: enhanced choline metabolism and reduced choline-ether-phospholipid synthesis. *Cancer Res.* 62, 1966–1970.

17. Franks, S.E., Smith, M.R., Arias-Mendoza, F., Shaller, C., Padavic-Shaller, C., Kappler, F., et al. (2002) Phosphomonoester concentrations differ between chronic lymphocytic leukemia cells and normal human lymphocytes. *Leuk. Res.* 26, 919–926.

18. Beloueche-Babari, M., Jackson, L.E., Al-Saffar, N.M., Eccles, S.A., Raynaud, F.I., Workman, P., et al. (2006) Identification of magnetic resonance detectable metabolic changes associated with inhibition of phosphoinositide 3-kinase signaling in human breast cancer cells. *Mol. Cancer Ther.* 5, 187–196.

19. Glunde, K., Jie, C., and Bhujwalla, Z.M. (2007) Mechanisms of indomethacin-induced alterations in the choline phospholipid metabolism of breast cancer cells. *Neoplasia.* 8, 758–771.

20. Glunde, K., Ackerstaff, E., Natarajan, K., Artemov, D., and Bhujwalla, Z.M. (2002) Real-time changes in 1H- and 31P-NMR spectra of malignant human mammary epithelial cells during treatment with the anti-inflammatory agent indomethacin. *Magn. Reson. Med.* 48, 819–825.

21. Flogel, U., Niendorf, T., Serkova, N., Brand, A., Henke, J., and Leibfritz, D. (1995) Changes in organic solutes, volume, energy state, and metabolism associated with osmotic stress in a glial cell line: a multinuclear NMR study. *Neurochem. Res.* 20, 793–802.

22. Maxwell, R.J., Martinez-Perez, I., Cerdan, S., Cabanas, M.E., Arus, C., Moreno, A., et-al. (1998) Pattern recognition analysis of 1H-NMR spectra from perchloric acid extracts of human brain tumor biopsies. *Magn. Reson. Med.* 39, 869–877.

23. Gribbestad, I.S., Sitter, B., Lundgren, S., Krane, J., and Axelson, D. (1999) Metabolite composition in breast tumors examined by proton nuclear magnetic resonance spectroscopy. *Anticancer Res.* 19, 1737–1746.

24. Jordan, B.F., Black, K., Robey, I.F., Runquist, M., Powis, G., and Gillies, R.J. (2005) Metabolite changes in HT-29 xenograft tumors following HIF-1α inhibition with PX-478 as studied by MR spectroscopy in vivo and ex vivo. *NMR Biomed.* 18, 430–439.

25. Sitter, B., Sonnewald, U., Spraul, M., Fjosne, H.E., and Gribbestad, I.S. (2002) High-resolution magic angle spinning MRS of breast cancer tissue. *NMR Biomed.* 15, 327–337.

26. Sitter, B., Lundgren, S., Bathen, T.F., Halgunset, J., Fjosne, H.E., and Gribbestad, I.S. (2006) Comparison of HR MAS MR spectroscopic profiles of breast cancer tissue with clinical parameters. *NMR Biomed.* 19, 30–40.

27. Bathen, T.F., Jensen, L.R., Sitter, B., Fjosne, H.E., Halgunset, J., Axelson, D.E., et al. (2007) MR-determined metabolic phenotype of breast cancer in prediction of lymphatic spread, grade, and hormone status. *Breast Cancer Res. Treat.* 104, 181–189.

28. Burns, M.A., He, W., Wu, C.L., and Cheng, L.L. (2004) Quantitative pathology in tissue MR spectroscopy based human prostate metabolomics. *Technol. Cancer Res. Treat.* 3, 591–598.

29. Cheng, L.L., Burns, M.A., Taylor, J.L., He, W., Halpern, E.F., McDougal, W.S., et al. (2005) Metabolic characterization of human prostate cancer with tissue magnetic resonance spectroscopy. *Cancer Res.* 65, 3030–3034.

30. Swanson, M.G., Zektzer, A.S., Tabatabai, Z.L., Simko, J., Jarso, S., Keshari, K.R., et al. Quantitative analysis of prostate metabolites using 1H HR-MAS spectroscopy. *Magn. Reson. Med.* 55, 1257–1264.

31. Valonen, P.K., Griffin, J.L., Lehtimaki, K.K., Liimatainen, T., Nicholson, J.K., Grohn, O.H.J., et al. (2005) High-resolution magic-angle-spinning 1H-NMR spectroscopy reveals different responses in choline-containing metabolites upon gene therapy-induced programmed cell death in rat brain glioma. *NMR Biomed.* 18, 252–259.

32. Tugnoli, V., Schenetti, L., Mucci, A., Nocetti, L., Toraci, C., Mavilla, L., et-al. (2005) A comparison between in vivo and ex vivo HR-MAS 1H-MR spectra of a pediatric posterior fossa lesions. *Int. J. Mol. Med.* 16, 301–307.

33. Sitter, B., Bathen, T., Hagen, B., Arentz, C., Skjeldestad, F.E., and Gribbestad, I.S. (2004) Cervical cancer tissue characterized by high-resolution magic angle spinning MR spectroscopy. *MAGMA.* 16, 174–181.

34. Lyng, H., Sitter, B., Beathen, T.F., Jensen, L.R., Sundfor, K., Kristensen, G.B., et-al. (2007) Metabolic mapping by use of high-resolution magic angle spinning 1H-MR spectroscopy for assessment of apoptosis in cervical carcinomas. *BMC Cancer.* 7, 11–23.

35. Tate, A.R., Foxall, P.J., Holmes, E., Moka, D., Spraul, M., Nicholson, J.K., et al. (2000) Distinction between normal and renal cell carcinoma kidney cortical biopsy samples using pattern recognition of 1H magic angle spinning (MAS) NMR spectra. *NMR Biomed.* 13, 64–71.

36. Morvan, D., Demidem, A., Papon, J., De Latour, M., and Madelmont, J.C. (2002) Melanoma tumors acquire a new phospholipid metabolism phenotype under cystemustine as revealed by high-resolution magic angle spinning proton nuclear magnetic resonance spectroscopy of intact tumor samples. *Cancer Res.* 62, 1890–1897.

37. Sullentrop, F., Moka, D., Neubauer, S., Haupt, G., Engelmann, U., Hahn, J., et al. (2002) 31P-NMR spectroscopy of blood plasma: determination and quantification of phospholipid classes in patients with renal cell carcinoma. *NMR Biomed.* 15, 60–68.

38. Bathen, T.F., Engan, T., Krane, J., and Axelson, D. (2000) Analysis and classification of proton NMR spectra of lipoprotein fractions from healthy volunteers and patients with cancer or CHD. *Anticancer Res.* 20, 2398–2408.

39. Chen, H., Pan, Z., Talaty, N., Raftery, D., and Cooks, R.G. (2006) Combining desorption electrospray ionization mass spectrometry and nuclear magnetic resonance for differential metabolomics without sample preparation. *Rapid Commun. Mass Spectrom.* 20, 1577–1584.

40. Serkova, N.J., Gamito, E.J., Jones, R.H., O'Donnell, C., Hedlund, T., and Crawford, E.D. (2008) Validation of citrate and derivatives in expressed prostatic secretions to predict prostate cancer: high-resolution 1H-NMR study. *Prostate* 68, 620–628.

41. Kline, E.E., Treat, E.G., Averna, T.A., Davis, M.S., Smith, A.Y., and Sillerud, L.O. (2006) Citrate concentrations in human seminal fluids and expressed prostatic fluid determined via 1H nuclear magnetic resonance spectroscopy outperform prostate specific antigen in prostate cancer detection. *J. Urol.* 176, 2274–2279.

42. Dunne, V.G., Bhattachayya, S., Besser, M., Rae, C., and Griffin, J.L. (2005) Metabolites from cerebrospinal fluid in aneurismal subarachnoid haemorrhage correlate with vasospasm and clinical outcome: a pattern-recognition 1H NMR study. *NMR Biomed.* 18, 24–33.

43. Boss, E.A., Moolenaar, S.H., Massunger, L.F.A.G., Boonstra, H., Engelke, U.F.H., deJong, J.G.N., et al. High-resolution proton nuclear magnetic resonance spectroscopy of ovarian fluid. *NMR Biomed.* 13, 297–305.

44. Pilatus, U., Aboagye, E., Artemov, D., Mori, N., Ackerstaff, E., and Bhujwalla, Z.M. (2001) Real-time measurements of cellular oxygen consumption, pH, and energy metabolism using nuclear magnetic resonance spectroscopy. *Magn. Reson. Med.* 45, 749–755.

Chapter 21

MRI and MRS of Human Brain Tumors

Bob L. Hou and Jiani Hu

Summary

The purpose of this chapter is to provide an introduction to magnetic resonance imaging (MRI) and magnetic resonance spectroscopy (MRS) of human brain tumors, including the primary applications and basic terminology involved. Readers who wish to know more about this broad subject should seek out the referenced books (1. Tofts (2003) Quantitative MRI of the brain. Measuring changes caused by disease. Wiley; Bradley and Stark (1999) 2. Magnetic resonance imaging, 3rd Edition. Mosby Inc; Brown and Semelka (2003) 3. MRI basic principles and applications, 3rd Edition. Wiley-Liss) or reviews (4. Top Magn Reson Imaging 17:127–36, 2006; 5. JMRI 24:709–724, 2006; 6. Am J Neuroradiol 27:1404–1411, 2006). MRI is the most popular means of diagnosing human brain tumors. The inherent difference in the magnetic resonance (MR) properties of water between normal tissues and tumors results in contrast differences on the image that provide the basis for distinguishing tumors from normal tissues. In contrast to MRI, which provides spatial maps or images using water signals of the tissues, proton MRS detects signals of tissue metabolites. MRS can complement MRI because the observed MRS peaks can be linked to inherent differences in biochemical profiles between normal tissues and tumors.

The goal of MRI and MRS is to characterize brain tumors, including tumor core, edge, edema, volume, types, and grade. The commonly used brain tumor MRI protocol includes $T2$-weighted images and $T1$-weighted images taken both before and after the injection of a contrast agent (typically gadolinium: Gd). The commonly used MRS technique is either point-resolved spectroscopy (PRESS) or stimulated echo acquisition mode (STEAM).

Key words: MRI, MRS, Brain tumor, MRI signal, Imaging contrasts, Brain metabolites, Transverse magnetization, Longitudinal magnetization, Spin echo, radient echo, STEAM, PRESS.

1. Introduction

To locate a tumor in the brain, we need to obtain MRI signals from both the tumor and the normal tissue. The MRI signal originates from resonance energy absorption of a nuclear spin, such as a proton (1H) in brain tissue, in the presence of a magnetic field,

Michael A. Tainsky, *Methods in Molecular Biology, Tumor Biomarker Discovery, Vol. 520*
© Humana Press, a part of Springer Science+Business Media, LLC 2009
DOI: 10.1007/978-1-60327-811-9_21

magnetic gradient, and emission of a radio frequency (RF). The signal is acquired using an MRI scanner, which consists mainly of a magnet, receiver, gradient, RF transmitter, and shim coils with corresponding systems connected to a computer console. A diagrammatic plot of the MRI scanner is shown in **Fig. 1**.

The magnet (B_0) used for a clinical whole body scanner is usually superconductive, possessing high field homogeneity and strength, most commonly 1.5 T. The magnet (B_0) along the z-axis is used to split energy levels of a nuclear spin (such as a proton in brain tissue) for being ready of a resonance energy adsorption. The gradient coils generate linear magnetic fields along the x-, y-, and z- axes so that the location of the spin can be determined. The magnetic field generated by the gradient coil is much smaller than B_0. The shim coils adjust the magnetic field so as to make it as homogeneous as possible. The RF coil transmits RF energy, which matches the difference between energy levels, allowing resonance energy absorption of the spin. The receiver coil and the system (i.e., amplifier) acquire and amplify the absorption signal. The computer console is used to carry out the commands for acquisition, processing, and storage of the signal and/or an image reconstructed from the signal.

The contrast in MRI images is the key to distinguish healthy tissues from tumors. Four major contrasts are applied in MRI: $T1$, $T2$, $T2*$, and 1H density. $T1$ is the longitudinal relaxation time or spin-lattice relaxation time, caused by the interaction between the spin and its environment. $T2$ is the transverse relaxation time or spin-spin relaxation time in a homogeneous local magnetic field, caused by the interaction between the spin and other nearby spins. $T2*$ is the transverse relaxation time or spin-spin relaxation time in a nonhomogeneous local magnetic field, and 1H density is the number of protons (or spins) per unit volume.

The $T1$, $T2$, $T2*$, and 1H density contrasts correspond to $T1$-, $T2$-, $T2*$-, and 1H density-weighted MRI images. $T1$, $T2$, and $T2*$ images are employed to distinguish lesions from tissues in the brain. Usually $T1$- and $T2$-weighted images are used for anatomical studies, i.e., displaying tissue and/or tumor structures in the brain. $T2*$-weighted images are used for investigating brain function and distinguishing tumors from normal brain

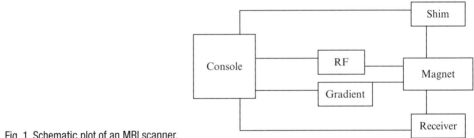

Fig. 1. Schematic plot of an MRI scanner.

tissues. 1H density-weighted images are not very useful for the diagnosis of brain tumors or investigation of brain function in a patient with a brain tumor.

Rather than providing images of water 1H in brain tissues and/or tumors, 1H MRS offers spectra of 1H metabolites in tissues and/or tumors using the same equipment as MRI (**Fig. 1**) by suppressing the strong water signals in the tissues and/or tumors. Thus 1H MRS can provide completely independent biochemical information to complement MRI, such as determining tumor grade or identifying tumor extension beyond the region scanned by MRI.

2. Methods of MRI and MRS for Brain Tumor Patients

2.1. Methods of MRI

To detect a brain tumor, the magnetic field must be adjusted ("shimmed") to obtain a uniform field, and the transmitter and receiver in the MRI scanner must be adjusted to optimum gain levels for the resonance frequency band. All of these tasks can be accomplished by applying an auto prescan mode in the MRI scanner. Then a series of pulse sequences such as $T1$- and $T2$-weighted MRI with associated acquisition parameters must be selected as having the necessary imaging contrasts to differentiate the tumor from the surrounding normal brain tissue.

The most commonly used contrasts for brain tumor imaging are $T1$, $T2$, and $T2^*$. The raw data for generating $T1$- and $T2$-weighted images can be acquired using a spin echo (SE) pulse sequence (PS). $T2^*$-weighted images are obtained from the raw data using a gradient echo (GE) pulse sequence. There are two RF pulses in the SE pulse sequence. The first one, with a flip angle of 90°, is an excitation pulse used for transverse magnetization, and the second (180°) is a refocusing pulse to reverse the spin phase and generate the SE. The most important acquisition parameters for the pulse sequence are echo time (TE), which extends from the end of the excitation pulse to the middle of the acquisition window (i.e., the time point corresponding to the maximum value of SE), and repetition time (TR), which is the interval between two successive excitation pulses for an acquired volume. The MRI signal (I) obtained from the SE pulse sequence follows **Eq. 1**:

$$I = M(0) \exp\left(-TE/T2\right)\{1 - 2\exp[-(TR - TE/2)T1] + \exp(-TR/T1)\}, \tag{1}$$

where $M(0)$ is a constant and represents the maximum MRI signal. If a short TR and TE are selected, the signal intensity I is proportioned to $\{1 - \exp(-TR/T1)\}$, providing $T1$-weighted images, in which the tissues with longer $T1$ values display hypointensity, such as cerebrospinal fluid (CSF) in the ventricle and water in the tumor craniotomy site as shown in **Fig. 2a**.

If a long TR and medium TE are selected, **Eq. 1** will be shortened to $\exp(-TE/T2)$. The image generated from the signal will be a $T2$-weighted image, in which areas of high molecular mobility (i.e., long $T2$) such as CSF in the ventricle, water in the edema associated with the tumor and at the edge of the craniotomy site, will display hyperintensity, as shown in **Fig. 2b**.

A GE pulse sequence has only one RF pulse with a flip angle of α for excitation of the signal and uses gradient pulses to refocus the spin phase and generate an echo (i.e., "gradient echo"). The GE signal (I) follows **Eq. 2** and is a function of $T2^*$.

$$I = M(0)\exp(-TE/T2^*)\sin\alpha\,[1-\exp(-TR/T1)]/ \\ [1-\cos\alpha\exp(-TR/T1)]. \qquad (2)$$

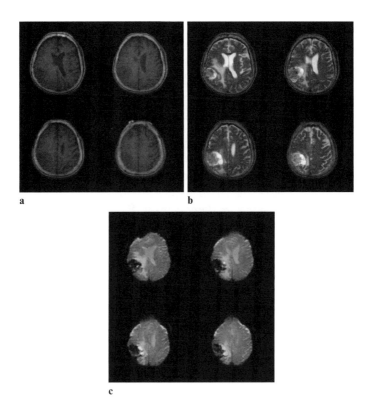

Fig. 2. (**a**) SE $T1$-weighted images (main acquisition parameters: TR/TE/flip angle = 567 ms/14 ms/ 90°) from a 3 T scanner for a patient with a tumor in the right frontal lobe. (**b**) SE $T2$-weighted images (main acquisition parameters: TR/TE/flip angle = 3,800 ms/102 ms/ 90°) from a 3 T scanner for a patient with a tumor in the right frontal lobe. (**c**) GE $T2^*$-weighted images (main parameters: TR/TE/flip angle = 4,000 ms/30 ms/90°) from a 3 T scanner for a patient with a tumor in the right frontal lobe.

Table 1
$T1$ and $T2$ values in brain for a 1.5-T or a 3.0-T scanner

1.5 T	WM	GM	Blood
$T1$	884 ± 50	1,124 ± 50	1,441 ± 120
$T2$	72 ± 4	95 ± 8	290 ± 30
3 T	WM	GM	BLOOD
$T1$	1,084 ± 45	1,820 ± 114	1,932 ± 85
$T2$	69 ± 3	99 ± 7	275 ± 50

If a long TR and α near 90° are used, the signal (I) is proportional to $\exp(-TE/T2^*)$, i.e., $T2^*$ for a short TE. The following figure shows $T2^*$-weighted images, in which highly nonhomogeneous magnetic field areas with short $T2^*$ including the edge of the frontal lobe and the craniotomy site, are not only distorted but have also lost signal intensity.

$T1$ and $T2$ values of protons (1H) in the human brain depend on tissues and/or fluids such as gray matter (GM), white matter (WM), CSF, blood, etc. In general, the more mobile the protons, the longer $T1$ and $T2$; hence $T1$ and $T2$ are longest in CSF, followed by GM, and shortest in WM. Usually $T1$ is magnetic field strength dependent, while $T2$ is not. In the following table, we list mean ± SD values of $T1$ and $T2$ for 1H in the brain (7) for a 1.5-T or a 3.0-T scanner (*see* **Table 1**).

$T2^*$ depends not only on 1H $T2$ in tissues, fluids, and tumor, but also on the additional relaxation time resulting from a nonhomogeneous local magnetic field coming from the magnet, gradient field, boundaries of brain structures, and/or contrast agent such as Gd.

Since $T1$, $T2$, and $T2^*$ values differ among brain tissues, fluids and/or lesions, $T1$-, $T2$-, and $T2^*$-weighted images have been applied routinely for the diagnosis of brain tumors. For low-grade tumors [i.e., grades I and II based on the criteria of the World Health Organization (WHO)], the $T1$- and $T2$-weighted images show a small area of edema, slight expansion of the affected area, and lack of contrast enhancement. For high-grade tumors (i.e., WHO grades III and IV), the images will display a large area of edema with a hyperintensity that extends beyond the enhanced core. $T2$-weighted images will show further infiltration and expansion into the surrounding brain (referred to as a large tumor mass effect), seen as moderate-to-intense heterogeneous enhancement. $T1$ images may reveal a central nonenhanced zone representing necrosis. Metastases will be seen as one or more discrete masses with a clear ring boundary that are hyperintense on T2-weighted images and also contain large amounts of edema that may seem disproportionate to the size of the tumor (4).

Besides T1-, T2-, and T2*-weighted images, there are other MRI methods for diagnosis of brain tumors. T2-weighted fluid attenuated inversion recovery (FLAIR) is mainly used to suppress the signal from CSF and increase the ratio of contrast to noise in the tumor area. Diffusion-weighted images (DWI) are used to measure water diffusion in tumor and brain tissues as well as in CSF. DWI can aid in differentiating herpes encephalitis, normal brain tissue, and infiltrative tumors, since the tumor will exhibit a higher diffusion coefficient. DWI is the only MRI modality with the ability to differentiate abscesses such as edema from tumor. Edema similar to an acute infarct with restricted water diffusion is hyperintense on DWI. This may be due to the high viscosity of pus, which results in restriction of water within the edematous area (4). In contrast, most brain tumors will have a hypointense signal on DWI. Perfusion-weighted imaging (PWI) is usually used to acquire data during IV injection of a contrast agent, including dynamic susceptibility enhancement (DSE), a T2*-weighted method, and dynamic contrast enhancement (DCE), a T1-weighted method. PWI relies on the assessment of blood with the injected gadolinium flowing into the mass and is used to obtain cerebral blood volume (CBV), cerebral blood flow (CBF), and fractional blood volume (fBV), which is proportional to the density and permeability of the blood vessels. Most high-grade gliomas demonstrate high regional CBV (rCBV) values, so that the tumor areas look "hot" on a color rCBV map. In contrast, non-neoplastic lesions (e.g., abscesses and subacute infarction) usually have much lower rCBV values, so that tumor areas appear "cold" on the rCBV map. DCE PWI demonstrates a high correlation between the degree of perfusion of a given lesion and its grade. Tumors with high perfusion (high permeability and fBV values) are usually high grade. There is a correlation between rCBV, tumor vessel permeability, and glioma grade that allows the surgeon to discriminate between low-grade (I and II) and high-grade lesions (III and IV) (4). If T1-weighted imaging is employed after administering a contrast agent, the images are called T1-POST, which is useful to demonstrate the enhanced portion of a malignant lesion. The enhancement results from either high blood vessel density, marked leakage from the vessels, or both. The region corresponds histologically to areas of tumor that have dense cellularity and neovascularization. Another T1-weighted imaging method that can provide high spatial resolution in a short scanning time is named three-dimensional spoiled gradient echo (3D SPGR) and is usually performed after T1POST for high resolution and large brain coverage in a short acquisition time to display anatomical structures of both brain and tumors.

2.2. Methods of MRS

There are four basic steps in performing 1H MRS (1) suppression of undesired strong signals (water, lipid, or both), (2) localization, (3) shimming or adjusting the magnetic field, and (4) detection.

1. *Suppression of undesired strong signals.* The signal from protons (1H) of metabolites of interest is typically many orders of magnitude below that of water or lipid (up to 10,000 times less). Therefore, water or lipid signals have to be sufficiently suppressed to prevent digitizer overflow or distorted metabolite signals. Water suppression is usually accomplished by a frequency-selective saturation technique called CHESS, which selectively excites and then destroys the water signal by dephasing it with spoiling gradients. Lipid suppression can also be accomplished using CHESS; however, for in vivo brain 1H MRS, it is usually achieved by selective excitation of the volume of interest (VOI) within the brain to prevent strong lipid signals from the scalp, because brain tissue itself contains few MR-detectable lipids.

2. *Localization.* Two widely used techniques to obtain selective excitation of the VOI are stimulated echo acquisition mode (STEAM) and point-resolved spectroscopy (PRESS). STEAM uses three perpendicular 90° slice selection pulses to determine the VOI, while PRESS utilizes one 90° and two 180° slice selection pulses. Generally, STEAM provides sharper localization, while PRESS offers a better signal-to-noise ratio. Another important concept in localization is single-voxel versus multivoxel techniques. Single-voxel STEAM or PRESS technique acquires one spectrum from a given area (VOI). Multivoxel STEAM or PRESS technique obtains multiple spectra from multiple spatial areas (voxels) within the VOI simultaneously in one measurement. Multivoxel spectroscopic technique is also called magnetic resonance spectroscopic imaging (MRSI) or chemical shift imaging (CSI), because the metabolite distribution can be represented as a map. MRSI offers several advantages over single-voxel techniques, including simultaneously acquiring spectra from a lesion and contralateral control areas, detecting tumors beyond Gd-enhanced MRI area and studying the heterogeneous nature of a tumor.

3. *Shimming.* Shimming is an MRI terminology which simply means to make the magnetic field as homogeneous as possible. The importance of shimming over the VOI cannot be overemphasized. Shimming can not only enhance the signal-to-noise ratio but also determine the success or failure of water suppression. In fact, it is because of the difficulty of shimming

that most in vivo 1H MRS studies have been performed on the brain, where shimming is the easiest.

4. *Detection.* Any coil that is suitable for MRI can be used for in vivo 1H MRS. Thus in vivo 1H MRS can be integrated with a routine MRI protocol without repositioning the patient or changing any hardware.

Conventional In vivo brain 1H MR spectroscopy can detect *N*-acetylaspartate (NAA), total choline (Cho), total creatine (Cr), myo-inositol (MI), lactic acid (Lac), and lipid (Lip). Of these, NAA, which is exclusively localized to neurons in the healthy adult brain, is a neuronal and axonal marker that decreases with neuronal loss or dysfunction. Cho, consisting of free choline, phospho-, glycerophospho-, and phospholipid-choline, is a marker for membrane synthesis. Cell proliferation, inflammation, or demyelination can elevate Cho. Cr, consisting of creatine and phosphocreatine, is a marker for intact brain energy metabolism. Dramatic elevation of Cho and reduction of NAA and Cr are classic 1H spectral characteristics of brain tumors. MI, an osmolyte located in astrocytes, increases as a result of glial proliferation. Significant elevation of MI generally suggests a low-grade brain tumor. Lac accumulates as a result of anaerobic glycolysis or hypoxia. Lac is not usually present in healthy adult brain tissue at 1.5 T. Elevation of Lip is often observed in the presence of necrosis. Significant elevation of Lac and Lip in untreated brain tumors generally suggests a poor prognosis. Measuring changes in these metabolites, which result from either abnormal function/ disease process or the effects of treatment, can provide valuable and unique biochemical information to complement MRI. 1H MRS is currently used as an adjunct to MRI in patients with brain masses. **Figure 3a** is a *T*2-weighted turbo spin-echo image showing the VOI from which the 1H MRS data were acquired using a two-dimensional (2D) PRESS pulse sequence. Because of the relatively long TE (135 ms), only signals from NAA (2.0 ppm), Cr (3.0 ppm), and Cho (3.2 ppm) are visible. **Figure 3b** shows a typical normal brain spectrum: signal amplitudes of Cr and Cho are roughly equal, while NAA is about twice of this value. **Figures 3c, d** illustrate the characteristics of a typical tumor spectrum: dramatic elevation of Cho and reduction of NAA and Cr compared to the normal pattern in **Fig. 3b**. In addition to the tumor spectral pattern, there was a higher percentage of dead tissue in the old tumor (**Fig. 3c**) than in the new lesion (**Fig. 3d**), as evidenced by the significant reduction in all three metabolites in Fig. 3c compared to **Fig. 3d**. A study of 58 brain tumors using 3D PRESS MRSI demonstrated that the sensitivity and the specificity for differentiating tumors from nontumor lesions were 96% and 70%, respectively, with a Cho/NAA ratio greater than 2.0 *(8)*. Moreover, because certain 1H metabolites are directly or

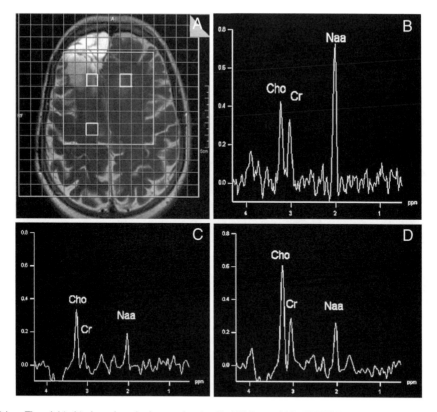

Fig. 3. (**a**) is a T2-weighted turbo spin-echo image showing the VOI from which 1H MRS images were acquired with a 2D PRESS pulse sequence. The three spectra (**b**, **c**, and **d**) labeled in **a** were extracted from the corresponding voxels in the normal brain tissue (**b**), and two Gd-enhanced area (**c**) and (**d**). The spectra were acquired with an echo time (TE) of 135 ms and an elliptical 16 × 16 phase encoding scheme. The acquisition time for the 2D data set was 4:45 min (*See Color Plates*).

indirectly involved in tumor metabolism such as rapid cell proliferation, 1H MRS can detect cancer earlier than MRI, as is well documented by abnormal 1H metabolite regions beyond contrast-enhanced MRI areas in brain tumors *(9)*. **Figure 4** shows two spectra from two different areas without Gd enhancement. The patient had glioblastoma multiforme (GBM) and received radiation treatment 2 months earlier. As clearly illustrated, both spectra had a typical tumor pattern.

Gln and Glu are two other important small molecules in tumor metabolism. In addition to their central significance in biosynthetic pathways of all living organisms *(10)* and their unique roles in neurochemistry, Gln and Glu are directly and indirectly involved in tumor proliferation and apoptosis *(11)*. Biochemical studies have demonstrated that malignant transformation of cells induces a profound change in Gln metabolism, because rapidly growing tumors require continuous nutrition, and Gln is the most

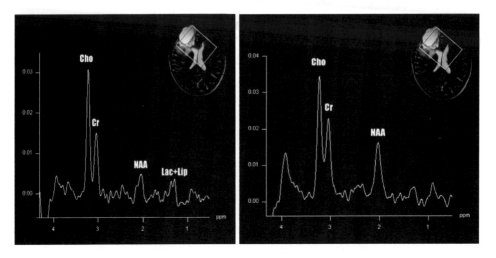

Fig. 4. Illustration of the capability of detecting tumors earlier than MRI. Both spectra from an area that appeared normal on MRI show high Cho, low NAA and Cr. The spectra were acquired with STEAM MRSI; TE = 80 ms, TM = 50 ms at 4 T.

abundant amino acid in the body as well as the main vehicle for circulation of ammonia in a nontoxic form *(12)*. Consequently, malignant transformation is accompanied by depletion of Gln in the host organism, but elevation of Gln in tumors. Because of this, tumors have been referred to as "Gln traps." Consistent with the biochemical findings, in vivo 1H MRS of human brain tumors using STEAM with optimized experimental parameters (TE = 80 ms, TM = 50 ms) at 4 T *(13)* suggests that dramatic elevation of Gln (from undetectable to clearly visible) is the in vivo hallmark of tumor as "Gln trap." **Figure 5a, b** show typical spectra of healthy brain tissue and tumor (biopsy confirmed the histological diagnosis of glioblastoma multiforme) using the technique. In addition to the typical tumor spectral pattern for the established markers (dramatic elevation of Ch and reduction of NAA and Cr as shown in **Fig. 3**), **Fig. 5b** illustrates a dramatic change in Gln/Glu pattern, with Gln going from undetectable (**Fig. 5a**) to clearly visible. All studies (nine patients so far) demonstrated consistent and remarkable increases in Gln, suggesting its diagnostic value as a tumor indicator. Figure 5c is the spectrum from another patient using the same technique and parameters. It illustrates a different spectral characteristic: a normal pattern for the established markers as in **Fig. 5a**, but a remarkable change in Gln/Glu just like **Fig. 5b**. Biopsy indicated that it was recurrent WHO grade IV glioma. These results suggest that the Gln and Glu could be an earlier indicator of malignant transformation than the established markers Cho, NAA, and Cr.

In summary, 1H MRS can help differentiate brain tumors from nontumor lesions, distinguish primary tumors from metastases, recommend biopsy sites, suggest tumor grade, assess progression *(14)*, and evaluate response to therapy *(8)*. Moreover,

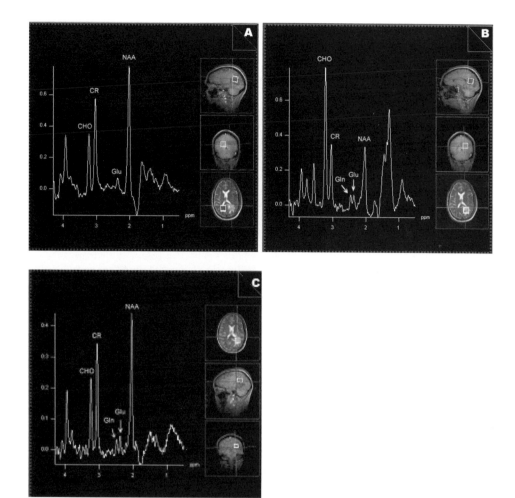

Fig. 5. Illustration of Gln/Glu as an earlier index for cancer detection than the established biomarkers Cho, Cr, and NAA. Spectra from (**a**) normal control brain tissue, (**b**) biopsy-proved tumor with a typical tumor spectral pattern for the established biomarkers and an abnormal Gln/Glu pattern, and (**c**) another biopsy-proved tumor with a normal spectral pattern for the established biomarkers but an abnormal Gln/Glu pattern.

in vivo 1H MRS can identify the extension of tumor beyond the area shown on MRI *(9)*.

2.3. An MRI/MRS Protocol for Brain Tumors

The methods mentioned in the above sections (a) and (b) are summarized in **Table 2**.

3. Examples

Images as shown in **Figs. 6–15** were obtained using the protocol in **Table 2**.

Table 2
A protocol for imaging brain tumors

Method (name)	Pulse sequence	Important acquisition parameters	Main applications for diagnoses
T1	SE	TR/TE/α/Matrix/NEX = ~600 ms/~14 ms/~90°/256 × 256/1	Anatomy: gray and white matter areas and tumor location(s)
T2	SE	TR/TE/α/Matrix/NEX = 3,800 ms/102 ms/90°/256 × 256/1	Anatomy: tumor, edema, and tumor location (s)
T2 IR FLAIR	IR	TR/TE/α/TI/Matrix/ NEX = 10,000 ms/165 ms/2,200/90°/256 × 192/1	Tumor mass (volume) and tumor edge. CSF suppression
DWI	SE	TR/TE/α/bvalue/Matrix/ NEX = 8,000 ms/90.3 ms/90/1,000/256 × 256/1	Tumor and edema
MRSI	PRESS	TR/TE/α/Matrix/FOV/ NEX = 1,500 ms/144 ms/90/8 × 8 × 8/1	Tumor and normal tissues. Tumor grade, necrosis in the tumor, primary or migrate brain tumor
PWI: DSE	GEEPI	TR/TE/α/Matrix/NEX/ number of phase (time points) = 1,000 ms/40ms/60/128 × 128/1/85	Tumor grades, necrosis in tumor, survival time of a patient with a tumor
PWI: DCE	3DSPGR	T1 map TR/TE/α/Matrix/NEX = 2.6 ms/0.9 ms/ 2°, 5°, 10°, 15°, and 26°/128 × 128/2 Perfusion data: TDEL/TR/ TE/α/Matrix/NEX = /5.6 s/3.1 ms/1.4 ms/30/128 × 128/1	Tumor grades and leakage areas of blood brain barrier (BBB)
T1 POST	SE	TR/TE/α/Matrix/NEX = 500 ms/10 ms/90/256 × 256/1	Tumor core area
SPGR POST	3DSPGR	TR/TE/α/Matrix/NEX = 22 ms/3.0 ms/30/512 × 512/1	Anatomy: high-resolution images for tumor and normal tissues

4. Notes

1) The main applications of MRI and MRS in patients with brain tumors are to detect the lesions; to guide tumor surgery or biopsy (15); to guide radiation treatment (RT) (16); to guide temperature treatment (TT) using ultrasound (17); to monitor chemotherapy (18), to follow the effects of surgery (19)

Fig. 6. $T1$-weighted image of a glioblastoma multiforme (GBM) in the right frontal lobe. The tumor area is hypointense. The image was used to show the location of the mass within the brain and its spatial relationship to various neuroanatomical structures. Since there is very little $T1$ contrast for the tumor area, this method is not helpful for this case.

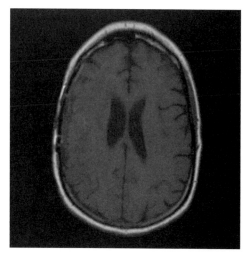

Fig. 7. $T2$-weighted image of the GBM in the right frontal lobe shown in **Fig. 6**. The tumor area is hyperintense. The image shows a large area of mild hyperintensity surrounding the enhanced hyperintense tumor core, representing peritumoral edema and a mass effect. Both tumor and edema are clearly localized.

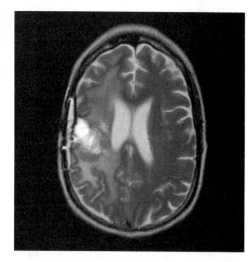

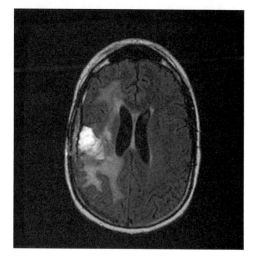

Fig. 8. $T2$-weighted FLAIR image of the GBM in the right frontal lobe shown in **Fig. 6**. The tumor is hyperintense. The high degree of hyperintensity was related to the high vascularity of the GBM and the poor integrity of the intratumoral vessels due to break down of the blood-brain barrier (BBB). The CSF signal in the ventricle was suppressed so that the tumor and edema could be seen clearly.

Fig. 9. Diffusion-weighted image (DWI) of the GBM in the right frontal lobe shown in **Fig. 6** The tumor core is hypointense and the area of edema is hyperintense. The DWI image clearly differentiates the tumor core and abscess (edema).

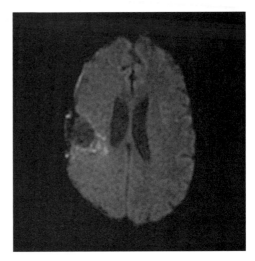

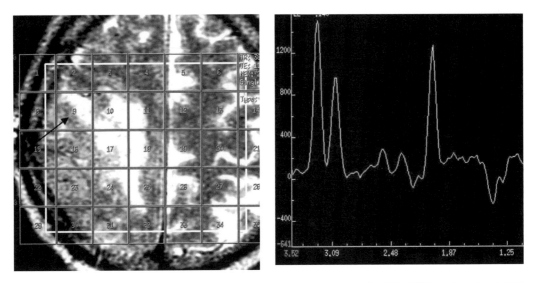

Fig. 10. MRS image of the GBM in the right frontal lobe. It is not the case shown in **Fig. 6**. The MRS spectrum for pixel #9 in the tumor area is shown on the right. The GBM has a characteristic spectrographic signature for a malignant tumor, demonstrating an increase in the choline (CHO) peak (3.2 ppm), a decrease in the n-acetylaspartate (NAA) peak (2.02 ppm), an increased CHO/creatine (3.0 ppm) ratio, and double inversed lactate peaks (1.35 ppm) in the left end of the spectrum (*See Color Plates*).

and RT *(20)*; and to monitor tumor progression and treatment-related damage and toxicity *(21–22)*.

2) The main advantages of MRI as a means of imaging brain tumors include (1) nondestruction, (2) high spatial resolution, and (3) multicontrast imaging presentation. The main limitation of MRI is its relatively poor temporal resolution. For example, the total acquisition time for running the protocol in **Table 2** is approximately 70 min, and a 3D SPGR

Fig. 11. rCBV image generated from perfusion-weighted DSE for the GBM in the right frontal lobe shown in **Fig. 10**. Usually a GBM will show a high rCBV, displayed as "hot" *red* color in the tumor core. In this case, due to prior surgical removal of the tumor, the high rCBV signal in the area was lost for the susceptibility artifact by using the $T2^*$-weighted GE pulse sequence. (*See Color Plates*)

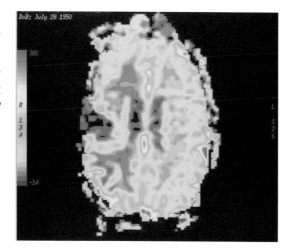

Fig. 12. $T1$-POST image of the GBM in the right frontal lobe shown in **Fig. 6**. The edge of the tumor is enhanced. The infiltration into and enlargement of surrounding brain structures, as well as the more marked enhancement, is suggestive of a high-grade glioma, in this case GBM. This image demonstrates that $T1$- POST is better than $T1$ (**Fig. 6**) for showing the tumor core and the infiltrated area.

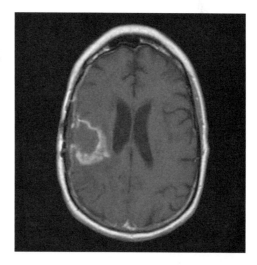

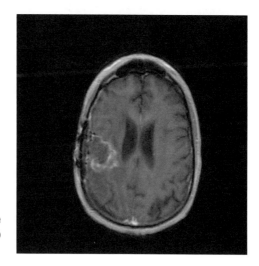

Fig. 13. $T1$-weighted (3DSPGR-POST) image of the GBM in the right frontal lobe shown in **Fig. 6**. The appearance is similar to **Fig. 12** but has higher spatial resolution.

Fig. 14. Ktrans map (~permeability map) generated from PWI DCE for a GBM in the left frontal lobe. The tumor core shows "hot" *yellow* color in the middle of the WM (the "cold" *pink*) area. The vessels serving the GBM exhibit poor integrity due to angiogenesis and there is marked leakage, seen as a hyperintense signal on the map (*See Color Plates*).

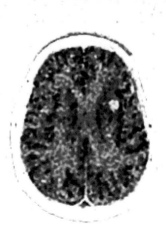

Fig. 15. fBV map generated from PWI DCE for the GBM in the left frontal lobe shown in **Fig. 14**. The portion of the GBM seen as hyperintense on the fBV map has a higher vascular density, resulting from angiogenesis. The center of the tumor is hypointense and may correspond to necrosis, which is always present in GBM (*See Color Plates*).

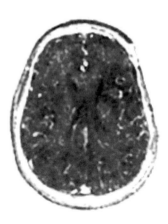

whole brain coverage with $1 \times 1 \times 1.5$ mm resolution takes about 9 min. Some patients with brain tumors cannot tolerate such a long scanning time. Also, since patients will be scanned in a closed and narrow MRI bore hole (~80 cm), some may refuse to undergo MRI due to the "claustrophobia feeling."

When running MRI scans on patients with brain tumors, we need to consider the following aspects:

1. A 1.5-T MRI scanner is a high magnetic field. Any metal in the field either feels a strong force and/or interferes with the

field. Hence any metal should be removed from the patient before an MRI scan. Otherwise it will produce artifacts and could lead to possible damage to the patient and/or scanner. Any patients having metal inside their body should be carefully dealt with and may have to be excluded from MRI.

2. The scanner is easily affected by interference from outside RF frequencies which are in the resonance band, so that the room with the magnet has to be shielded to avoid RF penetration, and the door of the suite has to be closed during an MRI scan.

3. MRI is very sensitive to motion of the head. Hence every effort should be made to reduce movement. Informing the patient beforehand how long the scan will take is a good way to reduce anxiety and allow him to feel more relaxed.

4. $T2^*$ MRI is limited by its susceptibility to artifacts in areas close to holes such as the nose, ears, eyes, or surgical site after tumor resection *(23)*.

5. When attempting to locate tumors of the skull during surgery, MRI markers (plastic buttons which can provide a strong MRI signal) should be put on the head before the scans. To avoid the uncertainty of high-grade tumor location and volume due to rapid growth of the brain, MRI using the protocol in Table 2 should be performed in the 24–48 h before tumor resection or other treatment.

6. It is worth noting that MRI appearance depends not only on contrasts $T1$, $T2$, and $T2^*$, but also on the strength of the magnetic field. **Figure 16** demonstrates $T1$ contrast differences in 1.5 T and 3.0 T fields.

1.5T   **3.0T**

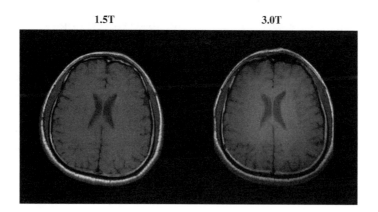

Fig. 16. *T*1-weighted images in a 1.5-T and a 3.0-T field. The 3.0-T field provides better quality for both contrasts with regard to WM, GM, and signal-to-noise ratio.

References

1. Tofts, P. (2003) Quantitative MRI of the brain. Measuring changes caused by disease. Wiley, Chichester, UK.

2. Bradley, W. G., and Stark, D. D. (1999) Magnetic resonance imaging, 3rd Edition. Mosby Inc, St. Louis.

3. Brown, M. A., and Semelka, R. C. (2003) MRI basic principles and applications, 3rd Edition. Wiley-Liss, New York.

4. Newton, H. B., Ray-Chaudhury, A., and Cavaliere, R. (2006) Brain tumor imaging and cancer management: the neuro-oncologists perspective. Top Magn Reson Imaging. 17(2):127–136.

5. Young, R. J., and Knopp, E. A. (2006) Brain MRI: tumor evaluation. JMRI. 24:709–724.

6. Hollingworth, W., Medina, L. S., Lenkinski, R. E., Shibata, D. K., Bernal, B., Zurakowski, D., Comstock, B., and Jarvik, J. G. (2006) A systematic literature review of magnetic resonance spectroscopy for the characterization of brain tumors. Am J Neuroradiol. 27(8):1404–1411.

7. Stanisz, G. J., Odrobina, E. E., Pun, J., Escaravage, M., Graham, S. J., Bronskill, M. J., and Henkelman, R. M. (2005) T1, T2 relation and magnetization transfer in tissue at 3T. Magn Reson Med. 54:507–512.

8. Nelson, S. (2004) Magnetic resonance spectroscopic imaging: evaluating response to therapy for gliomas. IEEE Eng Med Biol Mag, 23(5):30–39.

9. McKnight, T., von Dem Bussche, M., Vigneron, D., Lu, Y., Berger, M., McDermott, M., Dillon, W., Graves, E., Pirzkall, A., and Nelson, S. (2002) Histopathological validation of a three-dimensional magnetic resonance spectroscopy index as a predictor of tumor presence. J Neurosurg. 97:794–802.

10. Kovacevic, Z., and McGivan, J. (1983) Mitochondrial metabolism of glutamine and glutamate and its physiological significance. Physiol Rev. 63:547–605.

11. Mates, J., Perez-Gomez, C., Castro, I., Asenjo, M., and Marquez, J. (2002) Glutamine and its relationship with intracellular redox status, oxidative stress and cell proliferation /death. Int J Biochem Cell Biol. 34:439–458.

12. Medina, M. (2001) Glutamine metabolism: nutritional and clinical significant. J Nutr. 131:2539–2542.

13. Hu, J., Yang, S., Xuan, Y., Jiang, Q., Yang, Y., and Haacke, E. (2007) Simultaneous detection of resolved glutamate, glutamine, and g-aminobutyric acid at 4 Tesla. J Magn Reson. 185:217–226.

14. Brandao, L., and Domingues, R. (2004) MR spectroscopy of the brain. Chapter 10. Lippincott Williams & Wilkins, Philadelphia, PA.

15. Jung, T. Y., Jung, S., Kim, I. Y., Park, S. J., Kang, S. S., Kim, S. H., and Lim, S. C. (2006) Application of neuronavigation system to brain tumor surgery with clinical experience of 420 cases. Minim Invasive Neurosurg. 49(4): 210–215.

16. Nakasu, Y. (2007) Current strategies in radiation therapy for brain metastases. No Shinkei Geka. 35(1):7–16.

17. Ram, Z., Cohen, Z. R., Harnof, S., Tal, S., Faibel, M., Nass, D., Maier, S. E., Hadani, M., and Mardor, Y. (2006) Magnetic resonance imaging-guided, high-intensity focused ultrasound for brain tumor therapy. Neurosurgery. 59(5):949–955.

18. Lichy M. P., Bacher, P., Henze, M., Lichy, C. M., Debus, J., and Schlemmer, H. P. (2004) Monitoring individual response to brain-tumour chemotherapy: proton MR spectroscopy in a patient with recurrent glioma after stereotactic radiotherapy. Neuroradiology. 46(2):126–9.

19. Ulmer, S., Braga, T. A., Barker, T. A., Barker, F. G. II., Lev, M. H., Gonzalez, R. G., and Henson, J. W. (2006) Clinical and radiographic features of peritumoral infarction following resection of glioblastoma. Neurology. 67(9):1668–1670.

20. Saunders, D. E., Phipps, K. P., Wade, A. M., and Hayward, R. D. (2005) Surveillance imaging strategies following surgery and/or radiotherapy for childhood cerebellar low-grade astrocytoma. J Neurosurg. 102(2 Suppl):172–178.

21. Mabbott, D. J., Noseworthy, M. D., Bouffet, E., Rockel, C., and Laughlin, S. (2006) Diffusion tensor imaging of white matter after cranial radiation in children for medulloblastoma: correlation with IQ. Neurooncology. (3):244–252.

22. Genc, M., Genc, E., Genc, B. O., and Kiresi, D. A. (2006) Significant response of radiation induced CNS toxicity to high dose steroid administration. Br J Radiol. 79(948):e196–e199.

23. Kim, M. J., Holodny, A. I., Hou, B. L., Peck, K. K., Moskowitz, C. S., Bogomolny, D. L., and Gutin, P. H. (2005) The effect of prior surgery on blood oxygen level-dependent functional MR imaging in the preoperative assessment of brain tumors. Am J Neuroradiol. 26(8):1980–1985.

Chapter 22

Magnetic Resonance Spectroscopy of Living Tissues

Natalie J. Serkova, Kendra M. Hasebroock, and Susan L. Kraft

Summary

The comprehensive work of both clinical and basic science colleagues has demonstrated a clear proof of concept for "in vitro discovered- in vivo validated" biomarkers in translational metabolic profiling research using magnetic resonance techniques. Major tissue metabolites (initially discovered by high-resolution in vitro techniques on cancer specimens) can be translated into in vivo protocols based on noninvasive magnetic resonance spectroscopy (MRS). Using ^{1}H- and ^{31}P-MRS on living animals or patients, a decrease in citrate and polyamines in prostate cancer, an increase of cholines in breast cancer, as well as a decreased NAA and an increased lactate in gliomas during cancer progression can be assessed noninvasively. MRS can be used to follow up conventional cytotoxic as well as targeted anticancer therapies, which has been extensively done in animal models of cancer. This review focuses on applications and protocol development for in vivo ^{1}H- and ^{31}P-MRS on small animal models as well as on larger animals in cancer research, diagnosis, and treatment.

Key words: Localized MRS, Magnetic resonance spectroscopical imaging, Choline, Citrate, Tumor energy state, Tumor pH.

---

1. Introduction

There are clear advantages in using noninvasive methods for studying living systems. There are many areas of biomedical research, including oncology, where noninvasive studies of biochemistry can add significantly to the information provided by more traditional, invasive techniques. Magnetic resonance spectroscopy (MRS) is widely used as a noninvasive technique to assess metabolic markers noninvasively in the body (*see* **Note 1**). It is performed using animal or clinical MRI scanners to study animal or human metabolism without taking biopsy specimens or body fluids. Over the years, in vivo MRS and magnetic resonance spectroscopic imaging (MRSI) have been used to interrogate biochemistry of living tissue for cancer-related prognostic and diagnostic markers *(1–5)*. MRS allows

Michael A. Tainsky, *Methods in Molecular Biology, Tumor Biomarker Discovery, Vol. 520*
© Humana Press, a part of Springer Science+Business Media, LLC 2009
DOI: 10.1007/978-1-60327-811-9_22

for noninvasive quantitative assessment of tissue major metabolites such as lactate, lipids, total choline, total creatine, N-acetyl aspartate (NAA) and myo-inositol (brain only), citrate and polyamines (prostate only) by proton (^{1}H-) MRS as well as phosphomonoesters, phosphodiesters, nucleoside phosphates (NTP), inorganic phosphate and phosphocreatine by phosphor (^{31}P-) MRS (**Table 1**)

Table 1
Major metabolites, detectable by in vivo ^{1}H- and ^{31}P-MRS, and their biochemical significance for cancer (for a comprehensive review on metabolic significance please refer to (1–4))

Metabolite	Chemical shift (ppm)	Biochemical significance
Total Choline (Cho)	3.22 ppm (^{1}H)	Contains free choline, phosphocholine, and glycerophosphocholine. Increased in the majority of tumors, including brain, breast, and prostate. Choline concentrations are highly sensitive to antitumor treatment
Citrate	2.53 and 2.66 ppm (^{1}H)	A highly abundant metabolite in the prostate gland. Decreased in prostate cancers
Lactate	1.33 ppm (^{1}H)	The end-product of glycilysis, which is highly upregulated in tumors. Often is not present in normal tissues, but highly increased in tumors. Overlaps with lipid peaks
Lipids	**1.32** (major $(CH_2)_n$), 0.9, 1.6, 2.0, 2.3, 2.8 and 5.4 ppm (^{1}H)	Highly concentrated in a variety of tissues. Often increased in liposarcomas or during apoptosis development due to anticancer treatment
NAA in Brain	**2.02**, 2.5 and 2.6 ppm (^{1}H)	The most abundant (after water) metabolite in neurons and, thus, in the brain. Decreased in gliomas and majority of brain tumors
Nucleotide Phosphates	α:-7.7; β: –18.0; γ: –2.5 ppm (^{31}P)	Major energy source in the cell. Decreased during chemotherapy treatment
Phosphocreatine	3.03 and 3.9 ppm(^{1}H) 0 ppm (31P)	Major energy storage molecule. Often decreased in tumor tissues. Highly decreased during chemotherapy treatment
Inorganic Phosphate	pH dependent (^{31}P)	Its chemical shift can be used for noninvasive calculations of tumor pH (often acidic). Increased in hypoxic tumors and after radiation
Phosphodiesters	2.3–3.5 ppm (^{31}P)	Contains glycerophosphocholine and glycerolphosphoethanolamine, major catabolic products of membrane phospholipids. Often decreased in tumors and increased upon anticancer treatment
Phosphomonoesters	6.2–7.3 ppm (^{31}P)	Contains phocholine and phosphoethanolamine, major precursors of membrane phospholipids. Often increased in tumors and decreased upon anticancer treatment

(1, 4). These metabolites are closely associated with cancer progression, such as decrease in citrate and polyamines in prostate cancer, increase of total choline in breast cancer, decreased NAA, and increased lactate in gliomas *(6–12)*. The majority of these biomarkers have been initially discovered in vitro using cell, specimen, and biofluid analysis by high-resolution nuclear magnetic resonance spectroscopy (NMR, *see* Chap. 20 on "Metabolomics in Cancer") *(2–4)*. One of the major advantages of magnetic resonance techniques is the translational compounds, since it allows for noninvasive detection of established metabolic biomarkers in vivo. These characteristics are why MRS has been compared to a "noninvasive biopsy," which is currently the only way to obtain an expanded biochemical profile in a living tissue (*see* **Notes 1 and 2**). The majority of clinical in vivo MRS has been done, as mentioned earlier, in brain tumors *(6–8)*, breast cancer *(9, 10)*, and prostate cancer *(11, 12)*. Single clinical studies have been reported on MRS application for cervical and thyroid cancers *(5)*, as well as bone sarcomas *(13)*. An extensive amount of preclinical work has been done for monitoring metabolic response in xenograft tumors to conventional cytostatics (chemotherapy) and, more recently, to targeted anticancer agents *(4, 14)*. A significant decrease in cholines, especially phosphocholine and other phosphomonoesters, as a marker of inhibited membrane synthesis and cell proliferation, a decrease in NTP, as a marker of cell death and cytotoxicity, as well as an increase in polyunsaturated fatty acids (PUFA) as a marker for apoptosis, has been reported from animal models by in vivo MRS *(15–18)*.

This chapter focuses on MRS application, subject preparation, data acquisition and interpretation on animal models for cancer research and diagnosis.

2. Materials

2.1. Anesthesia

1. Ketamine
2. Xylazine
3. Isoflurane
4. Gas anesthesia machine
5. Physiological monitoring system

2.2. MRS Procedure

1. Many options are available for the coil. For most sizes of dog heads, commercial quadrature transmits receive coils designed for the knee and extremities work very well. For the largest dog head (giant dog breeds) the human head coil is appropriate. The important thing is to get the best filling factor and to prop the head up on pads so as to center the brain within the coil volume. A surface coil for receiving and use of body coil

for transmit can work well for a cat brain, but due to limited depth penetration is less ideal for a dog brain. Many facilities use specially designed custom coils with appropriate Q factors for optimal MRS.

2. Most standard commercial MR instruments now have automated software packages available for MR spectroscopy. Hardware and software suitable to acquire nonlocalized and 3D chemical shift imaging (3D-CSI) localized spectroscopy are helpful. For ^{31}P-MRS, proton-decoupling capabilities are required (*see* **Notes 3–5**).

3. Methods

All the MR protocols, described here, are developed and validated for 4.7 T (small animal MRS) and 1.5 T (larger animals). Due to considerable variations in software and hardware of the specialized higher field strength instruments (7–11.4 T for small rodents and 3–9.4 T for larger animals), it is not possible to provide specific enough instructions that would be relevant for those systems. However the general procedural principles are applicable across the different instruments *(19, 20)* (*see* **Notes 6–8**).

3.1. Animal Preparation

For all rodent species as well as for larger animals, general anesthesia is necessary for adequate immobilization for MR spectroscopy (*see* **Note 7**). There are many options for inducing general anesthesia in mice, rats, rabbits, dogs, and cats (*see* **Table 2**). This is most often done by intravenous injection of an ultrashort-acting barbiturate such as thiopental or propofol as needed to induce an animal to a plane of anesthesia to enable intubation (for larger animals). For dogs and cats, premedication prior to anesthetic induction lessens the total dose needed of the induction agent (therefore is more economical), gives a smoother induction and recovery, and can provide analgesia when needed. One common method is premedication with an analgesic drug (e.g., hydromorphone) and, if necessary, a sedative (e.g., medetomidine) prior to intravenous induction of anesthesia. Premedication is followed by an anesthetic induction agent, usually given intravenously. Following orotracheal intubation, the animal may be maintained with either a constant rate infusion of an injectable (e.g., propofol: 0.1–0.4 mg/kg/min) or with an inhaled anesthetic agent (e.g., isoflurane: 1–3%).

For small animals, a mixture of ketamine and xylazine is recommended for short-time scans (less than 30 min). General

Table 2
Recommended anesthetic agents and their doses for small and larger animals undergoing in vivo MRS examinations

A. Small animal

Mice	Ketamine/Xylazine	80–100 mg/kg Ketamine + 10 mg/kg Xylazine IP
Mice	Pentobarbital	50–90 mg/kg IP, dilute w/Nacl sol to give 0.1 ml/10 g bwt
Mice	Isoflurane	3–4% induction, then 1–2% maintenance via vaporizer
Mice	Halothane	3–4% induction, 1–3% maintenance via vaporizer
Mice	Propofol	12–26 mg/kg IV, titrate to effect (short duration)
Mice	Avertiri	250 mg/kg IP of 1.2% SoT. Fresh stock solution must be made every 2 weeks!
Rats	Ketamine/Xylazine	40–80 mg/kg Ketamine + 5–10 mg/kg Xytazine IM
Rats	Pentobarbital	40–50 mg/kg IP
Rats	Thiopental	20–40 mg/kg IV (5–10 mm duration)
Rats	Isoflurane	2–5% induction, 1–3% maintenance
Rats	Halothane	3–4% induction, 1–3% maintenance
Rats	Mactin	80 mg/kg IP 1–4 h Surgical Time
Rats	Chioral hydrate	300–450 mg/kg IP (≤ 5%!! Sol.)
Rats	Propofol	7.5–10 mg/kg IV (5–10 duration)

B. Larger animals

Rabbits	Ketamine/Xylazine	22–50 mg/kg Ketamine + 3–10 mg/kg Xylazine IM
Rabbits	Pentobarbital	20–50 mg/kg IP or 20–50 mg/kg IV slow! (Do not repeat IV)
Rabbits	Isoflurane	3–4% induction, 1.2–3% maintenance
Rabbits	Aceprornazine	1 mg/kg IM Preanesthetic
Rabbits	Telazol	32–64 mg/kg IM
Rabbits	Halothane	3–5% Induction, 1–4% Maintenance
Rabbits	Propofol	7.5–15 mg/kg IV (short duration: 5–10 mm)
Dogs	Pentobarbital	20–30 mg/kg IV
Dogs	Ketamine/Valium	5.5 mg/kg/ 0.20 mg/kg IV (Can mix same synnge)
Dogs	Telazol	2.2 mg/kg IV induction or 7.5 mg IM
Dogs	Isoflurane	1.5–2.2% maintenance after injectable induction
Dogs	Halothane	1.5–2.0% maintenance after injectable induction

anesthesia is then maintained with a mixture of oxygen and isoflurane gas through mechanical ventilation with an MR-compatible gas anesthesia machine. Another option is use of a nonrebreathing anesthetic circuit in which the anesthetic chamber device is kept well outside the five gauss line. Repeated doses of sodium pentobarbital have been used in the past, but it is difficult to maintain normal blood pressure, oxygen status, and other physiological homeostasis; therefore, that technique is not desirable. Although repeated doses of IV propofol can be adequate for short procedures such as MR imaging, this is less than ideal for MRS because of the long scanning times (typically over an hour including setup) and need for continued even plane of deep anesthesia for proper immobilization. Therefore, gas maintenance of anesthesia is highly recommended.

1. Maintain and monitor normal blood pressure and oxygen status, temperature, electrolyte balance (for instance by using Lactated Ringers solution with 5% dextrose and 10 mEq/L KCl at 50 mL/h), heart rate, and ventilation.

2. Positioning: Typically the animal is positioned in sternal recumbency (prone) with wedge padding and tape or a strap system to immobilize the head. The head should be positioned symmetrically and rest on foam pads to place the brain in the center of the coil. Aim for consistent location of the head within the coil volume and also landmark on the same skull location routinely.

3.2. ¹H-MRS on Small Animal Models (Mice and Rats) (Fig. 1)

The procedures described for MR spectroscopy of mice and rats are limited to comments specific to proton (^{1}H) spectroscopy of the brain and abdominal xenograft tumors, and are most relevant to users of commercial small animal MR instruments at a minimum of 4.7 T field strength.

1. MRS can be very challenging in mice and rats. This is due to the small anatomy relative to the bones and sinuses. Interference from bones and sinuses included in the area of interest can increase the magnetic susceptibility effects and heterogeneity of the volume making it more difficult to shim when using a 3-mm³ voxel size.

2. Perform a localization scan in order to designate the voxel location for the MRS. An initial localizer is first done of the body part. On a Bruker Paravision 4.7 T scanner the following parameters can be utilized for a localizer. FOV: 4 cm, slice thickness: 1 cm, no interslice gap, one slice in axial orientation, TR: 2.000 ms, TE: 50.8 ms, one echo, one average, 180-° flip angle and a 128 × 128 matrix totaling a 32-s scan time. With most scanners, initiation of the localizer typically also involves an automated global shim that optimizes the magnetic field homogeneity over the receiver coil volume.

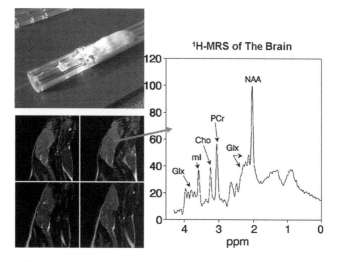

Fig. 1. Animal positioning, T$_2$-weighted brain MRI and localized ¹H-MRS of the brain. *Cho* Total cholines, *Glx* Glutamate + glutamine + GABA, *mI* myo-inositol, *NAA* N-acetyl aspartate, *PCr* Phosphocreatine + creatine (*See Color Plates*).

3. That localizer is then used to acquire a more detailed anatomic scan through the area of interest, usually a T$_2$ (brain) or proton-density (PD, abdominal) sequence 1-mm thick slices with no interslice gap in the transverse plane (which corresponds to the coronal plane for a human head). That scan plane will produce slice images showing the anatomy from dorsal to ventral, and right to left in each slice. Therefore a voxel can be located in the transverse plane with the least interference from bones (*see* **Note** 7).

4. Now designate the location of the single voxel (STEAM, PRESS) or chemical shift imaging (CSI) voxels in the region of interest. Size of the voxel should be as large as possible within a homogeneous tissue region for the best signal to noise, while avoiding interfaces from bones, sinuses, and major vessels. Proximity to the lateral ventricles is less problematic, although too much water contamination can drag the spectral peaks to the left. At 4.7 T, voxel sizes of 3 mm³ are best in order to have practical scan times. Water suppression can be achieved by CHESS sequence. The following parameters can be used with the PRESS-CHESS sequence on a Bruker Paravision scanner using a voxel size of 3 mm³: TR: 2,000 ms, TE1: 8.98 ms, TE2: 11.02 ms, and 1.5-mm outer volume suppression totaling an acquisition time of 13 min and 30 s. The scan parameters are designed based on what metabolites you are interested in detecting.

5. Check the two slices rostral and caudal to the voxel to assess proximity of sinuses and bones to the voxel and adjust the voxel location as necessary.

6. Apply saturation bands around margins of the voxel to suppress interference and magnetic susceptibility.

7. Once the voxel is designated and scan factors selected, a prescan (local shim) is performed. This varies the shim currents sequentially to produce the narrowest possible water peak. The aim is for the lowest possible value for the water full-width half-maximum (FWHM). The goal is less than 8 Hz (single voxel) or 15 Hz FWHM (multivoxel) for best S:N and homogeneity; with human brain the recommendation is 5 Hz (single voxel) and 10 Hz (multivoxel), but this may be difficult to achieve for mice and rats due to their smaller brain size and bones and sinuses in the area of interest.

8. Water peak suppression is performed next; water suppression > 97% is ideal.

9. If the water FWHM or suppression exceeds these values, try the following: Re-evaluate the voxel location and adjust to avoid heterogeneous anatomy or disease such as regions of hemorrhage. Make sure there is no motion (i.e., that the animal is immobilized and well anesthetized). Try swapping the frequency direction and gradient order of the shim. Reshim with autoshim. If values are still too high, repeat with a manual shim.

10. Record the FWHM for the water peak and the percent water suppression. Also save an image showing the voxel location for your records.

11. Proceed with the MRS scan. After the voxel spectrum has been acquired, repeat for the next desired voxel location.

3.3. MRS on Larger Animals (Cats and Dogs)

The procedures described for MR spectroscopy of dogs and cats are limited to comments specific to proton (^{1}H) spectroscopy of the brain, and are most relevant to users of commercial clinical MR instruments at 1.5-T field strength.

1. MRS of the dog or cat brain, when using a typical 1.5-T clinical scanner, is more challenging compared to human MRS. This is because their brains are relatively small, in combination with relatively larger frontal sinuses and thick bones of the calvaria. This increases the magnetic susceptibility effects and heterogeneity of the volume making it more difficult to shim, plus it is difficult to avoid interference from the skull and subcutaneous lipids and sinus air when using 2-cm³ voxel size.

2. Perform a localization scan in order to designate the voxel location for the MRS. An initial 3-plane localizer is first done of the entire brain. On most commercial scanners, initiation

of the 3-plane localizer typically also involves an automated global shim that optimizes the magnetic field homogeneity over the receiver coil volume.

3. That localizer is then used to acquire a more detailed anatomic scan through the area of interest, usually T_2-weighted series 5.0-mm thick slices (with no interslice gap) in the transverse plane (which corresponds to the coronal plane for a human head). That scan plane will produce slice images showing the anatomy from dorsal to ventral, and right to left in each slice. That plane is preferable particularly for the dog because the canine brain is longer than it is tall. Therefore a voxel can be located in the transverse plane with the least interference from the large frontal sinuses and surrounding skull.

4. Now designate the location of the single voxel or CSI voxels in the region of interest. Size of the voxel should be as large as possible within a homogeneous tissue region for the best signal to noise, while avoiding interfaces with the skull (especially the base of the brain and skull), sinuses, and major vessels. Proximity to the lateral ventricles is less problematic, although too much water contamination can drag the spectral peaks to the left. At 1.5 T, voxel sizes of 2 cm^3 (based on 20-mm slice thickness) are best in order to have practical scan times. A 1-cm^3 voxel size is possible in very homogeneous brain regions when the shim has been good, but the scan time will be longer.

5. Check the two slices rostral and caudal to the voxel to assess proximity of sinuses and skull to the voxel and adjust the voxel location as necessary.

6. Apply saturation bands around margins of the voxel at the skull interface and at sinuses to suppress lipid interference and magnetic susceptibility.

7. Select the MRS scan factors, including TR, TE, number of acquisitions, and number of data points for the time domain (vector size). The scan parameters are designed based on what metabolites you are interested in detecting.

8. Once the voxel is designated and scan factors selected, a prescan (local shim) is performed. This varies the shim currents sequentially to produce the narrowest possible water peak. The aim is for the lowest possible value for the water full-width half-maximum (FWHM). The goal is less than 8-Hz (single voxel) or 15-Hz FWHM (multivoxel) for best S:N and homogeneity; with human brains the recommendation is 5 Hz (single voxel) and 10 Hz (multivoxel), but this may be difficult to achieve for dogs due to their smaller brain size, larger sinuses, and thicker skull of the calvaria.

9. Water peak suppression is performed next; water suppression > 97% is ideal.

10. If the water FWHM or suppression exceeds these values, try the following: Re-evaluate the voxel location and adjust to avoid heterogeneous anatomy or disease such as regions of hemorrhage. Make sure there is no head motion (i.e., that the animal is immobilized and well anesthetized). Try swapping the frequency direction and gradient order of the shim. Reshim with autoshim. If values are still too high, repeat with a manual shim.

11. Record the FWHM for the water peak and the percent water suppression. Also save an image showing the voxel location for your records.

12. Proceed with the MRS scan. After the voxel spectrum has been acquired, repeat for the next desired voxel location.

3.4. Quantitation of MRS Scans (Fig. 2)

Presently, the most common type of numerical analysis on acquired MR spectra is computer analysis. In the simplest form a crude baseline is chosen, and the peak heights or peak areas (integrals) are calculated by the software provided by manufacturer (*see also* **Note 8**). There are three approaches to assess metabolite levels after integration: (1) report metabolite ratios normalized to total creatine (^{1}H-MRS) or inorganic phosphate (^{31}P-NMR) (Fig. 2); (2) report normal metabolite ratios; (3) absolute quantification.

1. Metabolite ratios normalized to creatinine or inorganic phosphate: Get a number for the "size" of each peak scaling it to a defined value of creatine or inorganic phosphate signal. In other words, the ratios measure the metabolites on a scale

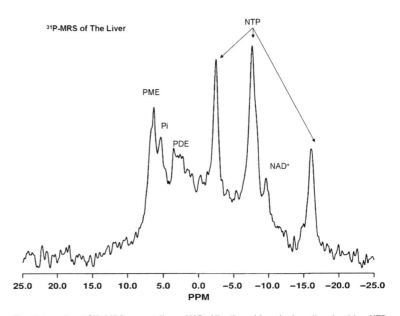

Fig. 2. Localized ^{31}P-MRS on rat liver. *NAD*$^+$ Nicotinamide adenine dinucleotide, *NTP* nucleoside triphosphates, *PDE* Phosphodiesters, *Pi* Inorganic phosphate, *PME* Phosphomonoesters.

that assumes that the measure of Cr = 1 (^{1}H-MRS) or Pi = 1 (^{31}P-MRS).

2. Normal metabolite ratios: Get a number for the "size" of each peak and calculate various ratios of various metabolites.

3. Absolute quantification: This method employs an internal (water) or external reference that is measured once for each animal; the signal from the reference combined with calibration values provides a scaling factor for the peak area. The scaled metabolite peak areas are then corrected for a number of NMR parameters including effects of T_1 and T_2 relaxation and J-coupling.

4. Notes

1. In general, magnetic resonance imaging (MRI) is a noninvasive imaging technique based on observation of physical properties of hydrogen in tissue water (H_2O), which is a major metabolite in living tissues. On the other hand, magnetic resonance spectroscopy (MRS) is a noninvasive chemical analysis on (mostly) hydrogen and phosphor nuclei of other than water, high-abundant endogenous metabolites in living tissues.

2. The major parameters of MRS include (a) chemical shift (due to slight differences in magnetic field which various nuclei experience based on their chemical environment), (b) spin-spin coupling (caused by an interaction between spins mediated by bonding electrons; this leads to the splitting of metabolite peaks), and (c) relaxation time (time, needed for the spin energy to revert to equilibrium after perturbation of the spin system caused by the resonance absorption). Each of these parameters allows for the simultaneous detection of major metabolites in a single in vivo MR spectrum (MRS) or for the spatial distribution of the selected metabolite in MR spectroscopical image (MRSI).

3. Single voxel techniques are simpler, easier, and faster to perform until experience is gained with MRS. The most useful single voxel techniques are the "single shot" methods stimulated echo acquisition mode (STEAM) and point-resolved spectroscopy (PRESS).

4. If using single voxels of normal brain vs. singular lesion, shim and scan for the normal brain first. This will produce a good prescan based on the normal brain first.

5. For diffuse disease consider using multiple single voxels (chemical shift imaging, CSI) located at different regions, or

ipsilateral and comparative contralateral single voxels for large solitary lesions. Higher-resolution CSI 2D or 3D multivoxel methods are particularly useful if the disease being studied is multifocal or if fine regional differences are of interest, and can also be used to compare normal to abnormal brain in a single acquisition. Spectral differences occur both regionally and between gray and white matter, so consistent voxel location is important.

6. The effects of T_1 and T_2 shortening due to gadolinium contrast agent on relative and absolute metabolite concentration can vary. Although it has been demonstrated that good-quality spectra can still be obtained postcontrast, it is generally recommended to obtain MR spectra before contrast agent injection. However, there may be an advantage in performing MRS after contrast enhancement if that helps to locate voxels in a particular area of a lesion based on its enhancement pattern. Consider using a FLAIR sequence for good lesion evaluation vs. a contrast-enhanced scan, prior to the MRS.

7. Even minor head motion such as caused by respiration needs to be controlled. Motion will negatively affect the acquired MR spectra because of contamination from tissues outside the desired volume. That can lead to a loss of signal:noise (S/N) and a bad shim, if motion leads to collecting data from outside the excited volume (single voxel) or corruption by extraneous phase differences (CSI) or incomplete cancellation of undesired signals (ISIS).

8. Establish a quality assurance program doing MRS with a phantom solution for repeated measures of FID amplitude. Do daily or prior to each experiment.

Acknowledgments

This work was supported by the grants from the National Institutes of Health, S10 RR019316 and P30 CA046934.

References

1. Gillies, R.J., and Morse, D.L. (2005) In vivo magnetic resonance spectroscopy in cancer. *Ann. Rev. Biomed. Eng.* 7, 287–326.

2. Gillies, R.J., Bhujwalla, Z.M., Evelhoch, J., Garwood, M., Neeman, M., Robinson, S.P., et al. (2000) Application of magnetic resonance in model systems: tumor biology and physiology. *Neoplasia.* 2, 139–151.

3. Evelhoch, J., Gillies, R.J., Karzcmar, G.S., Koutcher, J.A., Maxwell, R.J., Nalcioglu, O., et al. (2000) Application of magnetic resonance in model systems: cancer therapeutics. *Neoplasia.* 2, 152–165.

4. Glunde, K., and Serkova, N.J. (2006) Therapeutic targets and biomarkers identified in cancer choline phospholipid metabolism. *Pharmacogenomics.* 7, 1109–1123.

5. Mountford, C.E., Doran, S., Lean, C.L., and Russell, P. (1997) Cancer pathology in the year 2000. *Biophys. Chem.* 68, 127–135.

6. Howe, F.A., Barton, S.J., Cudlip, S.A., Stubbs, M., Saunders, D.E., Murphy, M., et al. (2003) Metabolic profiles of human brain tumors using quantitative in vivo 1H magnetic resonance spectroscopy. *Magn. Reson. Med.* 49, 223–232.

7. Nelson, S.J. (2001) Analysis of volume MRI and MR spectroscopic imaging data for the evaluation of patients with brain tumors. *Magn. Reson. Med.* 46, 228–239.

8. Balmaceda, C., Critchell, D., Mao, X., Cheung, K., Pannullo, S., DeLaPaz, R.L., et al. (2006) Multisection 1H magnetic resonance spectroscopic imaging assessment of glioma response to chemotherapy. *J. Neurooncol.* 76, 185–191.

9. Stanwell, P., Gluch, L., Clark, D., Tomanek, B., Baker, L., Giuffre, B., Lean, C., et al. (2005) Specificity of choline metabolites for in vivo diagnosis of breast cancer using 1H-MRS at 1.5 T. *Eur. Radiol.* **15**, 1037–1043.

10. Bolan, P.J., Nelson, M.T., Yee, D., and Garwood, M. (2005) Imaging in breast cancer; Magnetic resonance spectroscopy. *Breast Cancer Res.* 7, 149–152.

11. Schricker, A.A., Pauly, J.M., Kurhanewicz, J., Swanson, M., and Vigneron, D.B. (2001) Dualband spectral-spatial RF pulses for prostate MR spectroscopic imaging. *Magn. Reson. Med.* 46, 1079–1087.

12. Pucar, D., Koutcher, J.A., Shah, A., Dyke, J.P., Schwartz, L., Thaler, H., et al. (2004) Preliminary assessment of magnetic resonance spectroscopic imaging in predicting treatment outcome in patients with prostate cancer at high risk for relapse. *Clin. Prostate Cancer.* 3, 174–181.

13. Zakian, K.L., Shuka-Dave, A., Meyers, P., Gorlick, R., Healey, J., Thaler, H.T., et al. (2003) Identification of prognostic markers in bone marrow sarcomas using proton-decoupled phosphorus magnetic resonance spectroscopy. *Cancer Res.* 63, 9042–9047.

14. Rudin, M., Beckman, N., Porszasz, R., Reese, T., Bochelen, D., and Sauter, A. (1999) In vivo magnetic resonance methods in pharmaceutical research: current status and perspective. *NMR Biomed.* 12, 69–97.

15. McPhail, L.D., Chung, Y.L., Madhu, B., Clark, S., Griffiths, J.R., Kelland, L.R., et al. (2005) Tumor dose response to the vascular disrupting agent, 5,6-dimethylxantheone-4-acetic acid, using in vivo magnetic resonance spectroscopy. *Clin. Cancer. Res.* 11, 3705–3713.

16. Griffiths, J.R., McSheehy, P.M.J., Robinson, S.P., Troy, H., Chung, Y.L., Leek, R.D., et al. (2002) Metabolic changes detected by in vivo magnetic resonance studies of HEPA-1 wild-type tumors and tumors deficient in hypoxia-inducible factor-1β (HIF-1β): Evidence of an anabolic role for the HIF-1 pathway. *Cancer Res.* 62, 688–695.

17. Al-Saffar, N.M., Troy, H., Ramirez de Molina, A., Jackson, L.E., Madhu, B., Griffiths, J.R., et al. (2006) Noninvasive magnetic resonance spectroscopic pharmacodynamic markers of the choline kinase inhibitor MN58b in human carcinoma models. *Cancer Res.* 66, 427–434.

18. Griffin, J.L., Lehtimaki, K.K., Valonen, P.K., Grohn, O.H.J., Kettunen, M.I., Ula-Herttuala, S., et al. (2003) Assignment of 1H nuclear magnetic resonance visible polyunsaturated fatty acids in BT4C gliomas undergoing ganciclovir-thymidine kinase gene therapy-induced programmed cell death. *Cancer Res.* 63, 3195–3201, 2003.

19. Arias-Mendoza, F., Zakian, K., Schwartz, A., Howe, F.A., Koutcher, J.A., Leach, M.O., et al. (2004) Methodological standardization for a multi-institutional in vivo trial of localized 31P MR spectroscopy in human cancer research. In vitro and normal volunteer studies. *NMR Biomed.* 17, 382–391.

20. Clinical Applications. Ch6 in Clinical MR Spectroscopy by Nouha Salibi and Mark Brown. Wiley-Liss (New York), 1998. P 143–186.